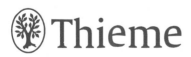

Pediatric Endoscopic Endonasal Skull Base Surgery

Harminder Singh, MD, FACS, FAANS
Clinical Associate Professor of Neurological Surgery
Director
Stanford Neuroanatomy and Simulation Laboratory
Stanford University School of Medicine
Stanford, California
Chief of Neurosurgery
Santa Clara Valley Medical Center
San Jose, California

Jeffrey P. Greenfield, MD, PhD
Vice Chairman of Academic Affairs
Associate Professor of Pediatric Neurological Surgery
Weill Cornell Medical College
New York, New York

Vijay K. Anand, MD, FACS
Clinical Professor of Otolaryngology
Otolaryngology—Head and Neck Surgery
Co-Director
Institute for Minimally Invasive Skull Base and Pituitary Surgery
Weill Cornell Medical College
New York, New York

Theodore H. Schwartz, MD, FACS
David and Ursel Barnes Professor in Minimally Invasive Neurosurgery
Director
Anterior Skull Base and Pituitary Surgery and Epilepsy Research Laboratory
Co-Director
Institute for Minimally Invasive Skull Base and Pituitary Surgery
Weill Cornell Medical College
New York, New York

Thieme
New York • Stuttgart • Delhi • Rio de Janeiro

Library of Congress Cataloging-in-Publication Data

Names: Singh, Harminder, editor. | Greenfield, Jeffrey P., editor. | Anand, Vijay K., editor. | Schwartz, Theodore H., editor.

Title: Pediatric endoscopic endonasal skull base surgery / [edited by] Harminder Singh, Jeffrey P. Greenfield, Vijay K. Anand, Theodore H. Schwartz.

Description: New York : Thieme, [2019] | Includes bibliographical references and index.

Identifiers: LCCN 2019030975| ISBN 9781626235014 (hardback) | ISBN 9781626235021 (ebook)

Subjects: | MESH: Skull Base Neoplasms–surgery | Neuroendoscopy | Child | Adolescent

Classification: LCC RD529 | NLM WE 707 | DDC 617.5/140597–dc23
LC record available at https://lccn.loc.gov/2019030975

© 2020 Thieme Medical Publishers, Inc.

Thieme Publishers New York
333 Seventh Avenue, New York, NY 10001 USA
+1 800 782 3488, customerservice@thieme.com

Thieme Publishers Stuttgart
Rüdigerstrasse 14, 70469 Stuttgart, Germany
+49 [0]711 8931 421, customerservice@thieme.de

Thieme Publishers Delhi
A-12, Second Floor, Sector-2, Noida-201301
Uttar Pradesh, India
+91 120 45 566 00, customerservice@thieme.in

Thieme Publishers Rio de Janeiro, Thieme Publicações Ltda.
Edifício Rodolpho de Paoli, 25º andar
Av. Nilo Peçanha, 50 – Sala 2508,
Rio de Janeiro 20020-906 Brasil
+55 21 3172-2297 / +55 21 3172-1896
www.thiemerevinter.com.br

Cover design: Thieme Publishing Group
Typesetting by Thomson Digital, India

Printed in The United States of America
by King Printing Co., Inc.

5 4 3 2 1

ISBN 978-1-62623-501-4

Also available as an e-book:
eISBN 978-1-62623-502-1

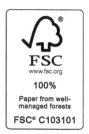

Important note: Medicine is an ever-changing science undergoing continual development. Research and clinical experience are continually expanding our knowledge, in particular our knowledge of proper treatment and drug therapy. Insofar as this book mentions any dosage or application, readers may rest assured that the authors, editors, and publishers have made every effort to ensure that such references are in accordance with **the state of knowledge at the time of production of the book.**

Nevertheless, this does not involve, imply, or express any guarantee or responsibility on the part of the publishers in respect to any dosage instructions and forms of applications stated in the book. **Every user is requested to examine carefully** the manufacturers' leaflets accompanying each drug and to check, if necessary in consultation with a physician or specialist, whether the dosage schedules mentioned therein or the contraindications stated by the manufacturers differ from the statements made in the present book. Such examination is particularly important with drugs that are either rarely used or have been newly released on the market. Every dosage schedule or every form of application used is entirely at the user's own risk and responsibility. The authors and publishers request every user to report to the publishers any discrepancies or inaccuracies noticed. If errors in this work are found after publication, errata will be posted at www.thieme.com on the product description page.

Some of the product names, patents, and registered designs referred to in this book are in fact registered trademarks or proprietary names even though specific reference to this fact is not always made in the text. Therefore, the appearance of a name without designation as proprietary is not to be construed as a representation by the publisher that it is in the public domain.

We would like to dedicate this book to the parents of the children on whom this work is based. These parents trusted us with the health of their children, which is perhaps the greatest gift bestowed upon a surgeon. Without their faith and willingness, this work could not have been accomplished. Hopefully, as a result, future generations of children will be helped by these innovative minimal access approaches. We would also like to dedicate this book to our wives and our families for encouraging us with our work.

Editors

To my parents, for embodying and instilling in their children the principles of hard work, gratitude, and love. To my brother, Jaspreet, who has always been there for me.

To my wife and best friend, Sawdie, who willingly sacrifices her own passions so I can pursue mine; who understands the time it takes to practice medicine, pursue research, and teach. I could not do this without you and your parents. To my children, Sofia, Sartaj and Kajal, whose wonder at the world fuels my own curiosity, and inspires me to become better every day.

To Waheguru, the Almighty, for placing me at this station in life, and blessing me with the grace and strength so that I can attempt to do it justice.

Harminder Singh, MD

Contents

Part III Skull Base Closure, Complication Management, and Postoperative Care

Video Contents

Foreword

In the past two decades, the advances in minimal access surgery to virtually all disciplines in procedural medicine have been transformative. Consider, for example, laparoscopic cholecystectomy, robotic prostatectomy, endovascular stent placement for coronary artery disease or cerebral artery aneurysms, and minimally invasive multi-level spinal decompression and fixation – all of these procedures are now performed with the expectation of diminished pain after surgery, shorter time to discharge, and, in many cases, enhanced quality of life. We can definitely now add to these examples the burgeoning field of endoscopic endonasal skull base surgery. Now, with "Pediatric Endoscopic Endonasal Skull Base Surgery", Drs. Singh, Greenfield, Anand and Schwartz demonstrate that the field of minimal access skull base surgery has recently developed to the point of impacting significantly on conditions of the skull base, and head and neck region that uniquely affect the pediatric population.

For quite some time now, pediatric neurosurgeons have become proficient in the use of intracranial endoscopy to perform endoscopic third ventriculostomy (ETV) for non-communicating hydrocephalus, cyst fenestration into the basal cisterns for symptomatic arachnoid cysts, removal of colloid cysts of the third ventricle, and septostomy for loculated lateral ventricular hydrocephalus. However, the application of advanced endoscopic techniques to the pediatric skull base was dependent, to a degree, on the development of these procedures in the adult population; and on the interest in these specialists in sharing "lessons learned" and best practices with their pediatric neurosurgery and otolaryngology colleagues.

There is a clear rationale and need to publish this multi-disciplinary and multi-authored book at this time. I was particularly pleased to see special chapters devoted to the operating room set-up, specific instrumentation required, combined approaches, and the important role of the pediatric anesthesiologist described in considerable detail. But perhaps the greatest purpose of this book is to provide a state-of-the-art approach to those skull base conditions that are somewhat unique to the pediatric population including arachnoid cysts, sincipital or basal frontal encephaloceles, and juvenile nasopharyngeal angiofibroma. I have been particularly impressed with the current results that can be obtained through the use of the endoscopic endonasal corridor in the removal of challenging lesions such as craniopharyngioma and Rathke's cleft cysts. For the former, these days, the endoscopic endonasal approach is quickly becoming the procedure of choice for the reasons mentioned above – less morbidity, earlier mobilization and discharge from hospital, and better endocrinologic outcomes.

Finally, it is clear that the best results for many of the complex pathologies described in this book come from the efforts of a dedicated multi-disciplinary team whose members share expertise and a common goal for the child. These efforts are well defined and clearly outlined in this book. As this is a "first of its kind" book in the field of skull base surgery, I truly look forward to seeing the continued developments and refinements of techniques which will naturally take place and be found in future editions of "Pediatric endoscopic endonasal skull base surgery". I congratulate the editors and authors on this timely compendium of knowledge in a most important area of active investigation.

James T. Rutka, MD, PhD, FRCSC, FAANS
Division of Pediatric Neurosurgery
The Hospital for Sick Children
RS McLuaghlin Professor and Chair
Department of Surgery
University of Toronto
Toronto, Ontario

Foreword

The benefits of endoscopic-assisted endonasal surgery are irrefutable and the practice of neurosurgery has moved well beyond an era of skepticism. Widened fields of view, optimized image resolution, enhanced illumination, greater extent of tumor removal, smaller surgical corridors, avoidance of brain retraction, and improved postoperative pain control, are just a sampling of the advantages of using high resolution optics through the nasal route for intracranial pathology.

Past contributions to the field by Dr. Schwartz and Dr. Anand are monumental. This team has exploited the transnasal corridor and taken the discipline from a one-size-fits-all to a compilation of approaches defined by specific anatomical goals. Surgeons that care for adults have traditionally evolved as experts in this domain owing to the frequency of pathologic substrates in the seller and parasellar region in older patients. On the contrary, there has been a slow adoption of these techniques in the pediatric sector because of the relative rarity of pathologic substrates in the pituitary region of children. Children have therefore lagged behind as beneficiaries of a well-proven surgical advance. While the transition of these children's care to "adult" specialists is one solution, it is simplistic, misguided, and potentially harmful.

It has long been recognized that the pediatric specialist is best suited to counsel and care for children due to age-specific pathologic entities, treatment-related impacts, contemporary disease management awareness, and understanding of development. Defining the goals of surgery for parasellar lesions such as craniopharyngioma, primary CNS germ cell tumor, Langerhan's cell histiocytosis (LCH), and hypothalamic hamartomas in children can be daunting. Integrating a surgeon versed in the appropriate goals of care is logical and in fact desirable. A need for a focus on children is also amplified by the distinct anatomy and the dynamic maturation of the nasal corridor and skull base in the young.

Dr. Jeffrey Greenfield, a highly talented and insightful pediatric neurosurgeon, has wonderfully bridged a technical advance with pediatric-specific elements, therefore filling a void. By serving as the pediatric nucleus for a talented group he is to be credited for defining the field of endoscopic assisted transnasal surgery for children. This accomplished group of authors have used lab-based research and an enriched patient experience to put forth an all-encompassing treatise that is a must read.

Beyond the masterful technical nuances, reading this book conveys a less apparent but equally meaningful message about the synergy of cross-disciplinary surgical practice. Both the fields of otolaryngology and neurosurgery have contributed immensely to this field. At no time and at no level of training should one discount the contributions that each field brings to the table. To work in isolation would be admitting inferiority and unfair from the patient's perspective.

This book not only serves as the first dedicated textbook on the topic but predictably will serve as a lasting reference for future generations of surgeons. It is essential reading for skull base surgeons who intend to care for children and have the prescience to be contemporary and the desire to possess a comprehensive repertoire.

Mark Souweidane, MD
Weill Cornell Brain and Spine Center
Weill Cornell Medicine
New York, New York

Foreword

I congratulate the lead editors, Drs. Singh, Greenfield, Anand, and Schwartz for their vision in this book, entitled *Pediatric Endoscopic Endonasal Skull Base Surgery*, which is the first of its kind to specifically highlight the nuances of pediatric endoscopic skull base surgery. Advances in endoscopic skull base surgery in adults and children have transformed our ability to treat complex skull base lesions via the transnasal approach. The unique pathology in the pediatric population requires a skill set that is highly collaborative between adult and pediatric neurosurgical and otolaryngologic skull base surgeons. Teamwork is imperative with these complex cases to achieve the best possible outcomes and to expand the adoption of this approach for complex skull base lesions in childhood.

Furthermore, the desire to perform minimally invasive surgery is attractive particularly in the pediatric population, although it does carry increased risk due to smaller corridors and the need for smaller endoscopic equipment with the same optics and light, lack of a pneumatized sella, and complex repair to avoid a CSF leak. There is also a learning curve during implementation, which requires careful planning, patience during every phase of opening, resection, and closure, as well as a valuable debrief after every case. The approach to these complex lesions needs to be rehearsed by the team in advance and studied in the skull base anatomy lab. At Stanford, we also use the Precision VR by Surgical Theater platform to plan together to optimize our exposure for safe resection. The patient-specific virtual tour in our Department 3D theater is also incredibly valuable in the training of our residents and fellows to rehearse the case step by step in advance of the case. Our team has also found 3D printing of the skull base anatomy, tumor, and vasculature helpful in this regard to understand the relationship of the tumor to surrounding neurovascular structures. A weekly multidisciplinary endoscopic skull base conference is also paramount to develop a consensus decision for each case reviewed.

Open skull base approaches have traditionally been limited to safely resect skull base lesions below the hypothalamus and optic chiasm and around neurovascular structures. We have used angled rigid endoscopes and mirrors to maximize the extent of resection while at the same time mitigating patient morbidity. Clearly, this is an ideal minimally invasive approach for intralesional resection of extradural skull base chordomas, but we are unable to perform an en bloc resection. So far, the surgical series combined with adjuvant radiotherapy in children are promising. How about craniopharyngiomas? The challenge of resecting these tumors up against the hypothalamus and optic chiasm and resultant morbidity has led to a more conservative debulking in the pediatric population followed by radiotherapy. However, the vivid ventral exposure we achieve with an endoscopic transnasal approach may now enable more safe and complete resection of these tumors with sharp microdissection and avoid upfront radiotherapy. We will need to continue to rigorously evaluate our results over time in children to achieve the best possible short term and long-term outcomes. Due to the rarity of these tumors in children, we will also need to closely collaborate with other expert centers to carefully track the outcomes of these children prospectively.

This book is a compendium of all of the collective wisdom of the authors. There are many technical pearls in every chapter which will serve as a wonderful resource for surgeons with all levels of training and varied disciplines. Thank you to the editors for putting together the first of its kind which will serve as the foundation for future editions.

Gerald A. Grant MD, FACS
Endowed Professor in Pediatric Neurosurgery
Professor, by Courtesy, of Neurology
Stanford University Medical Center
Stanford, California

Preface

Pediatric Endoscopic Endonasal Skull Base Surgery is intended to provide a comprehensive multimedia resource for neurosurgeons and otolaryngologists interested in this rapidly emerging field. Endonasal skull base surgery has become widely accepted as a technique to manage adult skull base tumors, however, there has been limited work done in the pediatric population. The developing pediatric sino-nasal and cranial base anatomy is much more restrictive than in adult patients and the pathology encountered is often unique to the pediatric population, which makes these surgeries more challenging.

As *adult* endoscopic skull base surgeons became facile with expanded endonasal approaches (EEAs) over the past two decades, they applied their surgical skill-set to address pediatric pathology, and learned several important lessons along the way. Several prominent groups around the globe have now published on their experience with *pediatric* endoscopic skull base surgery. However, there was a lack of a consolidated text on the subject that crystallized all their experience into a well-organized, easily referenceable book.

Pediatric Endoscopic Endonasal Skull Base Surgery aims to fulfill that knowledge gap, by providing a broad, yet detailed compendium of current knowledge and practice in this emerging field. The book is divided into three sections. *Section 1: Pediatric Anatomy, Approaches, and Surgical Considerations* lays the basic framework that practitioners should be familiar with before embarking on these cases, *Section 2: Pathology Specific to the Pediatric Skull Base* discusses management of pediatric skull-base pathology thru specific case examples, and *Section 3: Skull Base Closure, Complication Management and Postoperative Care* equips the surgeon to preempt complications or successfully tackle adversity should it arise in the peri-operative period.

Most surgeons are visual and spatial learners and for this reason, our book relies heavily on high-quality surgical illustrations and intra-operative pictures and videos to supplement the succinct text. Nurse-practitioners and physician-assistants will find this a valuable resource in helping them prepare pediatric patients for these surgeries, as well as take care of them in the perioperative period. Residents and fellows will benefit in understanding the developing pediatric skull-base anatomy and preparing for these cases. It will serve as a valuable reference for surgeons who infrequently performs these procedures, or as a "springboard" for those who want to delve deeper into this rewarding field.

This book is truly an international collaboration, and draws upon the experience of authors and thought-leaders in the field, both nationally and internationally, across five continents. Our hope is that this wealth of knowledge and aggregate experience, along with technological advancements in the field, will usher in a new surgical paradigm to use EEAs to successfully treat central skull base lesions in the pediatric population.

We invite you to join us on this journey.

Acknowledgements

We would like to acknowledge Timothy Hiscock, Executive Editor at Thieme Publishers, for believing in our team and greenlighting this project several years ago. We would also like to acknowledge the assistance of our editors at Thieme, Owen Zurhellen and Mary Wilson, for successfully shepherding this project along its various phases. Kimberly Taylor at Cornell also assisted in proof-reading and editing multiple chapters.

Specials thanks are also due to our Medical Illustrator, Matthew Holt (matthew@bodyrender.com), for beautifully rendering our rough sketches and intraoperative pictures into brilliant illustrations that you will find throughout this book.

And lastly, we would like to thank our fellows and residents, at Cornell and Stanford, for helping take care of our patients, and for their assistance in co-authoring our manuscripts and chapters.

Contributors

Andrew Alalade, MD
University College London Hospitals
NHS Foundation Trust
UCLH – Victor Horsley
Department of Neurosurgery
London, United Kingdom

Gustavo J. Almodóvar-Mercado, MD
Assistant Professor
Rhinology and Endoscopic Skull Base Surgery
Otolaryngology - Head and Neck Surgery Division
University of Puerto Rico, School of Medicine
San Juan, Puerto Rico

Vijay K. Anand, MD, FACS
Clinical Professor of Otolaryngology-Head and Neck
  Surgery
Weill Cornell Medical College
New York Presbyterian Hospital
New York, New York

Muaid I. Aziz-Baban, MD, FICMS
Unit of Otorhinolaryngology
Department of Biotechnology and Life Sciences (DBSV)
University of Insubria
Ospedale di Circolo e Fondazione Macci
Varese, Italy
Unit of Otorhinolaryngology – Head and Neck Surgery
Department of Surgery
University of Sulaimani
College of Medicine
Sulaymaniyah, Kurdistan, Iraq

Leonardo Balsalobre, MD
São Paulo Skull Base Center
São Paulo ENT Center
Professor Edmundo Vasconcelos Hospital
São Paulo, Brazil

Jeffrey R. Balzer, PhD
Associate Professor
Director, Clinical Services, Center for Clinical
  Neurophysiology
Director, Cerebral Blood Flow Laboratory
Department of Neurological Surgery
University of Pittsburgh Medical Center
Pittsburgh, Pennsylvania

Matei Banu, MD
Neurosurgery Resident
New York Presbyterian Hospital
Columbia University Medical Center
New York, New York

Paolo Battaglia, MD
Unit of Otolaryngology, Department of Biotechnology and
  Life Science (DBSV)
University of Insurbiria
Varese, Italy

Wenya Linda Bi, MD, PhD
Resident
Neurosurgery
Brigham and Women's Hospital
Boston, Massachusetts

Randall A. Bly, MD
Assistant Professor
Center for Clinical and Transitional Research
Otolaryngology, Cranial Base, Vascular Anomalies,
  Craniofacial
Seattle Children's Hospital
Seattle, Washington

Douglas L. Brockmeyer, MD, FAAP
Department of Neurosurgery
Primary Children's Medical Center
University of Utah School of Medicine
Salt Lake City, Utah

Paolo Cappabianca, MD
Department of Neurosciences and Reproductive
  and Odontostomatological Science
University of Naples Federico II
Division of Neurosurgery
Naples, Italy

Ricardo L. Carrau, MD, FACS
Department of Otolaryngology-Head & Neck Surgery
Department of Neurosurgery
The Ohio State University Medical Center
Columbus, Ohio

Paolo Castelnuovo, MD, FRCS (Ed), FACS
Division of Otorhinolaryngology
Department of Biotechnology and Life Science
University of Insubria,
Ospedale di Circolo e Fondazione Macchi
Varese, Italy

Luigi Maria Cavallo, MD
Division of Neurosurgery
Department of Neurosciences and Reproductive
    and Odontostomatological Science
University of Naples Federico II
Naples, Italy

Jason Chu, MD
Department of Neurosurgery
Emory University
School of Medicine
Atlanta, Georgia

Jeremy N. Ciporen, MD
Neurosurgery
Tuality Healthcare
Oregon Health and Science University
Hillsboro, Oregon

Vincent Couloigner, MD, PhD
Faculté de Médecine
Université Paris Descartes
Department of Pediatric Otorhinolaryngology
Hôpital Necker – Enfants Malades
Paris, France

Camila S. Dassi, MD
Research Fellow
The Ohio State University
Columbus, Ohio

Harley Brito da Silva, MD
Instructor
University of Washington
Bellevue, Washington

Maria Laura Del Basso De Caro, MD
Department of Advanced Biomedical Sciences
University of Napoli Federico II
Naples, Italy

Fara Dayani
Medical Student
UCSF School of Medicine
University of California
San Francisco, California

Onkar K. Deshmukh, PhD
Junior Consultant
Royal Pearl Hospital
Tiruchirappalli, Tamil Nadu, India

Georgiana Dobri, MD
Assistant Professor of Neuroendocrinology in Neurological
    Surgery
Department of Neurosurgery and Endocrinology
Weill Cornell Medical College
New York Presbyterian Hospital
New York, New York

Ian F. Dunn, MD
Associate Professor of Neurosurgery
Harvard Medical School
Brigham and Women's Hospital
Boston, Massachusetts

Charles S. Ebert, MD, MPH
University of North Carolina at Chapel Hill
Chapel Hill, North Carolina

Michael S.B. Edwards, MD
Lucille Packard Children's Hospital
Professor Emeritus
Pediatric Neurosurgery
Stanford University
Stanford, California

Jean Anderson Eloy, MD
Departments of Neurological Surgery
Otolaryngology-Head and Neck Surgery
Ophthalmology and Visual Sciences
Center for Skull Base and Pituitary Surgery
Rutgers Neurological Institute
Rutgers University
Newark, New Jersey

Mohamed El Zoghby, MD
Ain Shams University
Cairo, Egypt

Walid I. Essayed, MD
Weill Cornell Medical Center
New York, New York

James J. Evans, MD
Department of Otolaryngology-Head and Neck Surgery
Thomas Jefferson University
Philadelphia, Pennsylvania

Matthew G. Ewend, MD
Department of Neurosurgery
University of North Carolina at Chapel Hill
Chapel Hill, North Carolina

Paolo Farneti, MD
Department of Otorhinolaryngology
Sant' Orsola – Malpighi
University of Bologna
Bologna, Italy

Juan C. Fernandez-Miranda, MD
Professor of Neurosurgery and, by courtesy, of
   Otolaryngology Head and Neck Surgery at the
   Stanford University Medical Center
Stanford University
Stanford, California

Rafey A. Feroze, MD
MS3 Candidate
School of Medicine
University of Pittsburgh
Pittsburgh, Pennsylvania

Jonathan A. Forbes, MD
Department of Neurosurgery
Weill Cornell Medical College
New York Presbyterian Hospital
New York, New York

Sébastien Froelich, MD
Professor and Chairman
Department of Neurosurgery
Lariboisière University Hospital
Paris VII – Diderot University
Paris, France

Michelangelo Gangemi, MD
Division of Neurosurgery
Department of Neurosciences and Reproductive
   and Odontostomatological Science
University of Naples Federico II
Naples, Italy

Paul A. Gardner, MD
UPMC Center for Cranial Base Surgery
Department of Neurological Surgery
University of Pittsburgh Medical Center
Pittsburgh, Pennsylvania

Nurperi Gazioglu, MD
Department of Neurosurgery
Pituitary Center
Cerrahpasa Medical Faculty
Istanbul University
Istanbul, Turkey

Bernard George, MD
Department of Pediatric Otorhinolaryngology
Hôpital Necker – Enfants Malades
Paris, France

Gerald A. Grant, MD, FACS
Endowed Professor in Pediatric Neurosurgery
Stanford Health Care
Stanford University Medical Center
Stanford, California

Jeffrey P. Greenfield, MD, PhD
Pediatric Neurological Surgery
Department of Neurological Surgery
Weill Cornell Medical Center
New York, New York

Shunya Hanakita, MD
Department of Neurosurgery
Hôpital Lariboisière
Paris, France

Griffith R. Harsh IV, MD
Julian R. Youmans Endowed Chair in Neurological Surgery
Professor and Chair
Neurological Surgery
UC Davis Medical Group, Sacramento
Sacramento, California

Richard Harvey, MD, PhD, FRACS
Rhinology and Skull Base Research Group
St. Vincent's Center for Applied Medical Research
University of New South Wales
Sydney, New South Wales, Australia

Allen Ho, MD
Neurosurgery Resident
Stanford University School of Medicine
Stanford, California

Reid Hoshide, MD
The Center for Minimally Invasive Neurosurgery
Randwick, New South Wales, Australia

Peter H. Hwang, MD
Professor
Otolaryngology – Head and Neck Surgery
Stanford Sinus Center
Stanford University Medical Center
Stanford, California

Gianpiero Iannuzzo, MD
Division of Neurosurgery
Department of Neurosciences and Reproductive
   and Odontostomatological Science
University of Naples Federico II
Naples, Italy

Tiruchy Narayanan Janakiram, MD
Managing Director
Royal Pearl Hospital
Thillainagar, Trichy
Tamil Nadu, India

John Jane Jr., MD
University of Virginia School of Medicine
Charlottesville, Virginia

Ronak Jani, MD
School of Medicine
University of Pittsburgh
Pittsburgh, Pennsylvania

Douglas R. Johnston, MD
Pediatric Otolaryngology
Nemours Pediatric Specialists
Thomas Jefferson University
Philadelphia, Pennsylvania

Apostolos Karligkiotis, MD
Division of Otorhinolaryngology - Head & Neck Surgery
Forensic Dissection Research Center (HNS & FDRc)
DBSV
University of Insubria – Varese
Varese, Italy

Joseph R. Keen, DO
Department of Neurosurgery
Ochsner Medical Center
Gretna, Louisiana

John R.W. Kestle, MD
Department of Neurosurgery
Primary Children's Medical Center
University of Utah School of Medicine
Salt Lake City, Utah

Lily Kim, BA
MD Candidate
Stanford University School of Medicine
Stanford, California

Cristine N. Klatt-Cromwell, MD
Department of Otolaryngology
Head and Neck Surgery
University of North Carolina at Chapel Hill
Chapel Hill, North Carolina

Moujahed Labidi, MD, FRCSC
Department of Neurosurgery
Hopital Lariboisiere
Paris, France

Edward R. Laws Jr., MD, FACS
Department of Neurosurgery
Brigham and Women's Hospital
Boston, Massachusetts

James K. Liu, MD
Department of Neurological Surgery
Rutgers University-New Jersey Medical School
Rutgers Neurological Institute of New Jersey
Newark, New Jersey

Davide Locatelli, MD
Division of Neurological Surgery
Department of Biotechnology and Life Sciences
University of Insubria-Varese
Varese, Italy

Neil Majmundar, MD
Department of Neurological Surgery
Rutgers Neurological Institute of New Jersey
Rutgers University
New Jersey Medical School
Newark, New Jersey

João Mangussi-Gomes, MD
São Paulo Skull Base Center
São Paulo ENT Center
Professor Edmundo Vasconcelos Hospital
São Paulo, Brazil

Felipe Marconato, MD
São Paulo Skull Base Center
São Paulo ENT Center
Professor Edmundo Vasconcelos Hospital
São Paulo, Brazil

Ana B. Melgarejo, MD
The Ohio State University
Wexner Medical Center
Columbus, Ohio

Zachary Medress, MD
Neurosurgery Resident
Stanford University School of Medicine
Stanford, California

Kris S. Moe, MD, FACS
Professor
Facial Plastic and Reconstructive Surgery
Division of Facial Plastic Surgery
Department of Otolaryngology-Head and Neck Surgery
University of Washington School of Medicine
Seattle, Washington

Nelson M. Oyesiku, MD, PhD, FACS
Al Lerner Chair and Vice-Chairman
Department of Neurosurgery and Medicine
  (Endocrinology)
Program Director
Neurosurgical Residency Program
Emory University School of Medicine
Atlanta, Georgia

Ernesto Pasquini, MD
Ear, Nose, and Throat Metropolitan Unit
Surgical Department
AUSL Bologna, Bellaria Hospital
Bologna, Italy

Daniel M. Prevedello, MD
Department of Otolaryngology
Department of Neurological Surgery
The Wexner Medical Center
The Ohio State University
Columbus, Ohio

Jennifer L. Quon, MD, MHS
Resident
Stanford University School of Medicine
Stanford, California

Mindy R. Rabinowitz, MD
Department of Otolaryngology–Head and Neck Surgery
Thomas Jefferson University
Philadelphia, Pennsylvania

Khaled Radhounane, MD
Tunis Military Hospital
Medicine Faculty of Tunis
University of Tunis-El Manar
Tunis, Tunisia

Sanjeet V. Rangarajan, MD
Department of Otolaryngology
Head and Neck Surgery
Thomas Jefferson University
Philadelphia, Pennsylvania

Marc R. Rosen, MD
Department of Otolaryngology-Head and Neck Surgery
Thomas Jefferson University
Philadelphia, Pennsylvania

Seyed Mousa Sadrhosseini, MD
Associate Professor
Department of Otolaryngology-Head and Neck Surgery
Imam Khomeini Hospital
Tehran University of Medical Sciences
Tehran, Iran

Deanna M. Sasaki-Adams, MD
Department of Neurosurgery
University of North Carolina at Chapel Hill
Chapel Hill, North Carolina

Jacques H. Scharoun, MD
Assistant Professor of Clinical Anesthesiology
Weill Cornell Medical College
Weill Cornell Medicine Anesthesiology
New York, New York

Matthew J. Shepard, MD
Neurosurgery
University of Virginia Health System
Charlottesville, Virginia

Theodore H. Schwartz, MD, FACS
Professor of Neurosurgery, Neurology, and Otolaryngology
Department of Neurosurgery
Weill Cornell Brain and Spine Center
New York, New York

Vittorio Sciarretta, MD
Department of Otorhinolaryngology
Sant' Orsola – Malpighi Hospital
University of Bologna
Bologna, Italy

Aarti Sharma, MD
Associate Professor of Anesthesiology
Weill Cornell Medical College
New York Presbyterian Hospital
Weill Cornell Medical Center
New York, New York

Shilpee Bhatia Sharma, MD
Consultant Royal Pearl Hospital
Tiruchirapally, Tamilnadu, India

Harminder Singh, MD, FACS, FAANS
Clinical Associate Professor of Neurosurgery
Department of Neurological Surgery
Stanford University School of Medicine
Stanford, California

Alan Siu, MD
Department of Neurosurgery
Thomas Jefferson University
Philadelphia, Pennsylvania

Edward R. Smith, MD
Director
Pediatric Cerebrovascular Neurosurgery
Co-Director
Cerebrovascular Surgery and Interventions
Co-Director
Head, Neck, and Skull Base Surgery Program
Associate Professor
Harvard Medical School
Cambridge, Massachusetts

Carl H. Snyderman, MD, MBA
Center for Cranial Base Surgery
Eye and Ear Institute
University of Pittsburgh Medical Center
Pittsburgh, Pennsylvania

Domenico Solari, MD
Division of Neurosurgery
University of Naples Federico II
Naples, Italy

Aldo C. Stamm, MD, PhD
São Paulo ENT Center
São Paulo, Brazil

Amanda L. Stapleton, MD
Department of Otolaryngology
University of Pittsburgh School of Medicine
Pittsburgh, Pennsylvania

Charles Teo, MBBS, FRACS
Neurosurgeon
Duke Health
Durham, North Carolina

Parthasarathy D. Thirumala, MD
Associate Professor
Department of Neurological Surgery
Co-Director
Center of Clinical Neurophysiology
University of Pittsburgh Medical Center
Pittsburgh, Pennsylvania

Brian D. Thorp, MD
Department of Otolaryngology-Head and Neck Surgery
University of North Carolina at Chapel Hill
Chapel Hill, North Carolina

Mario Turri-Zanoni, MD
Department of Otorhinolaryngology
University of Insubria
Varese, Italy

Elizabeth C. Tyler-Kabara, MD, PhD
Department of Neurological Surgery
University of Pittsburgh
Pittsburgh, Pennsylvania

Eduardo Vellutini, MD
São Paulo Skull Base Center
DFV Neuro
Neurology and Neurosurgery Group
Sao Paulo, Brazil

Patrick C. Walz, MD
Nationwide Children's Hospital
Columbus, Ohio
Assistant Professor
Pediatric Otolaryngology–Head and Neck Surgery
Wexner Medical Center
The Ohio State University
Columbus, Ohio

Eric W. Wang, MD
Department of Otolaryngology
University of Pittsburgh
Pittsburgh, Pennsylvania

Kentaro Watanabe, MD
Department of Neurosurgery
Hôpital Lariboisière
Paris, France

Adam M. Zanation, MD
Department of Otolaryngology–Head and Neck Surgery
Department of Neurosurgery
University of North Carolina School of Medicine
Chapel Hill, North Carolina

Mehdi Zeinalizadeh, MD
Neurosurgeon
Department of Neurological Surgery
Iman Khomeini Hospital
Tehran University of Medical Sciences
Tehran, Iran

Nathan T. Zwagerman, MD
Department of Neurological Surgery
University of Pittsburgh
School of Medicine
Pittsburgh, Pennsylvania

Part I

Pediatric Anatomy, Approaches, and Surgical Considerations

I

1 Anatomy of the Developing Pediatric Skull Base

Matei Banu, Jeffrey P. Greenfield, Vijay K. Anand, and Theodore H. Schwartz

Abstract

Development of the pediatric skull base is an intricate process that starts in utero and spans the entire childhood. During development, endonasal endoscopic corridors change constantly. Some skull base targets are only accessible during the late stages of development, while others are safer to access in the early stages. Importantly, care must be taken not to transgress growth centers, as this will irreversibly disrupt the developmental process. Skull base growth is an asynchronous process, with delayed growth of its anterior portions. Thus, certain anterior corridors become available only once growth stages of the respective portion of the skull base are completed. The trajectories of important neurovascular structures undergo continuous alterations under the driving force of sphenoid sinus pneumatization, further impacting the surgical corridors for endoscopic endonasal approaches. Furthermore, pathology of the skull base, depending on its location and type, will have different effects on endonasal endoscopic corridors as the developmental process is delayed or distorted. Reconstructing the skull base with a nasoseptal flap after extended endoscopic endonasal approaches is only possible after the age of 10 years, or even later in children with long-standing pathology and delayed development. Thus, understanding the different steps of skull base development, as well as the impact of skull base pathology on this process should be an integral part in the surgical planning of endoscopic endonasal approaches for pediatric patients harboring skull base lesions.

Keywords: skull base, internal carotid artery, sphenoid sinus, pneumatization, expanded endonasal approach

1.1 Introduction

Development of the skull base begins at approximately 4 weeks in utero and continues throughout childhood. During development, the pediatric skull base is constantly molded from above, through growth of the cranial vault and from below, through aeration of the paranasal sinuses. This will directly influence growth of the craniofacial region, as well as trajectories of critical neurovascular structures. It is an asynchronous process, with the posterior skull base, a mesodermal structure, undergoing an accelerated growth process in early childhood, while the anterior portion, originating from neural crest cells, along with the midfacies, undergoes a growth spurt during puberty and finalizes the process after 14 years. Pneumatization of the sphenoid sinus begins at 2 years and is the main driving force of skull base development. Pneumatization of the sphenoid sinus also impacts the most important restriction site for endoscopic endonasal approaches (EEA), the intercarotid distance (ICD) at the level of the cavernous sinus, which reaches adult levels after 9 years. As the skull base grows in craniocaudal and anteroposterior direction, distances to specific target sites, such as the sella or the dens, have an abrupt growth trend, also directly correlated with the pneumatization process. The nasal septum reaches an adequate developmental stage for EEA

around 10 years. At this age, the nasoseptal flap will have the appropriate length to cover defects in the anterior skull base and sellar region. The nasoseptal flap may be insufficient for repair of transclival defects in the pediatric population, regardless of age group. Finally, certain tumors, such as suprasellar craniopharyngiomas can disrupt growth centers and significantly delay the developmental process. These aspects, along with certain technical aspects related to endonasal endoscopic surgery on the developing skull base, will be detailed in this chapter.

1.2 Considerations on Surgical Approaches to the Developing Skull Base

Pathology of the pediatric skull base is largely comprised of developmental anomalies. Skull base tumors are relatively uncommon in the pediatric population but can be particularly problematic due to the disruptive effects on the normal developmental process with inherent malformations and impact on long-term prognosis.[1,2] Invasive surgical procedures, open microsurgical approaches, and endoscopic procedures are generally reserved for severe debilitating pathology given the additional risk of transgressing growth centers and delaying the developmental process. Irreversible effects on skull base development can occur both due to tumor growth and as a result of aggressive surgical intervention. Finally, anatomical landmarks and restriction sites for surgical approaches change constantly during childhood as a result of the developing skull base. This will have a direct impact on surgical corridors, as well as surgical tools and instruments, which should be adjusted for age group as well as developmental stage. Therefore, knowing and understanding the developmental processes and patterns of the pediatric cranial base is essential in deciding the appropriate therapeutic approach as well as in planning surgical trajectories for pediatric skull base lesions.

Many lesions in the pediatric cranial base can lead to severe functional impairment.[2,3] Early intervention may help reset the growth process, thereby avoiding permanent damage.[4] However, accessing the skull base is not trivial in children. The cranial fossae are significantly smaller and shallower, while critical neurovascular structures are in close proximity to each other, making access particularly challenging.[2,4,5,6] The stage of tooth eruption or the aeration level of the paranasal sinuses can further hinder approaches, both transfacial approaches and endonasal interventions, and should be taken into consideration when deciding the type of surgical approach.[2,6]

In recent years, EEA have been advocated as the procedures of choice in this patient population. Feasibility of these approaches in children has been demonstrated in several modern case series.[7,8,9,10,11,12] Given its intrinsic magnification, the endoscope can provide superior visualization, an essential feature given the minute size of anatomical structures in children. Furthermore, endoscopic approaches can adapt more easily to the narrow anatomical corridors, thereby safely reaching areas that have thus far not been amenable to classical open routes.[5] Surgical interventions on the developing skull base can lead to disfigurement. Endonasal approaches are believed to have improved cosmetic outcomes, although inadvertent disruption of growth centers through endonasal routes can also lead to long-term disability. Navigation of growth centers during endoscopic surgery remains a major challenge. Knowledge of developmental patterns and age trends can be essential in perioperative planning for EEA.

The small pediatric skull base offers insufficient working space to accommodate both endoscope and instruments. Transitioning endoscopic approaches to the pediatric population has been delayed due to the inadequate working corridors. Choosing the appropriate trajectory to maximize your working space is a key factor in pediatric EEA and is largely based on developmental patterns that have emerged from recent radioanatomical studies. Several measurement systems have been developed over the last decade.[4,10,13,14] Quantitative parameters can guide preoperative planning, establishing optimal surgical routes, and anatomical limitations for the transsellar as well as expanded endoscopic approaches. Limitations for EEA corridors are primarily based on neurovascular structures with a constantly changing position during childhood.[5] Furthermore, certain anatomical structures can be reached more easily at certain points in skull base development, while other targets can only be safely accessed in the adult population.

Adequate closure of skull base defects after EEA is of utmost importance. The nasoseptal flap has been considered the most efficient method of reconstruction with a significant decline in cerebrospinal fluid (CSF) leak rates, both in the adult and in the pediatric patient population. The nasoseptal flap, a pedicled flap derived from the nasal septum and based on the nasoseptal artery, has been part of most multilayer reconstruction techniques. Development of the pediatric skull base is not a linear process. Certain parts of the skull base and the maxillofacial skeleton have a slower evolution. Importantly, skull base development appears to be accelerated in the first years of life, whereas parts of the nasal cavity lag behind. Thus, in certain age groups, especially in early childhood, the length or width of the harvested nasoseptal flap might be insufficient to repair large skull base defects. It is therefore important to have a complete understanding of the developmental process of both the pediatric skull base and the nasal cavity and to adjust exposure based on this. Radioanatomical measurements will further help tailor approaches based on developmental stage, individual anatomical characteristics, and pathology.

1.3 Brief Anatomy of the Skull Base

Skull base anatomy can be significantly distorted in children harboring skull base lesions given the deleterious effects of these lesions on the developmental process. A brief description of normal skull base anatomy is provided here for reference. The skull base is made up of several distinct bones and is comprised of the intracranial surface, subdivided into three distinct parts, and the exocranial surface. The intracranial surface has been traditionally divided into three fossae: the anterior, middle, and posterior fossa, each made up of individual bones and each with fairly distinct borders in adults. The frontal lobes rest in the anterior cranial fossa, made up of the sphenoid and ethmoid bones, paired bones that are formed after fusion of the metopic suture. An important bony structure for EEA at this level is the cribriform plate of the ethmoid bone that connects the nasal cavity and the intracranial cavity through a perforated bone traversed by olfactory nerve roots. The crista galli is an anterior bony prominence of the ethmoid bone that serves as an anchor point for the falx. The posterior border of the anterior cranial fossa is located at the level of the lesser wing of the sphenoid sinus.

The middle fossa forms through fusion of the squamous temporal bone and the parietal bone. The sella turcica is located in the center of the middle cranial fossa and harbors the pituitary gland. Immediately inferior to the sella turcica is the sphenoid sinus. The cavernous sinus, with its important anatomical structures, the carotid syphon of the internal carotids, and cranial nerves III, IV, V2, and VI, flanks the sella turcica. Neurovascular structures pass from the endocranium to the exocranium through distinct foramina. The superior orbital fissure allows passage for the oculomotor nerve, the trochlear nerve, the lacrimal, frontal and nasociliary branches of the ophthalmic nerve (V1), the abducens nerve, the superior and inferior divisions of the ophthalmic vein, and sympathetic fibers from the cavernous plexus. The maxillary nerve (V2) traverses the foramen rotundum, while the mandibular nerve (V3) traverses the foramen ovale.

The clivus is another important anatomical structure for EEA. The posterior border of the sella, along with the posterior aspect of the sphenoid bone and the basilar aspect of the occipital bone, forms the clivus. The abducens nerve runs along this sloped structure in its course toward the cavernous sinus. The posterior fossa is the largest cranial fossa and is delineated by the temporal and occipital bones laterally, as well as by the parietal bones posteriorly. The foramen magnum is located at this level and is a major passage point for the cervical spinal cord as well as vertebral arteries, anterior and posterior spinal arteries, and accessory nerve. The internal acoustic canal, part of the petrous part of the temporal bone, is also located at the level of the posterior fossa containing the facial and vestibular nerve. The jugular foramen, the third important passage point at this level, contains the glossopharyngeal nerve, the vagus nerve, and the accessory nerve along with the internal jugular vein.

The exocranial side of the skull base contains the palatine process, the zygomatic process, the palatine bone, the body of the sphenoid sinus, the petrous bones, the basioccipital bones, and the occipital condyles. An important anatomical structure of the exocranium in pediatric EEA is the pterygopalatine fossa, a cone-shaped structure in the infratemporal fossa posterior to the maxilla that is flanked by the pterygoid processes. It contains the pterygomaxillary fissure and communicates with the nasal cavity, the infratemporal fossa, the orbit, and the middle cranial fossa through different foramina: foramen rotundum, pterygoid canal, inferior orbital fissure, sphenopalatine foramen, pterygomaxillary fissure, and greater palatine canal. It contains the pterygopalatine ganglion, the terminal third of the maxillary artery, and the maxillary nerve.

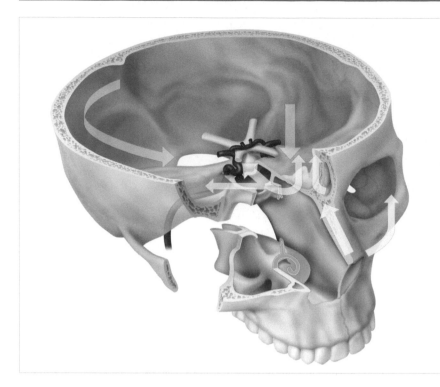

Fig. 1.1 The pediatric skull base is molded from above, through growth of the cranial vault (*yellow arrows*) and from below through aeration of the paranasal sinuses (*blue* and *green arrows*). Pneumatization of the sphenoid sinus is the main driving force of skull base development (*blue arrows*), which changes anatomical relationships between vital structures such as the internal carotids and the optic nerves.

1.4 Embryology of the Skull Base

The skull base undergoes a complex and highly intricate evolutionary process starting at approximately 4 weeks in utero and spanning the entire childhood. Skull base development, both in utero and postpartum, will directly impact development of the craniofacial region and the cerebrum. During this process, especially during early childhood, the cranial base is constantly being molded from above by the developing cranial vault and from below through progressive aeration of the paranasal sinuses (▶ Fig. 1.1). The cranium undergoes three distinct developmental stages: the membranous stage, the cartilaginous stage, and the ossification stage. The skull base, as well as the rostral portion of the neurocranium, originates from the rostral population of neural crest cells. At the level of the cranial vault, the coronal suture is the landmark between the structures of neural crest origin and those originating from cranial mesoderm. The developmental process is regulated by the interplay of several genes and transcription factors such as Indian hedgehog (Ihh), Sonic hedgehog (Shh), dickkopf family (Dkk1–3), Notch, Smad, Fgf, Msx, Wnt, and matrix metalloproteinases (Mmp9). Importantly, ossification of mesodermal structures occurs after formation of neurovascular elements traversing the cranial base.

Neural crest cells migrate to the embryonal pharynx before formation of the neural tube to form the embryonic arches, a mixture of ectoderm, endoderm, and mesenchymal mesodermal tissue. The cranium originates from the first two embryonic arches undergoing a gradual chondrification process, which starts at the level of the occipital bone. The anterior part of the skull base originates from neural crest cells, while the posterior skull base has mesodermal origin. The neurocranium and facial bones undergo intramembranous ossification, while the skull base undergoes endochondral ossification. The ossification process begins during week 5 of embryologic development. The notochord plays an important part, acting as the starting point of skull base development. During week 7, the cranial notochord located in the vicinity of the sella turcica induces the chondrification process of adjacent mesenchymal tissue with formation of the basioccipital bones and foramen magnum. This is followed by an ossification process. Subsequently, skull base components around the occipital bone undergo a similar chondrification and ossification process.

The rostral tip of the notochord also initiates development of the sella turcica and the anterior skull base elements. Hypophysial cartilages flanking the hypophysial pouch merge and form the primordium around the hypophysial stalk. The adenohypophysial pouch remains connected to the roof of the stomodeum, the primordial oral cavity, until the chondrification process is complete, with formation of the sella turcica. The body of the sphenoid bone forms by ossification of the presphenoid cartilages, the last portion of the median cranial base structures to undergo ossification. Thus, by the end of the third month in utero, the sphenoid region is connected with the cartilaginous nasal capsule, with almost complete formation of the cranial base. Several temporary passageways, such as the foramen cecum, the prenasal space, or the fonticulus frontalis, allow transit of other developing structures, such as dura, and normally close toward the end of the developmental process in utero.

The cartilaginous nasal capsule undergoes a similar ossification process during the fifth month of intrauterine life. This process leads to formation of the ethmoid bone, the ethmoidal labyrinth, the orbital floor, and the inferior concha. Several structures originating from the nasal capsule undergo intramembranous ossification with formation of the vomer and nasal bones, while several other portions do not undergo ossification and form the nasal septum. Similarly, mesenchymal condensation at the level of the otic capsule leads to formation of the cochlea and semicircular canals. Ossification of cartilaginous structures at these levels leads to formation of the internal acoustic meatus and the carotid canals.

1.5 Pneumatization of the Paranasal Sinuses: The Main Driving Force of Skull Base Development

The paranasal sinuses define endoscopic corridors. Aeration of the paranasal sinuses is a gradual process. Full aeration of the sinus is generally preferred prior to accessing the respective corridor. Moreover, this aeration process occurs simultaneously but in asymmetric fashion between the three main sinuses, the maxillary, ethmoid, and sphenoid sinus. The aeration process can be assessed by CT studies. More recently, thin-cut MRI scans have also been used to track the developmental process. The level of aeration will directly impact the drilling distance but will also affect neurovascular structures and restriction sites. Ultimately, safe drilling can be achieved through the soft immature bone regardless of pneumatization level especially when accessing lesions in the midline.[15] Thus, we consider pneumatization type to be a relative age-dependent limitation for EEA in children.

The sphenoid sinus is initially filled with red bone marrow. Between the ages of 7 months and 2 years, the red bone marrow is converted to yellow marrow, initially in the presphenoid plate and then extending posteriorly.[16] Effective pneumatization of the sphenoid sinus starts at 2 years and spans the entire childhood. It is thought of as the primary driving force of skull base development in children (▶ Fig. 1.1).[16,17] The progressive aeration of the sphenoid sinus directly impacts the transsphenoidal corridor. Certain parts of the corridor open up earlier than others and these anatomical differences can directly impact the endoscopic approach to the sinus. CT-based studies have shown that the aeration process follows a characteristic pattern, in inferior-to-superior and medial-to-lateral direction.[17] Volumetric studies using thin MRI cuts have shown that aeration occurs at a relatively slow pace.[1] Air first enters the sinus in a very exact location, namely the medial anteroinferior portion, and then expands laterally, inducing changes in both sphenoid and sellar width (▶ Fig. 1.2 and ▶ Fig. 1.3a). Access to the parasellar region is therefore optimal in older age groups. Significant volumetric and width changes at the sphenoid-sellar level occur slowly, around 11 to 13 years of age (▶ Fig. 1.2). There are no gender-dependent differences in sellar width or sinus volume. However, at the peak of the pneumatization process, higher variability in sphenoid sinus volume is also noted, due to changes in sinus width rather than length or height (▶ Fig. 1.2). The sphenoid sinus has been shown to predominantly expand in width during the aeration process, with little differences in drilling distances across age groups. Based on

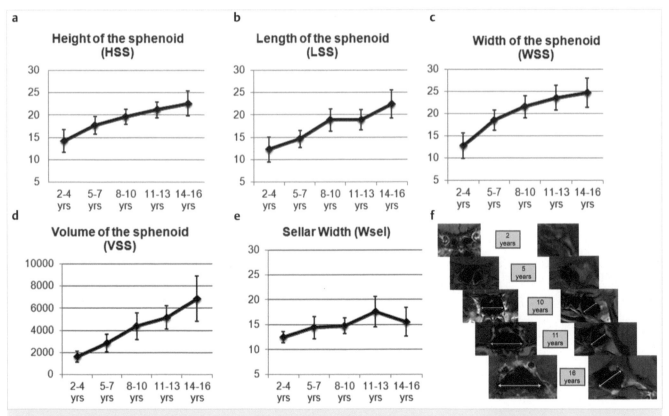

Fig. 1.2 Aeration of the sphenoid sinus is a progressive process, modifying the height, length, width, and overall volume as well as the width of the sellar area **(a-e)**. The process is finalized by 16 years of life. **(f)** The pneumatization process follows a characteristic pattern with predominant expansion in the lateral direction (inset).

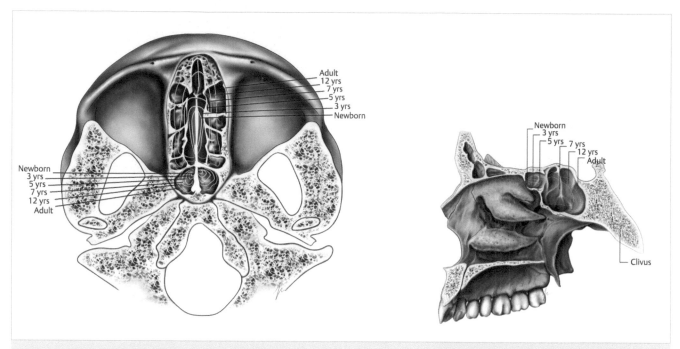

Fig. 1.3 Progressive aeration of the sphenoid sinus during skull base development (axial and sagittal depiction). Air first enters the sinus in the medial anteroinferior portion and then expands laterally, inducing changes in both sphenoid and sellar width.

these findings, we advocate for separation of pediatric surgical candidates in two distinct groups. Children 11 years or younger may require more drilling and, more importantly, have limited access to laterally extending lesions through the endonasal route. After the age of 12 years, air has sufficiently penetrated the lateral-most aspects of the sphenoid sinus, rendering access to the parasellar area easier and safer (▶ Fig. 1.3). Nonetheless, the pneumatization process can be frequently incomplete, with approximately 13 to 25% of adolescents and adults having a presellar pneumatization pattern at the end of the developmental process.[17] In such cases, air is solely localized in front of the sella turcica, requiring a more anterior entry point for transsphenoidal EEA.

The ethmoid sinus has a different pneumatization pattern, with air cells present immediately after birth at the anterior-most aspect of the sinus.[16] Air progressively penetrates posteriorly until puberty, for approximately 8 to 12 years, such that the medial and lateral walls of the sinus become parallel in anterior-to-posterior direction. The medial and inferior portions of the sinus are the last ones to become fully pneumatized, through extension of the anterior ethmoidal air cells. This inferomedial pneumatization process can also start at the level of the middle ethmoidal cells, creating a normal variant, the concha bullosa. The pneumatization process can also progress in an inferolateral direction, with extension along the roof of the maxillary sinus and the inferior lamina papyracea. During the normal pneumatization process, ethmoidal air can also be located at the level of the maxillary sinus ostium. Importantly, while the size of the ethmoid air cells changes with aeration, the relationship with the meatus does not change in evolution. During transethmoidal approaches, the pneumatization level and pattern of the ethmoid sinus can aid in adequate planning of the most appropriate surgical trajectory.

The maxillary sinus also undergoes a progressive aeration process, which will change its anatomical relationships. The rudimentary sinus has an initial volume of approximately $8\,cm^3$ and is located under the medial orbital wall. As it undergoes pneumatization, the sinus extends in lateral and inferior direction and reaches the maxillary bone and hard palate at approximately 9 years.[16] The final phases of the aeration process occur after the eruption of permanent teeth and push the floor of the sinus below the floor of the nasal cavity.

1.6 The Internal Carotid Arteries and Intercarotid Distance: Intracranial Restriction Sites

The posterolateral wall of the sphenoid sinus has a close anatomical relationship with the carotid and optic canals. Both structures are in direct contact with the sinus wall prior to sinus aeration. However, only the carotid artery location is changed by pneumatization of the sphenoid sinus. The optic canal has a constant position during skull base development.[3] Interestingly, clinoid pneumatization is believed to impact the position of both the optic nerve and the carotid canal.[14] Sphenoid aeration affects the internal carotid artery (ICA) at two levels: protrusion into the sinus and ICD at the level of the cavernous sinus (▶ Fig. 1.4). The level of ICA protrusion through the sphenoid sinus wall is directly related to the level of pneumatization. An overpneumatized sinus significantly increases the risk of ICA protrusion into the sinus and should be carefully assessed on imaging prior to planning the transsphenoidal trajectory. The pneumatization process further opens up endoscopic corridors while also constantly changing the location

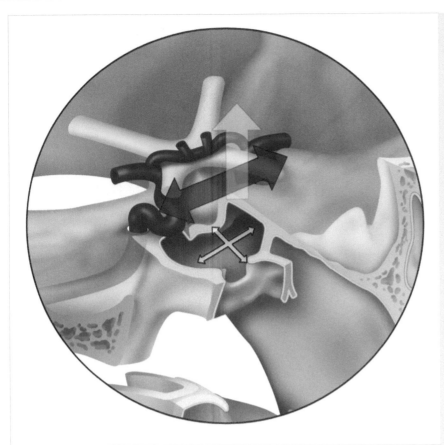

Fig. 1.4 Depiction of the relationship between the optic chiasm and internal carotid arteries and the impact of sphenoid sinus pneumatization on the intimate anatomical relationships between the two structures. The internal carotid arteries are pushed laterally (*red arrow*). These will impose the lateral limits of the endonasal endoscopic corridors. The optic chiasm is displaced cranially (*yellow arrow*).

and relationship of the ICAs. This will directly impact working trajectories and angles for the intradural dissection steps. Distance between the two ICAs will be a direct determinant of the lateral limits for EEA approaches in the pediatric population. Air enters the posterior and superior sections of the sphenoid sinus pushing the dorsal structures of the sinus superiorly and thereby modifying the anatomical relationships of the carotid canal[3] (▶ Fig. 1.1; ▶ Fig. 1.4).

However, whether the pneumatization process actually impacts the ICD at the level of the cavernous sinus and the clivus and whether there is a statistically significant difference in ICD between age groups remain controversial. Recent studies have revealed that incomplete pneumatization of the sphenoid sinus may indicate a narrow intercarotid corridor and a tight working angle at the level of the cavernous sinus, regardless of age group. In children still undergoing pneumatization, the cavernous ICD is 5 mm narrower compared to children with complete sphenoid aeration. Furthermore, the transsphenoidal angle, the working angle created by the two carotids at the level of the cavernous sinus, is 7° narrower in children with incomplete aeration of the sinus[1] (▶ Fig. 1.5). Other studies have found no statistically significant difference in cavernous ICD after 9 years or in clival ICD after 2 years.[17] In certain studies, an extreme medial course of the ICA was four times more common in adults compared to pediatric patients.[3] Differences in selection criteria, measurement techniques, and imaging studies may account for these incongruent findings.

The level of sphenoid sinus pneumatization can generally be predicted based on age group.[18] Indirectly, pneumatization pattern and age groups can be used to grossly predict the cavernous ICD. Nonetheless, recent studies have demonstrated that certain skull base lesions can delay or halt the aeration process. It is therefore important to assess the ICD whenever possible, regardless of age group, as the developmental process can be significantly altered by the presence of certain skull base lesions. This is especially true for the expanded EEA such as the transcavernous approach. Such approaches generally become feasible and safe after approximately 9 years of age, as the ICD reaches adult levels. In certain patients, this age cutoff may not directly correlate with the developmental stage. Direct measurements of the ICD and transsphenoidal angle (TA) may not be feasible due to tumor obstruction on MRI scans. Therefore, in cases where the ICD cannot be directly measured on imaging studies, we recommend using the sphenoid sinus pneumatization process as an indirect and accurate correlate for the ICD. Furthermore, patients with sellar pneumatization patterns, with air cells located along the entire width of the sella, are the best candidates for laterally expanded approaches. In such cases, the working TA is sufficiently wide to provide adequate freedom of movement and dissection. An ICD of 10 mm has generally been reported as the inferior safety limit.[19] Of note, recent studies in children without skull base lesions have demonstrated that the narrowest ICD is 11.3 mm, in the 2- to 4-year age group, thereby theoretically rendering expanded EEA safe in all pediatric age groups. Nonetheless, these distances are significantly altered in pediatric patients harboring skull base lesions and it is therefore important to be cognizant of this anatomical restriction site.

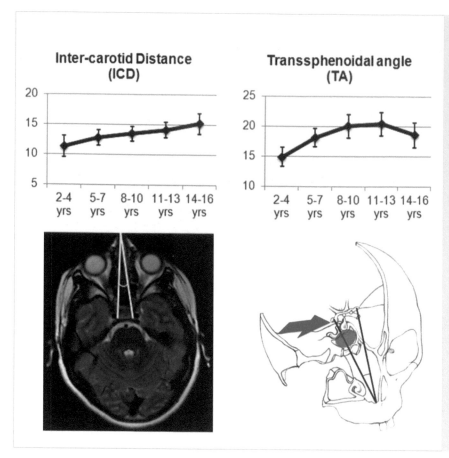

Fig. 1.5 Changes in intercarotid distance and transsphenoidal angle (TA) with age (in millimeters). The TA is defined at the level of the cavernous internal carotid artery. Insets depict measurement of the TA on MRI scans and schematic representation of the TA as an assessment of lateral extent of expanded endonasal approach corridors for sellar and suprasellar pathology.

1.7 Craniocaudal Skull Base Growth: Working Distances and Posteroinferior EEA Limits

Growth of the pediatric skull base is an asynchronous process: growth and development in certain areas of the skull base end before they even start in other regions.[20,21] This leads to significant asymmetry of skull base compartments during certain stages in childhood. Several areas of the face and skull have accelerated growth at the onset of puberty. Bones of the midfacies, including the piriform aperture and choanae, accelerate growth in late childhood, between 11 and 14 years of age.[22] This coincides with the peak of midsagittal craniocaudal expansion. Despite the relatively coordinated growth process of the anterior skull base during puberty, the dorsal portions have a more rapid development in earlier childhood, in the 5- to 7-year age group. This leads to asymmetry in both the anteroposterior and craniocaudal planes. The most dramatic changes occur at the most anterior and posterior areas of the skull base, the most active growth centers. Distances from the nasal aperture to various intracranial targets, such as the sella or the dens, have therefore a rather steep age-dependent growth trend. One exception is the maximal reachable zone of the dens (MaxRZD), measured from the platform of C2 to the naso-dens line. The MaxRZD changes little with age (▶ Fig. 1.6A–C). The nare-sellar distance has an accelerated growth trend in the first 12 years of life and then slow down 4 years before the completion of the developmental process, at approximately 16 years. Interestingly, in the extreme age groups, at 2 to 4 years and 14 to 16 years, there also appears to be a difference in this distance based on gender. In the 14- to 16-year age groups, the distance is approximately 8 mm shorter in girls compared to boys.[1]

On the other hand, several posterior areas of the skull base, such as the vomer and clivus, undergo insignificant location changes relative to the nasal aperture during development. The distance from the aperture to the vomer increases by only 8 mm from the start of skull base growth to puberty, when the growth process concludes. Similarly, the distance from the vomer to the clivus has a very mild growth slope, reaching a quick plateau at only 5 years of age (▶ Fig. 1.6d, e). Anterior skull base areas continue to expand throughout the entire childhood, whereas areas located more posteriorly finalize the developmental process early on. One notable exception to this rule is the craniovertebral junction (CVJ), described later. Overall, the craniocaudal and anteroposterior development of the skull base is an integrated process. Distance from the nasal aperture to the sella has been shown to directly correlate with distances to the vomer, clivus, and dens. Similarly, the sphenoid sinus pneumatization stage also directly correlates with distances to the sella and dens, demonstrating an aeration-driven developmental process. In children with a sellar pneumatization pattern, the mean distance from the nare to the sella is 13 mm longer compared to children with an incomplete, conchal pneumatization pattern. This relationship is much more evident for distances in the craniocaudal midsagittal plane but

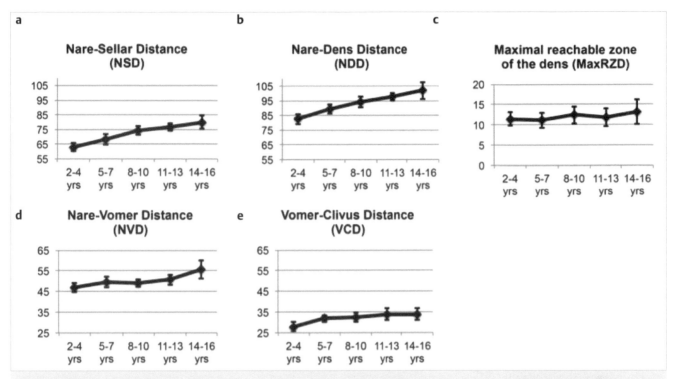

Fig. 1.6 Changes in working distances with age. Nare sellar and nare dens distance have a steep growth curve, while the maximal reachable zone of the dens changes little with age (**a-c**). Distances to the clivus quickly plateau by the age of 5 years (**d,e**).

becomes statistically insignificant for distances in the axial plane such as to the vomer to clivus distance. Pneumatization progresses in the posterosuperior direction and has, therefore, little effect on development and position of the clivus.

The EEA has been used to access the skull base from the cribriform plate to the CVJ. Accessing the posterior portions of the skull base in the pediatric population, especially the CVJ, is of particular importance given the preponderance of developmental pathology at this level. The CVJ, a complex anatomic region containing the clivus, the atlantoaxial complex, and the foramen magnum, harbors lesions frequently encountered in children such as basilar malformations and tumors. While the transoral route has been the approach of choice, recent studies have demonstrated the efficacy of EEA in accessing this region with minimal disruption of growth centers. Accessing the CVJ in the developing pediatric skull base has certain limitations, due to its posterior and, more importantly, inferior location in relationship to the initial EEA corridor. The inferior limit and working distance change constantly during development of the pediatric skull base and spine. The distance from the nasal aperture to the dens has a very steep growth curve based on age (▶ Fig. 1.6B). During the developmental process, the distance increases by approximately 20 mm, a much more abrupt increase compared to the more anterior target points via the transsphenoidal route. Interestingly, this increase mostly occurs during the first 6 years of development and is not significant past the 8- to 10-year age group. No gender-dependent differences have been reported for this target. This approach can be extended to the level of the C2 platform. Importantly, this MaxRZD has a relatively constant position during skull base development albeit with high individual variability and could therefore be accessed irrespective of age group (▶ Fig. 1.6c).

Development of the anterior elements will directly impact the working angle and, indirectly, the inferior limit for CVJ access. The length of the hard palate has been shown to be an accurate indirect predictor of the distance to the odontoid process.[23] In children without skull base pathology, an increase by 1 mm in the length of the hard palate has been shown to increase the distance from the nasal aperture to the CVJ by approximately 1.22 mm, further evidence of the asymmetry governing craniocaudal and anteroposterior skull base development. Based on age and developmental stage, the EEA has been shown in some studies to reach either the superior or the middle third of the odontoid process in children.[23] The relationship of the CVJ plane to the plane of the sphenoid sinus, the main EEA corridor, is the main factor in determining the inferior limit. This relationship changes constantly during normal growth, driven by several mechanical forces. Sphenoid sinus pneumatization occurs in anterior to posterior and inferior to superior fashion, pushing the clivus and atlantoaxial complex posteriorly and slightly superiorly, thereby increasing the working distance. At the same time, the pediatric spinal cord, undergoing a similarly complex growth process, influences the CVJ position from below. Spinal cord and spinal column development likely have the more important role as sphenoid sinus pneumatization preponderantly evolves in lateral direction. Therefore, since CVJ position is influenced by two independent developmental processes, the inferior limit cannot be simply predicted based on age. Importantly, developmental and neoplastic pathology at this level can throw normal patterns in disarray and make age-dependent predictions even less reliable. In such cases, CT- or MRI-based measurements can be of aid in perioperative planning.

1.8 The Piriform and Choanal Aperture: Extracranial Anatomical Restriction Sites and Skull Base Reconstruction

The piriform and choanal aperture, specifically the middle and inferior turbinates, are the most important superficial restriction points. The nasal aperture has a relatively independent developmental process from the rest of the skull base. Development of this region is predominantly influenced by the evolution of the midfacies and is a slow, gradual process without the earlier-described peaks and troughs. Furthermore, it is a process that reaches completion by mid-childhood. Some studies have found that the nasal aperture (NA) was significantly different only between extreme age groups, the 2- to 4-year and 11- to 13-year age groups.[1] Several studies have demonstrated that the NA concludes its growth process and reaches adult values by the age of 6 to 7 years.[17] Other studies have concluded that the NA continues its growth process well beyond 10 years of age.[23] Overall, the NA increases by only 3 to 5 mm throughout childhood. A 3-mm limit has been cited in the literature as being prohibitive for EEA.[17] Nonetheless, recent MRI-based studies, capable of adequate detection of local cartilaginous structures, have demonstrated that the minimal NA, in the 2- to 4-year age group, was approximately 6 mm, well beyond the restrictive limit. Furthermore, the cartilaginous structures of the developing NA can be easily manipulated to increase the workspace for EEA. Thus, we do not consider the inferior restriction points to be absolute contraindications for EEA in the pediatric population. Expanded EEA, both in anterior and posterior direction, have been safely performed in all pediatric age groups without the need for invasive facial approaches.[7,10,23] The overall volume of the piriform aperture is equally important, as it can directly impact working angles for EEA. Piriform aperture height increases by approximately 5 to 7 mm from the early childhood years (3–6 years) to the adolescent years (15–18 years). This increase in height along with increase in distance to various target sites described earlier increases the working distance as well as the access angle. Therefore, several approaches, especially expanded EEA, may in fact be more facile in younger children.

The next extracranial restriction site is located at the level of the turbinates, specifically the inferior and middle turbinates. The turbinates are bony structures, less malleable than the cartilaginous nasal aperture, and may be considered a true restriction site. Aeration of the sphenoid sinus progresses superiorly and has no impact on this area. Ethmoid sinus and maxillary sinus aeration may influence the relative position of the turbinates, but it is yet unclear to what extent. Thus, direct measurement of the maximal distance between the inferior and middle turbinates is necessary. The height and width of the choanae has been shown to be significantly different between the extreme pediatric age groups, 3 to 6 and 15 to 18 years. A difference of 5 mm in choanal height and 3 mm in choanal width was noted between these age groups.[23] Several authors have concluded that the 10.25-mm unilateral choanal aperture is a significant limitation for EEA corridors and that the uninostril approach is solely feasible in children 10 years or older. Other studies have shown that the maximal distance between the nasal turbinates, both the inferior and middle turbinates, is constant across age groups.[1] Importantly, high individual variability was noted for this region, demonstrating the need for perioperative measurements in order to assess the need for middle turbinate or posterior nasal septum resection as well as the need for a binostril versus uninostril approach.

Development of the nasal aperture can impact access to skull base lesions via endonasal endoscopic corridors as well as skull base reconstruction following the procedure. The nasoseptal flap, a neurovascular pedicled flap originating from the nasal septum, has become the gold standard in EEA, with significant reduction in CSF leak rates. The flap is harvested prior to the procedure and needs to provide sufficient coverage of the skull base defect (▶ Fig. 1.7). While the majority of the skull base has an accelerated growth trend in the first few years of life, the upper midfacies and, most importantly, the nasal septum trails behind. Cranium and skull base reach 95% of the adult measurements by 10 years of life, whereas facial measurements only reach 85% of their growth process by this age.[13] This asynchrony in development has little impact on the nasal and choanal aperture, as outlined earlier, but can affect skull base reconstruction. Using CT-based measurements, some authors have postulated that the nasoseptal flap may not be an adequate option for children 10 years or younger.[13] Between the ages of 10 and 13 years, the nasal septum undergoes a growth

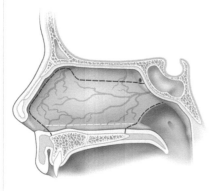
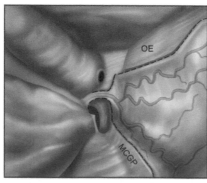

Fig. 1.7 Schematic representation of the nasoseptal flap. This pedicled flap has become the gold standard in skull base reconstruction after expanded endonasal approach. Dimensions of the nasoseptal flap change during the different stages of skull base development. The length of the nasoseptal flap is the most important limiting factor, while width has been shown to be appropriate irrespective of age group. For anterior skull base defects, the nasoseptal flap has adequate length and width after approximately 13 years, while for transsellar or expanded transplanar approaches it can be adequately used as early as 6 to 7 years. OE, olfactory epithelium; MCGP, maxillary crest growth plate.

spurt with significant increase in nasoseptal flap size reaching adult values by 14 years. Differences based on location of endonasal endoscopic corridor have also been described. Length of the nasoseptal flap is directly proportional to the size of the nasal septum and is the most important limiting factor. Width of the flap has been shown to be appropriate irrespective of age group. For anterior skull base defects secondary to expanded transcribriform approaches, the nasoseptal flap has both an adequate length and an adequate width after 13 years. On the other hand, the nasoseptal flap has appropriate dimensions for transsellar or expanded transplanar/transtubercular approaches as early as 6 to 7 years of age. The nasoseptal flap is insufficiently long for the transclival approach in all pediatric age groups. While this is an important limitation that should be taken into account when planning EEA in the pediatric patient, several other methods of skull base reconstruction have been described that can be used to complement the nasoseptal flap.

1.9 Impact of Skull Base Pathology on Skull Base Development

Development of the skull base is a highly regulated process with well-timed periods of acceleration and plateaus throughout childhood. Certain areas halt growth to allow other areas of the skull base to develop while also remotely influencing trajectories of neurovascular structures. This process can be significantly altered in children with skull base pathology. Skull base lesions delay the developmental process and significantly attenuate age-dependent differences by canceling the pneumatization-dependent growth trends of the sellar region. Certain types of lesions, such as tumors, are more likely to throw this process into disarray. Expansive suprasellar craniopharyngiomas, common pediatric tumors, have been shown to have the most dramatic effect.[1] Tumors of the skull base invade into the cranial cavity from below by eroding through bone and growth centers. Expansion into the sphenoid sinus of either skull base tumors or craniopharyngiomas and aggressive pituitary adenomas will block the pneumatization process, thereby canceling out the main driving force of skull base development. On the other hand, skull base lesions can also increase the maximal width between the inferior turbinates, providing easier access through the endonasal corridor. Location of the lesion is also important and will lead to significant alterations in development of certain areas. Lesions of the clivus or odontoid, two regions of active growth, significantly delay the growth process and can thereby shorten the distance to the sella by a maximum of 14 mm. Similarly, lesions located in the suprasellar region, such as craniopharyngiomas, have been shown to significantly delay the expansion of the CVJ complex and shorten the distance from the nasal aperture to the dens by approximately 27 mm. Furthermore, lesions in the maxillary or ethmoid sinus as well as lesions in the sellar region affect growth in the anteroposterior axial plane. Width of the sellar floor is significantly expanded in children harboring skull base lesions, especially in children with pituitary or suprasellar masses, thus expanding the EEA corridor laterally. Such differences are particularly evident around 11 to 13 years, the peak time for development of skull base and midfacies. Overall, skull base pathology has surprisingly little impact on neurovascular structures. Lesions located in the sellar region or at the clivus can nonetheless narrow the transsphenoidal intercarotid angle by 4.5° and 6°, respectively. Finally, skull base lesions can mask important anatomic landmarks, making perioperative planning particularly difficult. MRI- or CT-based skull base measurement systems can be particularly useful in such cases.[1,13,17,23]

These radioanatomical measurements cannot be simply predicted based on age in children with skull base lesions. MRI- or CT-based measurements have been described, assessing sphenoid sinus pneumatization patterns, volume of the sphenoid sinus, drilling distances, distances to various intracranial targets, restriction sites, and nasoseptal flap dimensions.[13,16,17,23] CT-based measurements can adequately assess bony anatomy, especially in eroding tumors, but can miss cartilaginous structures of the incompletely developed pediatric skull base. Recent studies have employed MRI-based measurements to overcome these limitations. These parameters have been proposed for perioperative planning to establish the safest surgical trajectory while also allowing optimal skull base reconstruction. However, most studies have demonstrated that, in the normal population, restriction parameters previously thought to be rate-limiting for EEA in children, such as the intercarotid cavernous distance or the choanal width, are well beyond the limiting threshold across all age groups after 5 years of age. The 2- to 4-year age group may be the only one with truly narrow corridors. Nonetheless, recent studies also suggest that these measurements can be significantly altered due to skull base pathology. Thus, performing these measurements prior to surgery is recommended regardless of age group, especially when assessing restriction parameters. Distances such as the nare–sellar distance, the nare–dens distance, the nare–vomer distance, or the vomer–clivus distance are correlated to the level of pneumatization. Other measurements such as the MaxRZD, the hard-palatine line, the choanal width and length, or the nasal aperture do not correlate with the aeration stage. The nare–sellar distance has been shown to accurately correlate with other working distances and can be used as an indirect measurement to predict these working distances. It can be used to obtain an overview of the skull base developmental stage and grossly assess restriction parameters in cases where other measurements are impeded by skull base pathology. Ultimately, narrow working corridors but short working distances are to be expected in children harboring skull base lesions, especially in those with aggressive tumors transgressing growth centers. Measurements can be used for planning but intraoperative navigation and knowledge of local anatomy and growth centers is recommended to increase safety in pediatric EEA.

References

[1] Banu MA, Guerrero-Maldonado A, McCrea HJ, et al. Impact of skull base development on endonasal endoscopic surgical corridors. J Neurosurg Pediatr. 2014; 13(2):155–169

[2] Tsai EC, Santoreneos S, Rutka JT. Tumors of the skull base in children: review of tumor types and management strategies. Neurosurg Focus. 2002; 12(5):e1

[3] Başak S, Karaman CZ, Akdilli A, Mutlu C, Odabaşi O, Erpek G. Evaluation of some important anatomical variations and dangerous areas of the paranasal sinuses by CT for safer endonasal surgery. Rhinology. 1998; 36(4):162–167

[4] de Divitiis E, Cappabianca P, Gangemi M, Cavallo LM. The role of the endoscopic transsphenoidal approach in pediatric neurosurgery. Childs Nerv Syst. 2000; 16(10–11):692–696

[5] Munson PD, Moore EJ. Pediatric endoscopic skull base surgery. Curr Opin Otolaryngol Head Neck Surg. 2010; 18(6):571–576

[6] Teo C, Dornhoffer J, Hanna E, Bower C. Application of skull base techniques to pediatric neurosurgery. Childs Nerv Syst. 1999; 15(2–3):103–109

[7] Chivukula S, Koutourousiou M, Snyderman CH, Fernandez-Miranda JC, Gardner PA, Tyler-Kabara EC. Endoscopic endonasal skull base surgery in the pediatric population. J Neurosurg Pediatr. 2013; 11(3):227–241

[8] Locatelli D, Massimi L, Rigante M, et al. Endoscopic endonasal transsphenoidal surgery for sellar tumors in children. Int J Pediatr Otorhinolaryngol. 2010; 74(11):1298–1302

[9] Kassam A, Thomas AJ, Snyderman C, et al. Fully endoscopic expanded endonasal approach treating skull base lesions in pediatric patients. J Neurosurg. 2007; 106(2) Suppl:75–86

[10] Banu MA, Rathman A, Patel KS, et al. Corridor-based endonasal endoscopic surgery for pediatric skull base pathology with detailed radioanatomic measurements. Neurosurgery. 2014; 10 Suppl 2:273–293,–discussion 293

[11] Stapleton AL, Tyler-Kabara EC, Gardner PA, Snyderman CH. Endoscopic endonasal surgery for benign fibro-osseous lesions of the pediatric skull base. Laryngoscope. 2015; 125(9):2199–2203

[12] Ma J, Huang Q, Li X, et al. Endoscopic transnasal repair of cerebrospinal fluid leaks with and without an encephalocele in pediatric patients: from infants to children. Childs Nerv Syst. 2015; 31(9):1493–1498

[13] Shah RN, Surowitz JB, Patel MR, et al. Endoscopic pedicled nasoseptal flap reconstruction for pediatric skull base defects. Laryngoscope. 2009; 119(6):1067–1075

[14] Tatreau JR, Patel MR, Shah RN, et al. Anatomical considerations for endoscopic endonasal skull base surgery in pediatric patients. Laryngoscope. 2010; 120(9):1730–1737

[15] Cavallo LM, de Divitiis O, Aydin S, et al. Extended endoscopic endonasal transsphenoidal approach to the suprasellar area: anatomic considerations–part 1. Neurosurgery. 2008; 62(6) Suppl 3:1202–1212

[16] Scuderi AJ, Harnsberger HR, Boyer RS. Pneumatization of the paranasal sinuses: normal features of importance to the accurate interpretation of CT scans and MR images. AJR Am J Roentgenol. 1993; 160(5):1101–1104

[17] Tatreau JR, Patel MR, Shah RN, McKinney KA, Zanation AM. Anatomical limitations for endoscopic endonasal skull base surgery in pediatric patients. Laryngoscope. 2010; 120 Suppl 4:S229

[18] Hamid O, El Fiky L, Hassan O, Kotb A, El Fiky S. Anatomic variations of the sphenoid sinus and their impact on trans-sphenoid pituitary surgery. Skull Base. 2008; 18(1):9–15

[19] Wolfsberger S, Neubauer A, Bühler K, et al. Advanced virtual endoscopy for endoscopic transsphenoidal pituitary surgery. Neurosurgery. 2006; 59(5):1001–1009, discussion 1009–1010

[20] Szolar D, Preidler K, Ranner G, et al. The sphenoid sinus during childhood: establishment of normal developmental standards by MRI. Surg Radiol Anat. 1994; 16(2):193–198

[21] Szolar D, Preidler K, Ranner G, et al. Magnetic resonance assessment of age-related development of the sphenoid sinus. Br J Radiol. 1994; 67(797):431–435

[22] Barghouth G, Prior JO, Lepori D, Duvoisin B, Schnyder P, Gudinchet F. Paranasal sinuses in children: size evaluation of maxillary, sphenoid, and frontal sinuses by magnetic resonance imaging and proposal of volume index percentile curves. Eur Radiol. 2002; 12(6):1451–1458

[23] Youssef CA, Smotherman CR, Kraemer DF, Aldana PR. Predicting the limits of the endoscopic endonasal approach in children: a radiological anatomical study. J Neurosurg Pediatr. 2016; 17(4):510–515

2 Pediatric Rhinologic Considerations

Gustavo J. Almodóvar-Mercado and Vijay K. Anand

Abstract

The developing sinonasal anatomy in children may differ from the adult patient; therefore, the rhinologist must play an important role in the endoscopic endonasal approach to the skull base in the pediatric patient. In this chapter, the developmental anatomy of the nasal cavity and four sets of paired paranasal sinuses are discussed in detail, and functional and comparative anatomy to that of adult sinuses will also be discussed. The location of the facial growth centers inside the nasal cavity should be carefully addressed during this approach to avoid facial growth abnormalities, in particular reference to posterior removal of the nasal septum. Understanding these concepts is integral for performing effective, safe, and appropriate pediatric endoscopic endonasal skull base surgery.

Keywords: pediatric endoscopic skull base surgery, sinonasal development, facial growth centers

2.1 Sinonasal Embryology and Developmental Anatomy

A clear knowledge of the embryologic and developmental anatomy of the nasal cavity, paranasal sinuses, and surrounding structures is integral to performing safe and appropriate pediatric endoscopic endonasal skull base surgery. In addition, an understanding of the embryologic development of the nasal cavity and paranasal sinuses allows for better comprehension of the spatial involvement of structures addressed during endoscopic approaches. Since the nasal and paranasal sinus structures develop from multiple bones rather than a single bone, the approaches to the targeted site have to be carefully considered in the surgical planning and execution.

The primary bones from which the nasal cavity and paranasal sinus structures develop are the maxillary, ethmoid, sphenoid, and frontal bones, with lesser contributions to paranasal sinus development from the lacrimal and zygomatic bones. The nasal septum develops from four sources: the perpendicular plate of the ethmoid bone, the maxillary bone or crest, the vomer, and the quadrangular cartilage.

2.1.1 Nasal Cavity

The development of the nasal cavity is heralded by the appearance of a series of ridges or folds on the lateral nasal wall between the fourth and eighth weeks of fetal life (▶ Fig. 2.1). During this time, the nasal septum can be seen dividing the right and left sides of the future nasal cavity as the frontonasal and maxillary processes join. The frontonasal process grows over developing forebrain, contributing to nasal olfactory placodes. At 8 weeks' gestation, the nasal septum arises as a posterior midline growth of the frontonasal process and midline extensions of mesoderm from the maxillary processes that are partially differentiated into cartilage.[1] The descending septum merges with the fused palate to create two distinct nasal cavities.

Beginning at 8 weeks, several ridges that persist throughout fetal development and into later life begin to develop along the lateral nasal wall.[1] These are traditionally called ethmoturbinals. The ethmoturbinals are considered to be ethmoid and

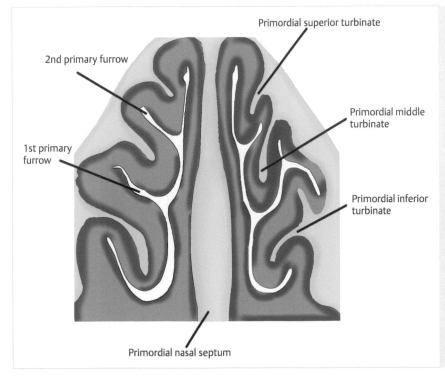

Fig. 2.1 Illustration of the nasal cavity at 8 to 12 weeks of embryological development.

Primordial superior turbinate

2nd primary furrow

Primordial middle turbinate

1st primary furrow

Primordial inferior turbinate

Primordial nasal septum

maxillary bone in origin and eventually develop into the agger nasi region of the ethmoid sinuses (superior portion of first ethmoturbinal or nasoturbinal), middle turbinate (second ethmoturbinal), superior turbinate (third ethmoturbinal), and supreme turbinate (fourth and fifth ethmoturbinals).[2,3] Between 9 and 12 weeks' gestation, a separate cartilaginous and soft-tissue bud corresponding to the uncinate process forms between the developing middle and inferior turbinates.[1,3] At 15 to 16 weeks' gestation, the inferior, middle, and superior turbinates are clearly formed and easily visible in embryologic sections.[3]

Around the same period, three furrows form between the ethmoturbinals and ultimately establish the primordial nasal meatuses and recesses that separate the adult turbinates.[4,5] The first furrow forms between the first and second ethmoturbinals. Its descending aspect forms the ethmoidal infundibulum, hiatus semilunaris, and middle meatus in the adult. Its ascending aspect can contribute to the frontal recess. The second furrow forms between the second and third ethmoturbinals developing into the superior meatus, while the third furrow forms between the third and fourth ethmoturbinals developing into the supreme meatus.

2.1.2 Olfactory Mucosa

At 8 weeks' gestation, a hypercellular mesenchymal capsule forms around the developing nasal structures and olfactory epithelium can be seen in the superior portion of the nasal cavity,

with the cribriform plate presenting in a cartilaginous form at 14 to 16 weeks. Postnatally, there is partial regression of the olfactory epithelium such that it occupies the area located in the nasal vault, the upper portion of the nasal septum, the medial surface of the superior turbinate, sectors of the medial surface of the middle turbinate, and the region of the cribriform plate.[6] The overall area averages 1 to 2 cm^2 in adults, but covers a much larger region in infants.[7]

2.1.3 Paranasal Sinuses

The extent of paranasal sinus pneumatization and development differs greatly from person to person as a result from the extent of invagination and evagination between the developing turbinates and their intervening furrows.[4] All paranasal sinuses are present to varying degrees in the newborn, each one having specific periods of significant growth. The ethmoid sinuses are the first to fully develop, followed in order by maxillary, sphenoid, and frontal sinuses (▶ Fig. 2.2).

Ethmoid Sinuses

As previously mentioned, the ethmoid sinus is the first to develop into detectable pneumatized cells in the fetus. Around the 11 to 12 weeks of fetal life, early anterior ethmoid cells, including the cartilaginous beginnings of the ethmoid bulla, form as a result of budding from the middle meatus.[1,5] At 14 to

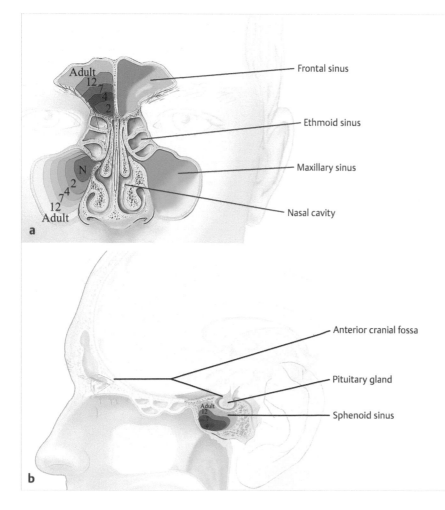

Fig. 2.2 (a) Coronal illustration of the nasal cavity, frontal, ethmoid, and maxillary sinuses. Note the pattern of development of the frontal and maxillary sinuses. N, newborn. (b) Sagittal illustration of the anterior cranial fossa, pituitary gland, and sphenoid sinus. Note the pattern of development of the sphenoid sinus. The numbers depict approximate years of age of the patient.

Frontal sinus

Ethmoid sinus

Maxillary sinus

Nasal cavity

Anterior cranial fossa

Pituitary gland

Sphenoid sinus

16 weeks, some anterior ethmoid cells are well formed.[1] Later, the posterior ethmoid buds begin to develop from the superior meatus by 17 to 18 weeks. Ossification of the ethmoid sinuses and lamina papyracea occurs by 20 to 24 weeks' gestation.[1,5]

At birth, the ethmoid sinuses are the most developed paranasal sinuses, having a complete number of cells in varying stages for development.[8] They undergo significant growth during the first decade of life, reaching their adult size by 12 years of age.[8,9] However, these cells can expand beyond the boundaries of the ethmoid bone to extend into the frontal recess (frontal cells, suprabullar cells, and frontal bullar cells), sphenoid bone (sphenoethmoid [Onodi] cell), and maxillary bone (infraorbital ethmoid [Haller] cell).

It is important to recall that the ethmoid bone contains more than the ethmoid sinuses. Other structures that are derived from the ethmoid bone include the middle turbinate, superior turbinate, supreme turbinate, cribriform plate, and the posterosuperior portion of the nasal septum (perpendicular plate of the ethmoid).

Maxillary Sinuses

The maxilla begins ossification at 11 to 12 weeks' gestation, as the early anterior ethmoid sinuses are developing.[1] The maxillary infundibulum becomes evident at 14 to 16 weeks of fetal life as an invagination of the maxillary bone, found lateral to the uncinate ridge. However, at this point, there is still no true maxillary sinus cavity. By 17 to 18 weeks' gestation, an air space is clearly seen lateral to the developing uncinate process, protruding toward the woven bone of the maxilla.[3] The developing maxillary sinus can be differentiated from the nasolacrimal duct at this stage as well.[3] Over the second and third trimesters, the maxillary sinus continues to enlarge from the maxillary infundibulum.

The maxillary sinuses are present at birth, although their small size typically precludes their radiologic appearance. Conspicuous growth in the maxillary sinuses begins by approximately 3 years of age, but inferiorly directed expansion does not occur until eruption of the permanent dentition, when the child is 7 to 8 years of age. The floor of the maxillary sinus approximates the inferior meatus at 8 years of age and reaches the level of the floor of the nose by 12 years of age. Adult size is reached by mid-adolescence.

Sphenoid Sinuses

Development of the sphenoid sinuses begins during the third to fourth months of gestation. The nasal cavity mucosa invaginates into the posterior portion of the cartilaginous nasal capsule to form a pouch-like cavity referred to as the cartilaginous cupolar recess of the nasal cavity.[10] The wall surrounding this cartilage is ossified in the later months of fetal development, and the complex is referred to as the ossiculum Bertini or "Bertini bone."[4,8] At this stage, the sphenoid bone has 2 ossification centers, separated by the canalis pharyngeus.[8] In the second and third years of life, the intervening cartilage is resorbed, and the ossiculum Bertini becomes attached to the body of the sphenoid bone.

The sphenoid sinus does not begin clinically significant pneumatization until 4 to 5 years of age with progression by 6 or 7 years. By 12 years of age, the anterior clinoids and pterygoid process can become pneumatized. Sphenoid sinus pneumatization is typically completed between 9 and 12 years of age, although it is highly variable in terms of the final extent of sphenoid bone pneumatization that can continue during adulthood.

Frontal Sinus

The last paranasal sinuses to begin, and complete development, are the frontal sinuses. The frontal recess originates as an outgrowth of the middle meatus in the frontal recess regions, at the superior aspect of the groove between the first and second ethmoturbinals.[2]

The frontal sinuses are typically not present at birth; growth begins during the fourth year of age of age and continues well into adolescence. Similarly to the sphenoid sinus, its pneumatization is highly variable, is of limited clinical significance until the early adolescent years, and continues to aerate until early adulthood. The thin posterior table and floor of the frontal sinuses have important anatomic relationship to the anterior cranial fossa and orbital structures, respectively.

2.2 Applied Anatomy and Facial Growth

The relatively small size of the child's nose has traditionally made endonasal endoscopic sinus surgery comparatively risky because of limited surgical exposure. Although still challenging, this situation has improved with the development of instrumentation and telescopes of appropriate size for the application of endoscopic endonasal surgery directed at the skull base region in the pediatric population.

Concerns of interruption to the patient's facial growth secondary to endoscopic sinus and skull base surgery has been described in the literature. Studies in piglets led to the suspicion that endoscopic sinus surgery could lead to an interruption of facial growth.[11,12] The first study to mention facial growth as an issue in children undergoing sinus surgery was that of Wolf in 1995, which noted no interruption of facial growth in children.[8] In one study, facial growth in children who had endoscopic sinus surgery at a mean of 3.1 years of age were examined 10 years later and compared with patients who did not have surgery.[13] A facial plastic surgeon performed both qualitative facial analysis and quantitative anthropomorphic analysis. His conclusion led to there being no evidence of malformations in facial growth in children undergoing surgery. This concept can be applied to pediatric endoscopic endonasal skull base surgery, since it employs sinus surgery techniques and procedures.

When harvesting the nasoseptal flap and performing removal of the posterior nasal septum for access during pediatric endoscopic skull base surgery, special consideration must be paid to preserve the adjacent facial growth centers. The growth centers of the nose have been designated as the sphenodorsal zone and the sphenospinal zone (▶ Fig. 2.3).[14] The length and height of the nasal bones are increased by growth of these zones along with the outgrowth of the maxilla. Trauma to these centers has been shown experimentally to interrupt growth of the nose and face in a predictable pattern, thus leading to progressive nasal deformity.[14,15,16]

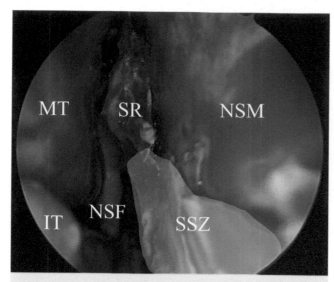

Fig. 2.3 Intraoperative picture showing the sphenospinal zone (SSZ), shaded in yellow, after harvesting of the nasoseptal flap (NSF) and removal of the posterior septum. MT, middle turbinate; IT, inferior turbinate; SR, sphenoid rostrum; NSM, contralateral nasal septum mucosa.

When performing endoscopic endonasal approaches in the pediatric patient, the techniques are similar to those employed in adult surgery. Special attention needs to be paid in evaluating the respective pneumatization pattern of the sinuses that will be involved during the procedure according to the patient's age, as previously described. For example, when performing an endoscopic endonasal approach for resection of a congenital encephalocele in a 3-year-old patient, no frontal sinus pneumatization will be encountered, and therefore the skull base will be more anteriorly located and inadvertently penetrated if this is not taken into consideration. In the same patient, the sphenoid sinus will most likely be underdeveloped, and special attention needs to be paid near the opticocarotid recesses since they will not be clearly demarcated at this age due to the poor pneumatization of the sphenoid at this age.

2.3 Conclusion

It is clear from these developmental anatomic changes in children that the structural anatomy can vary, and the complex mechanisms involved in sinonasal development will need to be carefully considered by the surgeon while performing pediatric endonasal endoscopic skull base surgery. Even though there is experimental evidence in the safety of certain approaches that have minimal impact on structural midfacial growth, the surgeon should be cognizant of the potential deformities at a later age in the young adults prior to the maturation of the midfacial area.

References

[1] Wake M, Takeno S, Hawke M. The early development of sino-nasal mucosa. Laryngoscope. 1994; 104(7):850–855

[2] Stammberger H. Functional Endoscopic Sinus Surgery: the Messerklinger Technique. Philadelphia, PA: B.C. Decker; 1991

[3] Bingham B, Wang RG, Hawke M, Kwok P. The embryonic development of the lateral nasal wall from 8 to 24 weeks. Laryngoscope. 1991; 101(9):992–997

[4] Wise SK, Orlandito RR, DelGaudio JM. Sinonasal development and anatomy. In: Kennedy DW, Hwang PH, eds. Rhinology: Diseases of the Nose, Sinuses, and Skull Base. New York, NY: Thieme; 2012:1–20

[5] Wang RG, Jiang SC, Gu R. The cartilaginous nasal capsule and embryonic development of human paranasal sinuses. J Otolaryngol. 1994; 23(4):239–243

[6] Escada PA, Lima C, da Silva JM. The human olfactory mucosa. Eur Arch Otorhinolaryngol. 2009; 266(11):1675–1680

[7] Naessen R. The identification and topographical localisation of the olfactory epithelium in man and other mammals. Acta Otolaryngol. 1970; 70(1):51–57

[8] Wolf G, Anderhuber W, Kuhn F. Development of the paranasal sinuses in children: implications for paranasal sinus surgery. Ann Otol Rhinol Laryngol. 1993; 102(9):705–711

[9] Shah RK, Dhingra JK, Carter BL, Rebeiz EE. Paranasal sinus development: a radiographic study. Laryngoscope. 2003; 113(2):205–209

[10] Vidić B. The postnatal development of the sphenoidal sinus and its spread into the dorsum sellae and posterior clinoid processes. Am J Roentgenol Radium Ther Nucl Med. 1968; 104(1):177–183

[11] Mair EA, Bolger WE, Breisch EA. Sinus and facial growth after pediatric endoscopic sinus surgery. Arch Otolaryngol Head Neck Surg. 1995; 121(5):547–552

[12] Carpenter KM, Graham SM, Smith RJ. Facial skeletal growth after endoscopic sinus surgery in the piglet model. Am J Rhinol. 1997; 11(3):211–217

[13] Bothwell MR, Piccirillo JF, Lusk RP, Ridenour BD. Long-term outcome of facial growth after functional endoscopic sinus surgery. Otolaryngol Head Neck Surg. 2002; 126(6):628–634

[14] Verwoerd CD, Verwoerd-Verhoef HL. Rhinosurgery in children: developmental and surgical aspects of the growing nose. GMS Curr Top Otorhinolaryngol Head Neck Surg. 2010; 9:Doc05

[15] Nolst Trenité GJ. Rhinoplasty in children. In: Papel ID, Frodel JL, Larrabee WF, et al., eds. Facial Plastic and Reconstructive Surgery. 3rd ed. New York, NY: Thieme; 2009:605–617

[16] Bae JS, Kim ES, Jang YJ. Treatment outcomes of pediatric rhinoplasty: the Asan Medical Center experience. Int J Pediatr Otorhinolaryngol. 2013; 77(10):1701–1710

3 Anesthetic Considerations in Pediatric Patients

Aarti Sharma and Jacques H. Scharoun

Abstract

Anesthesia for children undergoing endoscopic endonasal neurosurgical procedures presents an interesting challenge to the pediatric anesthesiologist. The endoscopic endonasal technique used in skull base surgery has evolved greatly in recent years and has become a well-established approach for resection of anterior skull base and pituitary tumors. Pituitary tumors can be functioning tumors with hormonal excess or nonfunctioning tumors with mass effect. The endoscopic surgical approach has been shown to significantly decrease the rate of complications, time in the operating room and length of hospital stay, and patient post-op discomfort. Successful surgical management of children with anterior skull base tumors requires a multidisciplinary approach and is critically dependent on the perioperative care of the pediatric patient. In this chapter, we address the preoperative assessment of these patients, intraoperative considerations related to the endoscopic endonasal surgical approach along with the postoperative complications related to the surgical approach, and the integrity of the hypothalamic–pituitary axis.

Keywords: pediatric anesthesia, endoscopic endonasal, pituitary tumors, neurosurgery, positioning, craniopharyngioma

3.1 Preanesthetic Considerations

3.1.1 General Considerations in Pediatric Patients

The child awaiting surgery will be anxious and may benefit from anxiolytic premedication. Excessive fasting will increase distress and cause dehydration and should be avoided. NPO (nil per os) guidelines should encourage drinking clear liquids until 2 hours before surgery. Blood loss is well tolerated until severe, and hypotension is a late sign of volume depletion.

3.1.2 Anatomical Considerations of Pediatric Skull Base Surgery

The sphenoid bone is solid at birth. Pneumatization is not complete until puberty.[1] The pediatric neurosurgeon must drill through a variable amount of solid sphenoid bone to reach the sella turcica.[1] Size considerations generally limit the fully endoscopic endonasal approach to children older than 3 to 4 years. The internal carotid arteries and cavernous sinus are in the middle skull base; any surgery in this area risks massive bleeding.[2]

3.1.3 Common Lesions

Craniopharyngioma, Rathke's cleft cyst, and pituitary adenoma are typical pediatric skull base lesions.[1] Multiple Endocrine Neoplasia 1 (MEN 1) causes both pituitary adenoma and hyperparathyroidism.[3]

3.1.4 Mass Effect of Skull Base Tumors

Skull base tumors can compress the third ventricle, causing hydrocephalus and elevated intracranial pressure (ICP).[4] Pressure on the optic chiasm leads to visual defects.[4] Compression of the pituitary can cause hyposecretion of one or more pituitary hormones and cause hypothyroidism, growth failure, secondary adrenal insufficiency, or diabetes insipidus (DI).[2]

3.1.5 Pituitary Hormone Excess

Pituitary adenomas may secrete excess hormones. The most common is prolactinoma, which is usually medically managed and does not impact anesthetic care significantly.[4]

Adrenocorticotropic hormone (ACTH) excess causes Cushing's disease, with many anesthetic implications.[4] The patient may have central obesity, with increased risk of gastroesophageal reflux disease (GERD) and aspiration. The Cushingoid face may impede mask ventilation. Hypertension is common, as is hyperglycemia. The skin is easily torn; care with tape and positioning is essential. Mild obstructive sleep apnea (OSA) is also common.[4]

Excess growth hormone may cause gigantism in a child or acromegaly in the teenager. Acromegaly causes macroglossia, hypertrophied pharyngeal tissue, and laryngeal stenosis; both OSA and difficulty with intubation are common. Hyperglycemia and hypertension are also common.[2] Thyroid-stimulating hormone (TSH) hypersecretion is rare in the pediatric population.[4]

3.1.6 Laboratory Investigations

Electrolytes should be assessed. Hyponatremia may occur with overzealous DI therapy, hypernatremia from undertreated DI. Hypercalcemia may occur with MEN 1. Hyperglycemia is common in Cushing's disease, and hypoglycemia occurs with ACTH deficiency.[3]

A type and screen, complete blood count, and coagulation studies should be checked due to the risk of massive intraoperative bleeding from large vascular structures.[4]

Pituitary functional assessment includes serum cortisol, ACTH, TSH, insulin-like growth factor 1 (IGF-1), and prolactin level. Any hormonal deficiency should be replaced.[4]

3.1.7 Imaging

MRI and CT are performed to evaluate hydrocephalus, invasiveness of lesion, compression or encasement of vital structures, and also as a component of neuronavigation.[1]

3.1.8 The Morning of Surgery

The patient with a hypopituitarism should continue the hormone replacement therapy (including glucocorticoid stress dosing).[4]

Physical examination should look for signs of Cushingoid facies or acromegaly, which may cause difficult mask ventilation or intubation, respectively.[2] Lethargy, emesis, and papilledema suggest elevated ICP, which may warrant rapid sequence intubation.[3]

Premedication can be useful after ruling out elevated ICP. Midazolam 0.5 mg/kg orally will facilitate parental separation, ease anxiety, and enhance patient compliance. Glycopyrrolate may be given for antisialagogue activity if difficult airway is anticipated.

3.2 Intraoperative Considerations

3.2.1 Induction

The endonasal endoscopic approach to skull base surgery avoids the potential injury caused by brain retraction and other complications associated with a transfrontal craniotomy.[5] This technique can be performed in children as young as 3 to 4 years, below which the naris is too small to allow successful instrumentation.

The choice between inhalation and intravenous induction can be jointly decided between the parent, child, and anesthesiologist, provided that ICP is not elevated. Unless the child has acromegaly or Cushing's disease, airway management is routine. A cuffed endotracheal tube is mandatory to prevent significant aspiration of blood and secretions from the nasal cavity. Two large bore peripheral intravenous catheters should be placed because of the risk of bleeding.

If the patient has hypopituitarism, stress dose glucocorticoids should be administered.

3.2.2 Monitoring

In addition to routine anesthesia monitors, the patient should also have continuous arterial blood pressure monitoring, first, to assist in monitoring extreme hemodynamic fluctuations, second, because of the risk of sudden massive blood loss, and, third, to monitor electrolytes in the event of DI. A Foley is essential because the patient may be receiving mannitol and also to monitor urine output because of the risk of DI. A central venous pressure (CVP) is generally not necessary.

3.2.3 Positioning

The patient will be positioned supine with head elevated approximately 30°, with the head slightly extended and turned to the left. The head is secured in a Mayfield clamp. The operating room table is then rotated 90° away from the anesthesiologist. The endotracheal tube should be well secured to prevent displacement during surgical manipulation. A throat pack is placed by the surgeon to help keep blood out of the stomach and lungs.

Maintenance of anesthesia may be accomplished by volatile agent alone, total intravenous anesthesia (TIVA), or more commonly a combination of the two. If the patient has elevated ICP, then TIVA is preferred.[6]

TIVA is easily accomplished using continuous infusion of propofol and remifentanil. TIVA also has the advantage of less postoperative nausea.

Visual evoked potentials (VEP), although not routine, are occasionally monitored to help preserve the integrity of the visual pathway. TIVA may increase the predictive value of VEP changes.[7]

Neuromuscular blockade is routinely used to prevent potentially disastrous patient movement.

The surgeon will begin preparing the nasal cavity with lidocaine and epinephrine to induce vasoconstriction. This may cause tachycardia and hypertension. This temporary problem can be treated by increasing the depth of anesthesia.

The surgeon may elect to place a lumbar spinal drain to detect (with intrathecal fluorescein) and decrease the incidence of cerebrospinal fluid (CSF) leak in select patients with high-risk settings.[8] Newer surgical closure techniques have greatly reduced the likelihood of the CSF leak.[9]

Antibiotic prophylaxis must provide coverage for gram-positive bacteria frequently found on the nasopharynx.

Normocapnia is ideal to prevent pituitary retraction upward and out of the sella turcica. Blood pressure should be maintained at preinduction levels. Hypotension may result in cerebral ischemia, while hypertension will increase the likelihood of bleeding.

3.2.4 Intravenous Fluid Management

Prevention of brain edema and hypovolemia are the primary goals of intravenous fluid (IVF) management. Hyponatremia must be avoided. Infusing Plasma-Lyte or normal saline will accomplish both of these goals; however, Plasma-Lyte has the additional advantage of avoiding hyperchloremic metabolic acidosis.[10] Dextrose-containing solutions are best avoided in the absence of hypoglycemia. Hyperglycemia may increase neurosurgical morbidity as in the ischemic areas of the brain, glucose metabolism may enhance the tissue acidosis.[11]

Mannitol may be requested by the surgeon to decrease brain edema.

3.2.5 Potential Intraoperative Complications

DI may occur during lengthy dissection of the pituitary but more commonly occurs postoperatively. DI is suggested by increased urine output greater than 4 mL/kg/h in the absence of diuretic administration or hyperglycemia, plasma sodium greater than 145, and plasma osmolarity greater than 300 with a urine osmolarity less than 300. If this occurs, the intravenous vasopressin infusion should be started at 0.5 mU/kg/h, and titrated upward until urine output decreases. Once this occurs, IVF should be restricted to two-thirds maintenance after initial hypovolemia has been corrected.

Venous air embolism, although rare in this procedure, is possible due to elevation of the head and should be considered in the differential diagnosis of unexplained hypotension.

Although oozing is expected, major bleeding is unlikely. However, due to the proximity of the internal carotid arteries and cavernous sinus, one should be prepared for massive transfusion.

3.2.6 Emergence

Post-op nausea and vomiting (PONV) is common and all patients should receive a 5HT3 antagonist. Additionally, dexamethasone is given to decrease PONV if the patient has not received stress-dose steroids.

The throat pack is removed, the stomach is suctioned with an oral gastric tube, and neuromuscular blockade is reversed.

The goals of emergence include avoidance of coughing or hypertension, both of which may cause bleeding at the surgical site. The oropharynx should be clear of blood and secretions before extubation. The patient should be able to follow commands soon after extubation to allow a neurological assessment.

3.3 Postoperative Considerations

These patients need to be followed up, preferably in the pediatric intensive care unit, for hemodynamic monitoring and postoperative complications. Complications after pituitary surgery can be related to its anatomical location and its role in regulating various endocrine axes. Disturbance in fluid and electrolyte balance can be seen in the immediate postoperative period. DI is a common complication, possibly due to compression or destruction of the posterior pituitary gland, interruption of the blood supply to the gland, or edema to the pituitary stalk. Meticulous assessment of volume status is made; frequent serum sodium levels are obtained to monitor the development of DI or syndrome of inappropriate antidiuretic hormone (SIADH) secretion or cerebral salt wasting (CSW) syndrome.

DI is often a transient phenomenon, and patients may be able to maintain neutral fluid balance by drinking to the stimulus of thirst. However, it may be beneficial to administer Desmopressin (1-deamino-8-D-arginine vasopressin, abbreviated DDAVP) prior to bedtime to allow patients to sleep comfortably i.e., not disturbed by the need to get up constantly to drink fluids.[12]

SIADH may develop later in the postoperative period and is defined by hyponatremia and hypo-osmolality due to inappropriate secretion of antidiuretic hormone, which results in impaired water excretion. SIADH causes water retention in the body; first line of treatment should be water restriction. If significant hyponatremia persists with Na levels less than 120 mmol/L, treatment with hypertonic saline may be considered.

CSW is a rare cause of hyponatremia and it should be distinguished from SIADH because restriction of water in CSW can be deleterious to patients. Clinical distinction between the two can be challenging. Patients with CSW have evidence of extracellular fluid depletion, such as negative fluid balance, low CVP, increased urea, and tachycardia; the treatment is replacement of sodium and fluid losses.

After transsphenoidal adenomectomy, new unplanned hypopituitarism may occur in a small number of patients. Various tests may be ordered to detect hormonal status of the pituitary gland, such as serum cortisol level, free thyroxin, TSH, IGF-1, growth hormone, follicle-stimulating hormone, luteinizing hormone, testosterone, and estradiol.

Patients undergoing surgical resection of pituitary adenomas are frequently given perioperative glucocorticoid therapy. In patients with proven ACTH deficiency preoperatively, it is recommended that the glucocorticoid therapy should be administered perioperatively up to 48 hours postoperatively. For patients with intact hypothalamic–pituitary–adrenal (HPA) axis function preoperatively, and in whom selective adenomectomy is possible, perioperative glucocorticoids are not necessary.

Early postoperative assessment depends on daily clinical assessment of the patient and morning plasma cortisol levels.

Vigilance in clinical monitoring of the patient's neurological and visual status is imperative, as patients may develop complications such as hematomas, epistaxis, ischemic events, hydrocephalus, CSF leak, and meningitis. Some nasal discharge in the immediate postoperative period may be expected. However, if excessive clear fluid drainage from the nose is encountered, if the patient reports a salty taste in the back of the throat with the discharge, and if the drainage is worse with the bending forward motion and is associated with the headache, then a CSF leak should be ruled out. Drainage should be collected and sent to the laboratory for the specific CSF markers. CT scan of the head should also be obtained to evaluate for pneumocephaly. CSF leak is treated with immediate re-exploration and repair. Intraoperative CSF leak has been identified as the risk factor for development of postoperative meningitis. When clinical suspicion of meningitis is high, lumbar puncture should be performed and empiric antibiotics should be started.[13,14]

Postoperative bleeding can result in hematoma at the operative site or intraventricular bleeding; the latter may result in postoperative hydrocephalus. Postoperative hematoma can be occasionally encountered in patients with pituitary apoplexy. This may result in neurological deterioration, stroke, and seizure, and needs to be addressed in a time-sensitive manner. Neurological deterioration due to any reason may warrant tracheal reintubation and mechanical ventilation.[15]

Postoperative bleeding resulting in hematoma may cause deterioration of the visual field. Other causes of visual loss could be direct injury to the optic apparatus, cerebral vasospasm, orbital fracture, pneumatocele, prolapse of the optic chiasm into empty sella, infectious process, or overgenerous fat or muscle packing.[16]

Postoperative nausea and vomiting (PONV) is frequently seen after neurosurgery. Incidence of PONV is lower following transsphenoidal surgery due to the less invasive nature of the procedure, resulting in minimal disturbance of the chemoreceptor trigger zone. Moreover, the smaller incision and minimal disruption of the surrounding structures may lead to less inflammation and pain with lower incidence of PONV. Some of the risk factors that may contribute to higher incidence of PONV are CSF leak, fat grafting, and lumbar drain placement. PONV may be treated with 5HT3 receptor antagonist.[17]

Postoperative analgesia is needed for pain at the operative site and for the headache. Postoperative opioid requirement in the transsphenoidal pituitary surgical patients is found to be minimal. The reason for this is thought to be because the pituitary has the highest concentration of endogenous opioids in the central nervous system, and it is possible that its manipulation during surgery releases these endogenous opioids, diminishing the need for postoperative opioid analgesia.[17]

References

[1] Khalili S, Palmer JN, Adappa ND. The expanded endonasal approach for the treatment of intracranial skull base disease in the pediatric population. Curr Opin Otolaryngol Head Neck Surg. 2015; 23(1):65–70

[2] Smith M, Hirsch NP. Pituitary disease and anaesthesia. Br J Anaesth. 2000; 85 (1):3–14

[3] Dunn LK, Nemergut EC. Anesthesia for transsphenoidal pituitary surgery. Curr Opin Anaesthesiol. 2013; 26(5):549–554

[4] Nemergut EC, Dumont AS, Barry UT, Laws ER. Perioperative management of patients undergoing transsphenoidal pituitary surgery. Anesth Analg. 2005; 101(4):1170–1181

[5] Chivukula S, Koutourousiou M, Snyderman CH, Fernandez-Miranda JC, Gardner PA, Tyler-Kabara EC. Endoscopic endonasal skull base surgery in the pediatric population. J Neurosurg Pediatr. 2013; 11(3):227–241

[6] Cole CD, Gottfried ON, Gupta DK, Couldwell WT. Total intravenous anesthesia: advantages for intracranial surgery. Neurosurgery. 2007; 61(5) Suppl 2: 369–377, discussion 377–378

[7] Nakagawa I, Hidaka S, Okada H, Kubo T, Okamura K, Kato T. Effects of sevoflurane and propofol on evoked potentials during neurosurgical anesthesia. Masui. 2006; 55(6):692–698

[8] Tien DA, Stokken JK, Recinos PF, Woodard TD, Sindwani R. Cerebrospinal fluid diversion in endoscopic skull base reconstruction: an evidence-based approach to the use of lumbar drains. Otolaryngol Clin North Am. 2016; 49 (1):119–129

[9] Garcia-Navarro V, Anand VK, Schwartz TH. Gasket seal closure for extended endonasal endoscopic skull base surgery: efficacy in a large case series. World Neurosurg. 2013; 80(5):563–568

[10] McFarlane C, Lee A. A comparison of Plasmalyte 148 and 0.9% saline for intraoperative fluid replacement. Anaesthesia. 1994; 49(9):779–781

[11] Rovlias A, Kotsou S. The influence of hyperglycemia on neurological outcome in patients with severe head injury. Neurosurgery. 2000; 46(2):335–342, discussion 342–343

[12] Nemergut EC, Zuo Z, Jane JA, Jr, Laws ER, Jr. Predictors of diabetes insipidus after transsphenoidal surgery: a review of 881 patients. J Neurosurg. 2005; 103(3):448–454

[13] Halvorsen H, Ramm-Pettersen J, Josefsen R, et al. Surgical complications after transsphenoidal microscopic and endoscopic surgery for pituitary adenoma: a consecutive series of 506 procedures. Acta Neurochir (Wien). 2014; 156(3): 441–449

[14] Dumont AS, Nemergut EC, II, Jane JA, Jr, Laws ER, Jr. Postoperative care following pituitary surgery. J Intensive Care Med. 2005; 20(3):127–140

[15] Naunheim MR, Sedaghat AR, Lin DT, et al. Immediate and delayed complications following endoscopic skull base surgery. J Neurol Surg B Skull Base. 2015; 76(5):390–396

[16] Magro E, Graillon T, Lassave J, et al. Complications related to the endoscopic endonasal transsphenoidal approach for nonfunctioning pituitary macroadenomas in 300 consecutive patients. World Neurosurg. 2016; 89:442–453

[17] Flynn BC, Nemergut EC. Postoperative nausea and vomiting and pain after transsphenoidal surgery: a review of 877 patients. Anesth Analg. 2006; 103 (1):162–167

4 Patient Positioning and Operating Room Setup

Fara Dayani, Zachary Medress, Vijay K. Anand, Theodore H. Schwartz, Harminder Singh

Abstract

Patient positioning and operating room setup are critical initial steps in ensuring the success of a pediatric endoscopic operation. Mask based registration systems are an alternative for pediatric patients who are too young for rigid cranial fixation in pins. Thoughtful positioning of the head allows for ergonomically efficient access to sellar, suprasellar, planum, and clival regions in endoscopic cases. Likewise, attentive organization of the surgical staff, operating room table, endoscopic tower, and operative adjuncts within the operating room play an important role in performing efficient and safe surgery. In this chapter, we discuss nuances in patient positioning and operating room set up that pave the way for achieving success in pediatric endoscopic operations.

Keywords: patient positioning, operating room set up, cranial fixation, neuro-navigation

4.1 Introduction

Patient positioning and operating room setup are critical steps in ensuring the success and safety of pediatric endoscopic skull base surgery. With recent technological advances in neuroendoscopic surgery, there has been an exponential increase in the skull base surgeon's armamentarium, with different instrument clusters vying for space and attention in the operating room. Therefore, it is vitally important to optimize operating room setup, patient positioning, and use of navigational technology to ensure a smooth workflow, improve ergonomics, and minimize clutter. This chapter will provide an updated overview of patient positioning and operating room setup specific to pediatric endoscopic skull base surgery.

4.2 Patient Positioning

Patient positioning is a critical component of each surgery, as it determines accessibility to the surgical target, visualization, and any potential harm done to the patient in this process. The patient's head may be secured using a clamp/pin-based system (▶ Fig. 4.1), which provides rigid fixation, or a mask-based system (▶ Fig. 4.2), which allows for free manipulation of the head during surgery. There are advantages and disadvantages associated with each method that make one more favorable than the other depending on the case.

The Mayfield clamp (three pins) or the Sugita head holder (four to six pins) allows for stabilization of the head by distributing the pressure at multiple pin sites. The more the number of pins used to fix the head, the less pressure on each individual pin site, making a calvarial breach less likely in younger patients. Upon fixation of the head in a certain position, any changes in the position of the head are not feasible during surgery. This could be a disadvantage if a wide range of maneuvers is required during surgery. Another drawback with rigid-pin fixation in pediatric patients is the increased risk of skull

fracture, scalp laceration, or development of a pin-site hematoma. Pin-site epidural hematoma in children has been reported to have an incidence of rate of 0.65%.[1] Currently, there are no guidelines in place for the application of cranial fixation pins, but it is often avoided in patients younger than 3 years of age.[2,3]

The major disadvantages of rigid head fixation are addressed in the mask-based system. The patient's head is placed in a soft headrest (▶ Fig. 4.2a,b), which allows for easy mobility of the head during surgery. This flexibility in head movement allows the surgeon to flex, extend, or rotate the patient's head to access varying regions of the skull base in an ergonomic fashion. This will be further discussed later in the chapter. A mask-based navigation system (▶ Fig. 4.2c) is placed on the patient's face/forehead to allow for accurate stereotactic localization of pathology. It is important to note that by not fixating the head, there is increased risk for unwanted head movements during the procedure. Another option for accurate stereotactic localization without cranial fixation is to screw the localization prong directly into the patient's skull. This, however, might not be an attractive option in younger patients with thin calvariums.

4.2.1 Head Positioning

The head can be positioned in a neutral position, or at different points along the sagittal plane in flexion or extension (▶ Fig. 4.3b), depending on the location of the lesion. Clival lesions require the head to be positioned in a neutral to slightly flexed position. Lesions located within the sella require the head to be positioned in a neutral or slightly extended position. Suprasellar and planum lesions require further extension of the head to about 15° from the neutral position. These variations in inclination of the head according to location of the lesion are necessary to improve ergonomics and facilitate direct access to the lesion. However, since the endoscope itself can be positioned at any angle, the main goal of head positioning is the surgeon's comfort rather than visualization. If a patient's head with a planum lesion is pinned neutral or in flexion, a 0-degree endoscope will be positioned too close to the patient's chest in

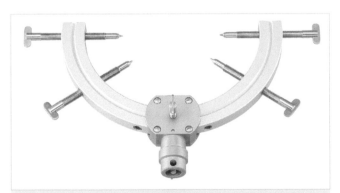

Fig. 4.1 Sugita head holder. This instrument demonstrates the basics of a clamp/pin-based system. The patient's head is placed inside the frame, and it is stabilized in a fixed position using 4 to 6 pins. (This image is provided courtesy of Mizuho.)

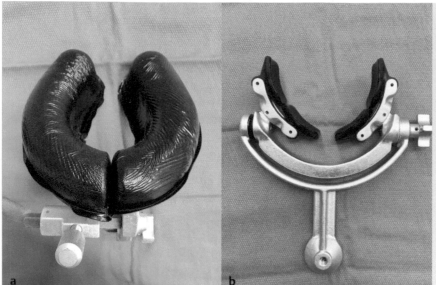

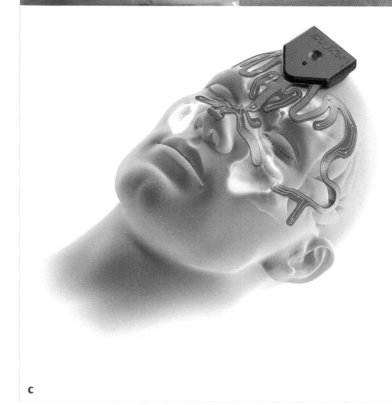

Fig. 4.2 Mask-based system for stereotactic endoscopic endonasal surgery. The patient's head is placed on the headrest **(a,b)** without the use of any pins and clamps, permitting wide range of movements during the operation. **(c)** The mask-based navigation system used for stereotactic localization. The Stryker cranial mask is placed on the patient's face to register the 3D position of the patient in order to match that to preoperative images. (These images are provided courtesy of Stryker.)

order to "look up," interfering with the maneuvering of the surgical instruments. Similarly, if a patient's head with a clival lesion is pinned in extension, the 0-degree endoscope will be positioned too high above the patient's chest in order to "look down," creating an awkward working angle for the surgeon.

Head rotation, which involves moving the head along the axial plane (▶ Fig. 4.3a), and head tilt, in which the head is rotated in the coronal plane (▶ Fig. 4.3c), are other ways to manipulate head positioning. Usually, the head is rotated and tilted 10-15° toward the side where the primary surgeon is standing to improve ergonomics. For right-handed surgeons, the head is rotated and tilted toward the right side and vice versa. Optimal head positioning is paramount in cases where

the patient's head is in rigid pin fixation, because that is the position that the head will remain throughout the case. More importantly, in order to minimize bleeding and reduce venous engorgement, it is important to try to elevate the head above the heart with flexion of the back or reverse Trendelenburg. In order to achieve adequate head elevation, the bed must often be positioned low to the ground.

4.3 Operating Room Setup

In today's practice, each operation entails participation of different team members at different stages of the operation.

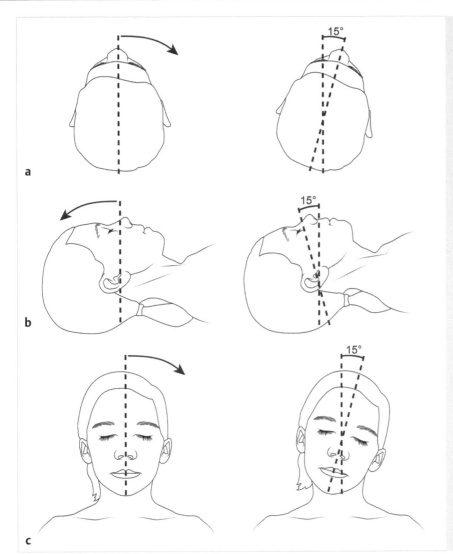

Fig. 4.3 Head positioning along three different axes to gain optimal access and visualization. (a) Head rotation (axial plane). (b) Head extension or flexion (sagittal plane). (c) Head tilt (coronal plane), respectively.

Moreover, technological advances have found their way into the operating room in the form of instruments, intraoperative imaging, stereotactic localization, neuromonitoring, surgical aspiration and ablation devices, and so forth (see Chapters 5 and 6). With the presence of multiple devices and personnel, it is of utmost importance to have a systematic way of setting up the operating room to promote organization, efficiency, and optimal performance.

Image guidance is a crucial component of endoscopic surgery. Surgeons could use previously acquired CT/MR imaging or utilize live intraoperative CT (iCT) or intraoperative MR imaging (iMRI). This variation requires a different operating room (OR) setup. OR setup with imaging guidance using previously obtained CT/MR imaging is shown in ▶ Fig. 4.4. The surgeon and the assistant stand on opposite sides of the operating table, both of them facing an imaging guidance monitor. The endoscope and image guidance monitors are placed toward the head of the patient. The infrared camera for tracking image guidance is also placed toward the patients' head. The anesthesia team sits behind the assistant.

The OR setup with image guidance using iCT is illustrated in ▶ Fig. 4.5. In this case, the CT scanner ring is placed close to the patient's head. Both the surgeon and the assistant stand on the same side of the operating table in order to accommodate the ring of the CT scanner. The endoscope and image guidance monitors are placed on the contralateral side to the surgeon and assistant. A disadvantage of this setup is that only one surgeon can operate at a time using the endoscope that is mounted on an endoscope holder contralateral to the surgeon and assistant. It is important to note that infrared camera is placed at the end of the bed, close to the patient's feet, so that it is in direct line of sight to the three-prong reference array, as well as the localization markers on the face of the CT scanner ring, to allow for image guidance registration in real-time. Finally, the anesthesia team is placed behind the ring of the CT scanner.[4]

In both these scenarios, if a fascia lata graft needs to be harvested from the thigh for skull base repair, it should be obtained from the contralateral thigh of the patient to where the primary surgeon is standing. In this way, the primary surgeon can continue the skull base portion of the case while the assistant harvests the graft.

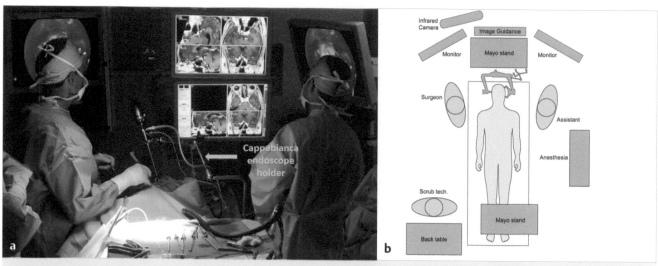

Fig. 4.4 (a) Photograph of the operating room setup for endonasal endoscopic cases using preoperative MRI/CT imaging for stereotactic localization. (b) Schematic of the operating room setup.

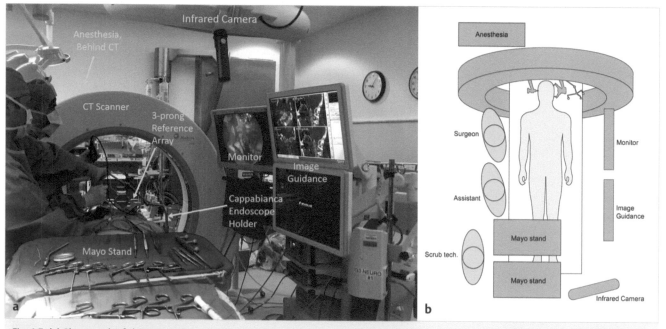

Fig. 4.5 (a) Photograph of the operating room setup for endonasal endoscopic cases with intraoperative CT image guidance for stereotactic localization. (b) Schematic of the operating room setup.

4.4 Conclusion

In pediatric endoscopic skull base procedures, patient positioning and OR setup are critical to ensure the safety and efficiency of the operation. In children, stereotactic localization can be achieved by utilizing a pins/clamp-based system or a mask-based system. Clamp-based systems with pins are not utilized in children younger than three years. Depending on the location of pathology, the patient's head can be moved along different axis to allow for easier access and better visualization. OR setup can differ depending on the type of image guidance used during the procedure.

References

[1] Vitali AM, Steinbok P. Depressed skull fracture and epidural hematoma from head fixation with pins for craniotomy in children. Childs Nerv Syst. 2008; 24 (8):917–923, discussion 925

[2] Berry C, Sandberg DI, Hoh DJ, Krieger MD, McComb JG. Use of cranial fixation pins in pediatric neurosurgery. Neurosurgery. 2008; 62(4):913–918, discussion 918–919

[3] Reavey-Cantwell JF, Bova FJ, Pincus DW. Frameless, pinless stereotactic neurosurgery in children. J Neurosurg. 2006; 104(6) Suppl:392–395

[4] Singh H, Rote S, Jada A, et al. Endoscopic endonasal odontoid resection with real-time intraoperative image guided computed tomography (CT). J Neurosurg. 2018; 128(5):1486–1491

5 Instrumentation

Walid I. Essayed, Khaled Radhounane, Theodore H. Schwartz, and Harminder Singh

Abstract
In this chapter, we describe instrumental advances in endoscopic endonasal surgery and their application in pediatric neurosurgery. After reviewing the technical innovations of endoscopes, we will describe the advances in instrumentation following their use at different surgical phases.

Keywords: instrumentation, endoscopic technology, skull base, 3D endoscopy, pediatric neurosurgery

5.1 Introduction

Over the last decade, endoscopic endonasal surgery (EES) progressively became the gold standard for approaching the anterior skull base in adults. As surgical instrumentation and techniques continue to evolve, the array of pathologies treatable through this route will continue to broaden. This surgery was mainly developed in adults, given the higher prevalence of midline skull base tumors and the wide aeration of the sinuses; however, with increasing experience and the development of smaller, specially designed instrumentation, application to pediatric EES is increasing.[1] The main principles of EES remain the same in both adults and children; however, potential anatomical and physiological limitations such as piriform aperture, sphenoid pneumatization, clival intercarotid distance, and maxillary crest growth plate preservation must be considered in pediatric endonasal skull base surgery.[2]

In this chapter, we will review the advances in instrumentation that allowed adaptation of endoscopic surgery to pediatric patients. These advances will be discussed according to the logic of their use during surgery, starting with the improvements of the endoscopes.

5.2 Endoscopes and Associated Tools

5.2.1 Endoscopes

Successive improvements in endoscopic technology progressively revolutionized skull base surgery. First generations of endoscopes required cumbersome large lenses, and provided low-definition images with poor illumination. These limitations were gradually surpassed by continuous technological advances, allowing currently available endoscopes and high-definition cameras to render an unprecedented wide, high-definition image of the operative field. Endoscope diameter can be as small as 2.7 mm, which can be extremely useful in young children given the small size of the nostrils and sinus cavities.[3]

Currently, most endoscopes used for skull base surgery are rigid rod-lens type and are 18 or 30 cm in length and 2.7 or 4.0 mm in diameter. As light is better transmitted through large-diameter endoscopes because of the larger lens, the

4-mm-diameter endoscopes are the most frequently used. Anatomically, when compared to adults, nasal aperture is significantly narrower in children younger than 7 years. This can significantly limit the endoscopic route in younger patients.[4] In these situations, the narrower 2.7-mm endoscope can be of use. Nonetheless, some authors have reported effective use of the 4-mm endoscope in infants whose body weight was in excess of 2.2 kg.[5] Given the small size of the nasal passages, when using a 4-mm endoscope, the instruments are generally passed solely through the contralateral nostril and not in the same nostril as the endoscope, as is often done in adults. The longer length (30 mm) of the endoscope is helpful in situations where an endoscopic holder is used. The holder arm usually attaches to the shaft of the endoscope, and the long length keeps the bulk of the holding apparatus away from the nares. This allows the surgeon adequate room to maneuver the surgical instruments without hindrance from the holder arm.

The lack of depth perception while using classical 2D endoscopes is now mendable using 3D endoscopes.[6] The visualization of spatial relationships between anatomical structures improves surgical dexterity while shortening the learning curve for endoscopic surgeons.[6] The first-generation 3D endoscopes suffered multiple limitations: large shaft diameter, lack of angled lenses, and decreased resolution. Currently, innovative technology is overcoming these limitations with new generation of endoscopes capable of rendering unprecedented 3D view of the surgical field.[6] The better depth perception facilitates anatomical understanding and safe maneuvering of instruments inside the nasal cavity, which is crucial in pediatric patients with unusual anatomic landmarks, and limited intranasal room. The Visionsense 3D-endoscope, (Visionsense, Philadelphia, PA) has been the most frequently used for endonasal surgery given its 4-mm diameter. However, a new 3D endoscope designed by Karl Storz offers a similar diameter with a dual-lens technology that may provide improved color and optics (▶ Fig. 5.1).

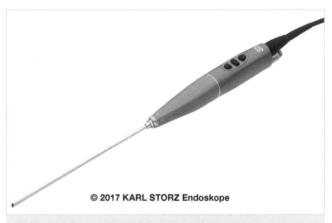

© 2017 KARL STORZ Endoskope

Fig. 5.1 The 30-degree Karl Storz Full HD 3D Endoscope. (This image is provided courtesy of KARL STORZ Endoscopy-America, Inc.)

Several angled endoscope lenses are commercially available. The standard set usually includes 0-, 30-, and 45-degree objective lenses. The 0-degree lens provides a frontal view of the operative field and is the most commonly used. The 30-degree lens is helpful to operate around corners, and rotating the lens brings a larger surface area of the operative field into view. The 45- and 70-degree endoscopes are mostly helpful for inspection. Operating at such acute angles is not only technically challenging, but also very disorienting for most surgeons. The development of adjustable viewing angle endoscopes, such as the EndoCAMeleon (Karl Storz, Tuttlingen, Germany), allows the surgeon to quickly change the lens angle from 0 to 120° by dialing an adjustment knob, providing instantaneous panoramic visualization of the surgical field (▶ Fig. 5.2).

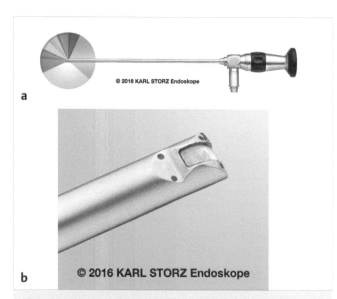

Fig. 5.2 **(a)** The EndoCAMeleon: the adjustable viewing angle endoscope from Karl Storz. **(b)** Close-up of the variable viewing angle lens. (These images are provided courtesy of KARL STORZ Endoscopy-America, Inc.)

For illumination, endoscopes are usually coupled to the light source via a fiberoptic cable. Different types of light sources are available (tungsten, halogen, xenon), although currently xenon is the preferred light source for endoscopic skull base surgery, as its spectral characteristics allow for a whiter light than the classic yellow halogen light.[3] The use of fluorescence imaging through the endoscope is possible to visualize fluorescein, 5-aminolevulinic acid (5-ALA), and indocyanine green (ICG). Fluorescein is often used to appreciate cerebrospinal fluid (CSF) leaks,[7,8,9] while 5-ALA and ICG have been used experimentally to distinguish tumor from the normal gland.[10,11,12]

5.2.2 Endoscope Holder

The use of endoscope holders is optional, as many centers prefer manual endoscope manipulation. However, a stable view of the operative field can be advantageous to facilitate bimanual microsurgical dissection. Therefore, endoscope holders can be a useful adjunct for the endoscopic equipment.[3] They must ensure a stable and secure hold, while having the ability to be easily and quickly adjustable throughout the surgery.

The mechanical holding arms, which are currently most widespread, may exhibit a tendency to drift after placement in their final desired position. However, their low profile makes setup easy (▶ Fig. 5.3). They are also considerably cheaper than the latest generation of pneumatic and electronic holding arms, which even though bulky, help ensure more stable positioning and smooth drive.[3] The most common is the Mitaka Arm (Mitaka, Inc., Denver, CO), which can either be mounted to the bed or rest on the floor (▶ Fig. 5.4).

The more common option is to have the endoscope held by an assistant during surgery. The dynamic movement of the 2D endoscope can help the surgeon receive feedback regarding the anatomy and depth of the operative field. The obvious drawback is assistant (holder) fatigue during long cases, as well as the clustering of hands (surgeon and assistant) near the nostrils. We have found it useful to use the endoscope free hand during the approach portion of the case, and then have it fixed during the delicate intracranial dissection of the pathology.

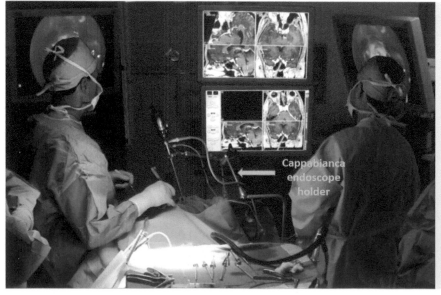

Fig. 5.3 The Cappabianca mechanical endoscope holding arm from Karl Storz.

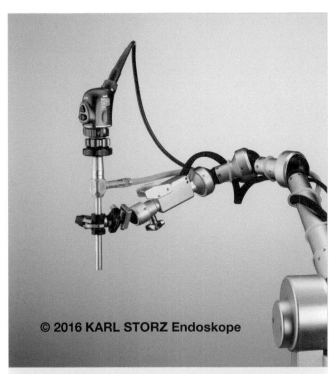

Fig. 5.4 The Mitaka Point Setter is a pneumatic endoscope holding arm. (This image is provided courtesy of KARL STORZ Endoscopy-America, Inc.)

5.2.3 Irrigation Systems

The close proximity of the endoscope lens to the surgical field exposes it to frequent soiling by blood, fluid, and bone dust. Multiple endoscope irrigation systems are commercially available that flush the lens to solve the problem of frequent blurred endoscopic vision, without having to remove the endoscope from the nostril. One of the available tools is the suction-irrigation sheath (CLEARVISION II/K-ENDOSHEATH) that allows simultaneous intraoperative irrigation and suctioning, controlled by a motorized pedal-activated pump.

A cheaper alternative is to flush the scope with a saline syringe and IV tubing attached to the sheath. Constant negative pressure is applied to the syringe (by gently drawing back on the plunger) to prevent water droplets from accumulating on the lens, and intermittent irrigation at varying intensity and duration can be controlled by the assistant to keep the lens clear. This technique also helps irrigate the surgical field, particularly when the bony surface becomes highly reflective and hot during skull base drilling. Another option is to drip fluid down the outside of the endoscope, which can also clean the scope, but less reliably.

5.3 Preoperative Planning and Surgery

5.3.1 Neuronavigation and Virtual Reality Systems

Pathology at the developing pediatric skull base can frequently distort the anatomy and obscure endonasal surgical landmarks.

A thorough preoperative evaluation of the anatomy is therefore necessary with thin slice CT and/or MRI (with angiography). Currently available software tools are able to merge information from CT, MRI, and angiogram for a comprehensive understanding of the encountered anatomy. Preoperative rehearsal of neurosurgical procedures has been shown to help with aneurysm surgery and may also be useful in endoscopic skull base procedures.[13,14] Augmented reality may also be useful for intraoperative planning and surgical navigation.[15]

Standard frameless neuronavigation is often extremely helpful during these approaches. It is particularly important in a pediatric setting given the less-predictable developing anatomy and the frequent necessity of extensive skull base drilling due to lack of sinus pneumatization. Registration of CT angiography (CTA) images is perhaps the most helpful when drilling out a nonpneumatized sinus to determine the location of the adjacent internal carotid artery (ICA) and the trajectory to the pathology. Real-time navigation of the drill or other surgical instruments can also be helpful.

5.3.2 Neuromonitoring

Intraoperative neuromonitoring (IONM) is often used in open skull base surgery to identify and preserve functionality in proximal cranial nerves. As EES gradually extended beyond the sella to encompass diseases craniocaudally from the cribriform plate to the cervicomedullary junction, and laterally to the cavernous sinus, Meckel's cave, and infratemporal fossa, comprehensive IONM has also become a helpful adjunct in extended EES.[16] Surgeons should be familiar with the currently available neuromonitoring techniques to better tailor the monitoring montage to the planned surgery and for more effective communication with the neurophysiologist (▶ Table 5.1). Straight-shafted monitored microdissecting instruments are now available that allow the surgeon to continually monitor cranial nerve activity while actively dissecting the tumor from the cavernous sinus or petrous apex.

5.3.3 Microdrills

Exposure and resection of skull base lesions often requires drilling in close proximity of critical neurovascular structures.

Table 5.1 Intraoperative neuromonitoring montages[29]

Midline		Lateral	Midline montage + EMG
Transethmoidal, transcribriform	EEG, SSEPs, MEPs	Orbital apex	CN III, IV, VI
Transsphenoidal, suprasellar, transplanum, transtuberculum		To cavernous sinus	CN III, IV, VI
Transclival		Transpterygoid	CN V
		Transclival/transpetrous	CN VI, VII
Cervicomedullary junction		Transcondylar/transjugular	CN IX, X, XI, XII

Abbreviations: CN, cranial nerve; EEG, scalp electroencephalography; EMG, electromyography; MEP, motor evoked potentials; SSEP, somatosensory evoked potentials.

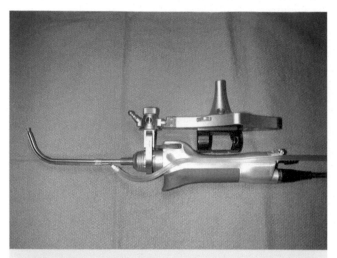

Fig. 5.5 Angled drill from Medtronic-Xomed, with navigation prong attached.

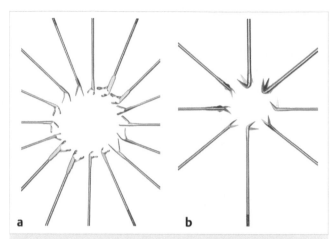

Fig. 5.6 Assortment of single-shaft graspers (a) and scissors (b) from the Evans Rotatable Set from Mizuho. (This image is provided courtesy of Mizuho America, Inc.)

Lightweight and ergonomic microdrills are now available for EES. Tapered hand pieces are particularly helpful as they offer better maneuverability through the nostril while allowing excellent visibility of their tips. Endonasal drills are now available with straight and angulated tips and can be used in conjunction with neuronavigation (▶ Fig. 5.5).

Drilling usually starts with cutting burrs in the nasal cavity, then switches to diamond burrs in the sphenoid sinus as the dura and ICA are approached. Cutting burrs are aggressive and can be used for rapid bone removal; however, they provide no hemostasis. Diamond burrs provide good bony hemostasis; however, they can be tedious to use and generate excessive heat. To avoid risk of direct soft-tissue damage from cutting burrs and diffused heat from diamond burrs, some authors advocate the use of coarse (or hybrid) diamond burrs.[17,18] This might be a good option in the pediatric population, where lack of sinus pneumatization may predispose the surgeon to drill through soft conchal bone. In our practice, we favor the use of Kerrison rongeurs to progressively extend the skull base exposure, once the midline dura is safely exposed and the surrounding bone egg shelled.

An alternative to the drill for removing bone is the Sonopet ultrasonic bone curette.[19] The Sonopet offers the ability for slow bone removal with less risk of damage to underlying dura or neurovascular structures. However, the progress of bone removal is often quite slow when removing thick bone.

5.3.4 Doppler Ultrasonography

In young children, the intercarotid distance is smaller compared to adults, and incomplete sphenoid sinus pneumatization might necessitate extensive drilling, resulting in the absence of classical anatomical landmarks. All these features expose the ICA to injury with potential catastrophic complications, emphasizing the importance of accurate ICA localization before dural opening.[20,21] Intraoperative micro-Doppler is a quick, easy, and reliable tool, as it offers accurate real-time data about the proximity of ICAs or any other major vessels.[20] The real-time

feedback is particularly helpful in cases where tumor debulking can lead to shifts in neuroanatomy, rendering the neuronavigation less accurate.

5.3.5 Endoscopic Microinstruments

Classic microsurgical instruments are ill-fitted for EES. These bayonetted dual-shaft instruments are difficult to maneuver inside the nasal cavity, which presents a narrow surgical corridor, and even more so in the pediatric population. Therefore, an assortment of variable length (11–25 cm), low-profile, single-shaft instruments have been developed for EES, which can be introduced into the nasal corridor along the same axis as the endoscope (▶ Fig. 5.6a,b) These instruments are ergonomically designed and proximally weighted so that their center of gravity lies in the surgeon's hand for better control and equilibrium.

Retractable blade lancets provide for a safer insertion, decreasing the risk of injuring the nasal mucosa, while traversing the blade through the narrow nasal corridor. Double-function curettes are commercially available that allow curettage and suction simultaneously, decreasing the need to constantly switch instruments. Rotatable, single-shaft instruments have been developed that can be adjusted to any desired angle without having to remove the instrument from the nasal cavity (▶ Fig. 5.7). Angled instruments and suction cannulas allow the surgeon to operate in areas of the surgical field only visible with angled endoscopes.

The EES instruments come with two different handle configurations: pistol grip and forceps grip. Pistol-grip instruments are robust and have higher torque and superior opening and closing force compared to their forceps-grip counterparts. Forceps-grip instruments, on the other hand, provide excellent tactile feedback and allow for delicate, sharp dissection through the endonasal corridor (▶ Fig. 5.8a,b). The most popular pistol-grip instruments are made by Karl Storz and Integra (Wormald), whereas forceps-grip instruments include Sepehrnia (Karl Storz) and Evans Rotatable Instruments (Mizuho America, Inc.). Further innovations have now led to the development of

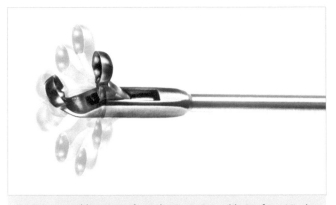

Fig. 5.7 Rotatable grasper from the Evans Rotatable Set from Mizuho. (This image is provided courtesy of Mizuho America, Inc.)

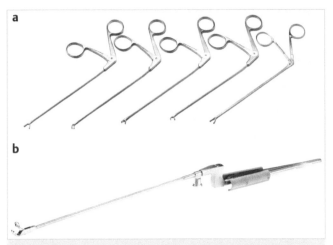

Fig. 5.8 Pistol grip (a) and forceps grip (b) instruments. Forceps grip grasper from the Evans Rotatable Set from Mizuho. (This image is provided courtesy of Mizuho America, Inc.)

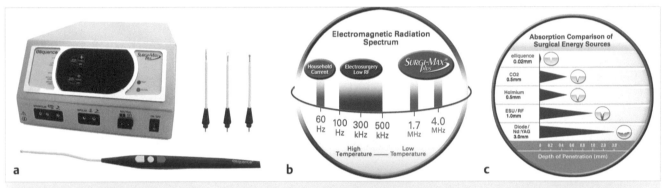

Fig. 5.9 (a) The Surgi-Max (Elliquence, LLC) uses high-frequency, low-temperature radio waves to vaporize fibrous tumors, with minimal heat spreading to surrounding tissues. (b) The electromagnetic radiation spectrum at which the Surgi-Max operates produces little to no heat, as compared to traditional Bovie electrocautery. (c) Absorption comparison of surgical energy sources. (These images are provided courtesy of Elliquence, LLC.)

malleable single-shaft forceps-grip instruments, which can be gently curved to adapt to patient-specific endonasal anatomy.

5.3.6 Tumor Debulking

Ultrasonic surgical aspirators (CUSA, Sonopet) have now been modified to be used for EES and allow for safe and quick tumor debulking, particularly fibrous ones. They are more compact, lighter, and slender than their microsurgical counterparts. Heat dispersion should, however, be accounted for, particularly during their use near critical neurovascular structures.

The side-cutting aspiration device (NICO Myriad, NICO, Indianapolis, IN) may be considered a useful alternative, as it is purely mechanical and does not generate heat at the resection site or along its shaft. Its rotating tip facilitates directing the cutting aperture away from critical neurovascular structures.[22] Caution should be exercised while using this instrument near close proximity to vascular structures, as they can be sucked into the cutting aperture inadvertently.[22,23]

Another option is the Surgi-Max (Elliquence, LLC, Baldwin, NY), which uses high-frequency, low-temperature radio waves to vaporize fibrous tumors, without significant heat spread and damage to adjacent structures.[23] It is particularly useful for central debulking of meningiomas, prior to the sharp dissection of their capsules. The shaft of the instrument can also be bent to adapt to endonasal anatomy, and it comes with different tip attachments (▶ Fig. 5.9).

5.3.7 Hemostasis

Bleeding during EES is frequently encountered and can be troublesome to manage. Monopolar cautery, incorporated with a suction cannula to aspirate smoke, can be used in the nasal cavity. However, its use inside the sphenoid sinus and in the intradural space is not recommended, because of the close proximity of critical neurovascular structures.

Single-shaft bipolar coagulation forceps with an array of diverse tips are now available to aid the surgeon with hemostasis during surgery.[17,24] Popular brands of pistol-grip bipolars include Take-Apart (Karl Storz) and Stammberger (Karl Storz). Popular forceps-grip bipolars include Stamm (Integra) and Calvian Endo-pen (Sutter). Low-flow bleeding (capillary,

Table 5.2 Summary of biomaterial agents commonly used in endoscopic endonasal surgery[25,26,30]

Biomaterial agent	Mechanism	Onset of action	Side effect
Topical antifibrinolytics (tranexamic acid)	Competitive binding with the lysine site on plasminogen	Improved quality of the surgical field at 2, 4, and 6 min	No significant adverse effects
Gelatin–thrombin matrix (SURGIFLO, FLOSEAL)	Provides tamponade of injured vessels and rapid clot formation on the tissue surface	Hemostatic effect at an average of 2 min	Loss of cilia on the epithelium, increased adhesion and granulation tissue formation
Microporous polysaccharide hemospheres (ARISTA)	Dehydrate blood and concentrate bloody components, including platelets, red blood cells, and clotting factors	Hemostatic effect at approximately 30–45 s	No significant adverse effects. Not indicated in neurologic and ophthalmic procedures
Oxidized methylcellulose (SURGICEL)	Activation of the intrinsic coagulation pathway, formation of a gel-like layer (matrix) that holds clots in place	Hemostasis is achieved between 2 and 8 min following application	No known adverse effects
Fibrin glue (TISSEEL)	Fibrin clot formation	Approximately 10 s	May expose to hepatitis virus, parvovirus B19, possible allergic or anaphylactic reactions
Microfibrillar collagen (INSTAT MCH, AVITENE)	Enhance platelet aggregation and release of proteins to form fibrin	Within 10 min	Potentiation of infection, adhesion formation, allergic reaction
Gelatin sponges (GELFOAM)	Formation of a mechanical matrix that facilitates clotting, release of thromboplastin from platelets	6 ± 2 min	Increase bacterial growth, can swell and cause potential problems in confined spaces

venous, and small arteries) can be inhibited by the topical application of absorbable biomaterials (▶ Table 5.2).[25,26]

5.4 Future Perspectives

As technology continues its inexorable progress, the armamentarium of tools available for endoscopic skull base surgeons will continue to grow, expanding with it the array of surgeries possible through this route. Virtual reality and surgical simulations have proven to be a helpful educational tools for anatomical evaluation and surgical rehearsal for trainees; however, implementation in the operative room is still limited.

Augmented reality might soon jump that bridge by becoming the next stage of neuronavigation, allowing the surgeon to superimpose previously segmented structures (nerves, vessels, bone, tumor, etc.) onto the surgical view in real time.[15] With heads-up displays, the surgeon will be able to access imaging, vital signs, references texts, etc., as needed during the case.

Robotic technology will progressively become inescapable in the operating room of the future. The use of voice-controlled robotized endoscope holders has already been reported.[27] Robotized flexible endoscopes and haptic instruments might enable surgeons to efficiently deal with some of the current surgical limitations of scale and degrees of freedom,[28] and even allow surgeons to remotely assist or coach a procedure.

The development of new biomaterials and 3D printing will also improve the quality of skull base reconstruction, customized to individual patient pathology. In this world of precision medicine and personalized care, it is not inconceivable that in the near future, even the surgical instruments will be custom printed for the individual surgeon operating on unique patient-specific pathology. The instruments will then truly become an extension of the surgeons' hands.

References

[1] Banu MA, Rathman A, Patel KS, et al. Corridor-based endonasal endoscopic surgery for pediatric skull base pathology with detailed radioanatomic measurements. Neurosurgery. 2014; 10 Suppl 2:273–293, discussion 293

[2] Banu MA, Guerrero-Maldonado A, McCrea HJ, et al. Impact of skull base development on endonasal endoscopic surgical corridors. J Neurosurg Pediatr. 2014; 13(2):155–169

[3] Gaab MR. Instrumentation: endoscopes and equipment. World Neurosurg. 2013; 79(2) Suppl:14.e11–14.e21

[4] Rastatter JC, Snyderman CH, Gardner PA, Alden TD, Tyler-Kabara E. Endoscopic endonasal surgery for sinonasal and skull base lesions in the pediatric population. Otolaryngol Clin North Am. 2015; 48(1):79–99

[5] Holzmann D, Bozinov O, Krayenbühl N. Is there a place for the endoscope in skull base surgery in children less than 5 years? J Neurol Surg A Cent Eur Neurosurg. 2014; 75(2):133–139

[6] Tabaee A, Anand VK, Fraser JF, Brown SM, Singh A, Schwartz TH. Three-dimensional endoscopic pituitary surgery. Neurosurgery. 2009; 64(5) Suppl 2:288–293, discussion 294–295

[7] Banu MA, Kim JH, Shin BJ, Woodworth GF, Anand VK, Schwartz TH. Low-dose intrathecal fluorescein and etiology-based graft choice in endoscopic endonasal closure of CSF leaks. Clin Neurol Neurosurg. 2014; 116:28–34

[8] Jakimovski D, Bonci G, Attia M, et al. Incidence and significance of intraoperative cerebrospinal fluid leak in endoscopic pituitary surgery using intrathecal fluorescein. World Neurosurg. 2014; 82(3–4):e513–e523

[9] Raza SM, Banu MA, Donaldson A, Patel KS, Anand VK, Schwartz TH. Sensitivity and specificity of intrathecal fluorescein and white light excitation for detecting intraoperative cerebrospinal fluid leak in endoscopic skull base surgery: a prospective study. J Neurosurg. 2016; 124(3):621–626

[10] Hide T, Yano S, Shinojima N, Kuratsu J. Usefulness of the indocyanine green fluorescence endoscope in endonasal transsphenoidal surgery. J Neurosurg. 2015; 122(5):1185–1192

[11] Litvack ZN, Zada G, Laws ER, Jr. Indocyanine green fluorescence endoscopy for visual differentiation of pituitary tumor from surrounding structures. J Neurosurg. 2012; 116(5):935–941

[12] Rapp M, Kamp M, Steiger HJ, Sabel M. Endoscopic-assisted visualization of 5-aminolevulinic acid-induced fluorescence in malignant glioma surgery: a technical note. World Neurosurg. 2014; 82(1–2):e277–e279

[13] Chugh AJ, Pace JR, Singer J, et al. Use of a surgical rehearsal platform and improvement in aneurysm clipping measures: results of a prospective, randomized trial. J Neurosurg. 2017; 126(3):838–844

[14] Kockro RA, Killeen T, Ayyad A, et al. Aneurysm surgery with preoperative three-dimensional planning in a virtual reality environment: technique and outcome analysis. World Neurosurg. 2016; 96:489–499

[15] Li L, Yang J, Chu Y, et al. A novel augmented reality navigation system for endoscopic sinus and skull base surgery: a feasibility study. PLoS One. 2016; 11(1):e0146996

[16] Elangovan C, Singh SP, Gardner P, et al. Intraoperative neurophysiological monitoring during endoscopic endonasal surgery for pediatric skull base tumors. J Neurosurg Pediatr. 2016; 17(2):147–155

[17] Vaz-Guimaraes F, Su SY, Fernandez-Miranda JC, Wang EW, Snyderman CH, Gardner PA. Hemostasis in endoscopic endonasal skull base surgery. J Neurol Surg B Skull Base. 2015; 76(4):296–302

[18] AlQahtani A, Castelnuovo P, Nicolai P, Prevedello DM, Locatelli D, Carrau RL. Injury of the internal carotid artery during endoscopic skull base surgery: prevention and management protocol. Otolaryngol Clin North Am. 2016; 49 (1):237–252

[19] Cappabianca P, Cavallo LM, Esposito I, Barakat M, Esposito F. Bone removal with a new ultrasonic bone curette during endoscopic endonasal approach to the sellar-suprasellar area: technical note. Neurosurgery. 2010; 66(3) Suppl operative:E118–, discussion E118

[20] Dusick JR, Esposito F, Malkasian D, Kelly DF. Avoidance of carotid artery injuries in transsphenoidal surgery with the Doppler probe and micro-hook blades. Neurosurgery. 2007; 60(4) Suppl 2:322–328, discussion 328–329

[21] Tatreau JR, Patel MR, Shah RN, et al. Anatomical considerations for endoscopic endonasal skull base surgery in pediatric patients. Laryngoscope. 2010; 120 (9):1730–1737

[22] McLaughlin N, Ditzel Filho LF, Prevedello DM, Kelly DF, Carrau RL, Kassam AB. Side-cutting aspiration device for endoscopic and microscopic tumor removal. J Neurol Surg B Skull Base. 2012; 73(1):11–20

[23] Dhandapani S, Negm HM, Cohen S, Anand VK, Schwartz TH. Endonasal endoscopic transsphenoidal resection of tuberculum sella meningioma with anterior cerebral artery encasement. Cureus. 2015; 7(8):e311

[24] Kassam A, Snyderman CH, Carrau RL, Gardner P, Mintz A. Endoneurosurgical hemostasis techniques: lessons learned from 400 cases. Neurosurg Focus. 2005; 19(1):E7

[25] Antisdel JL, Matijasec JL, Ting JY, Sindwani R. Microporous polysaccharide hemospheres do not increase synechiae after sinus surgery: randomized controlled study. Am J Rhinol Allergy. 2011; 25(4):268–271

[26] Sindwani R. Use of novel hemostatic powder MPH for endoscopic sinus surgery: initial impressions. Otolaryngol Head Neck Surg.. 2009; 140(2):262–263

[27] Nathan CO, Chakradeo V, Malhotra K, D'Agostino H, Patwardhan R. The voice-controlled robotic assist scope holder AESOP for the endoscopic approach to the sella. Skull Base. 2006; 16(3):123–131

[28] Cabuk B, Ceylan S, Anik I, Tugasaygi M, Kizir S. A haptic guided robotic system for endoscope positioning and holding. Turk Neurosurg. 2015; 25(4):601–607

[29] Singh H, Vogel RW, Lober RM, et al. Intraoperative neurophysiological monitoring for endoscopic endonasal approaches to the skull base: a technical guide. Scientifica (Cairo). 2016; 2016:1751245

[30] Gall RM, Witterick IJ, Shargill NS, Hawke M. Control of bleeding in endoscopic sinus surgery: use of a novel gelatin-based hemostatic agent. J Otolaryngol. 2002; 31(5):271–274

6 Intraoperative Neurophysiological Monitoring during Endoscopic Endonasal Skull Base Surgery

Parthasarathy D. Thirumala, Rafey A. Feroze, Ronak Jani, and Jeffrey R. Balzer

Abstract

Endoscopic endonasal approach (EEA) surgery in pediatric patients has become an alternative to open surgery for the treatment of cranial base tumors. However, EEA carries a risk of damage to neurovascular structures and cranial nerves resulting in transient or permanent neurological deficits. The use of intraoperative neurophysiological monitoring (IONM) has been shown to reduce the risk of neurological deficits in open skull base surgery. Multimodal IONM provides real-time continuous monitoring of neurovascular structures and cranial nerves during adult EEA. IONM has become a routine part of adult EEA procedures at our center and should be considered an integral part of pediatric EEA treatments based on its ability to detect and reduce perioperative injury. This chapter provides a brief introduction to four commonly used methods of IONM.

Keywords: neuromonitoring, somatosensory evoked potentials, brainstem auditory evoked potentials, motor evoked potentials, electromyogram, juvenile nasopharyngeal angiofibroma

6.1 Somatosensory Evoked Potentials

Somatosensory evoked potentials (SSEPs) are a common intraoperative neurophysiological monitoring (IONM) modality utilized in skull base surgery where there is a risk of neurovascular damage. During endoscopic endonasal approach (EEA), ulnar/median nerves from the upper extremities and tibial/peroneal nerves from the lower extremities are stimulated bilaterally via subdermal needle electrodes. Recordings are made along the ascending neural axis from the Erb's point, cervical spine, and contralateral somatosensory cortex from the scalp (International 10–20 system for scalp recording electrodes). This allows simultaneous assessment of the integrity of peripheral nerves, spinal cord dorsal column tracts, brainstem medial lemniscal pathways, and somatosensory thalamocortical connections.[1] Alterations in SSEP amplitude and latency have been noted secondary to patient positioning, ischemia/infarction of somatosensory pathways in the cervical spine or medial lemniscal pathways in the brainstem, and/or cortical generators of SSEPs including the somatosensory cortex and thalamus.[2] Thus, SSEPs are a sensitive diagnostic tool for the detection of neurovascular damage along the somatosensory pathway during EEA procedures.

While EEA has reduced the morbidity and mortality in pediatric skull base tumor resection relative to conventional open techniques, there is still a risk of vascular damage. Juvenile nasopharyngeal angiofibromas (JNAs), which are highly vascular tumors that are commonly treated via EEA in pediatric patients, carry the risk of significant hemorrhage and cerebral ischemia during resection (▶ Fig. 6.1). Tumors of the clival region, such as chordomas, can compress the brainstem and impair vascular perfusion.[3] SSEP monitoring during resection of such tumors helps identify intraoperative vascular compromise. In studies on adult EEA, SSEP monitoring was found to have positive and negative predictive values of 80% and 99.79%, respectively, in predicting neurological deficits.[2] SSEP changes indicative of deficits are manifested as real-time sudden or insidious changes in SSEP waveforms indicating neurological compromise.[2]

The parameters of interest in SSEP waveforms during IONM are response amplitude and latency of the cortical and subcortical waveforms.[1] The American Society of Neurophysiological Monitoring (ASNM) has recommended a 50% decrease in the amplitude and/or 10% increase in the latency of SSEP response as a significant change, which should be communicated to the surgical team as a sign of possible neurological compromise.[4] When significant changes in the SSEPs are noted, localization of the cause of change and appropriate surgical maneuvers can be performed to prevent neurological deficits. In our experience from adult EEA, patients who experienced significant changes that were reversed during the procedure had lower chance of neurological deficit. Factors affecting nerve conduction such as

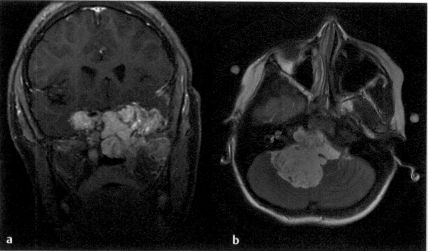

Fig. 6.1 (a) T1-weighted MRI with contrast of a 14-year-old patient diagnosed with juvenile nasopharyngeal angiofibroma treated with endoscopic endonasal approach (EEA) during which intraoperative neuromonitoring with somatosensory evoked potential (SSEP), brainstem auditory evoked potentials (BAEPs), and electromyograms (EMGs) was applied. (b) T2-weighted MRI of a 10-year-old patient diagnosed with a clival chordoma and treated with EEA during which intraoperative neuromonitoring with SSEP, BAEPs, and EMGs was applied.

nerve fiber diameter, degree of myelination, or synaptogenesis impact SSEP amplitude and latency.[5] These factors are in flux during the early years of life and must be considered in the pediatric patient population. Because of these physiological maturational effects, interpretation of baseline data as well as changes in SSEPs during the procedures should be evaluated, taking the factors into consideration.

Cortical and subcortical recordings obtained simultaneously can often differentiate the origin of SSEP changes. For example, cortical ischemia, which can occur secondary to surgical manipulation, manifests as a change in the cortically recorded potential without any major changes in SSEPs at the cervical level. In contrast, a change in patient positioning or perturbation of the surgical environment, such as drilling or dissection, may result in SSEP changes from both recording sites.

Sensitivity of SSEPs to cortical and subcortical ischemia has been well established in animal models. In animal experiments, a decrease in cerebral blood flow (CBF) below 10 to 20 mL/100 g/min has been shown to cause a reversible decrement in the amplitude of SSEP responses. Animal studies also show that an increase in mean arterial pressure (MAP) and, subsequently, CBF restores depressed SSEP amplitudes to normal.[6] Similarly, reduction in CBF in humans to approximately 14 mL/100 g/min has been shown to result in a 50% reduction in SSEP amplitude.[7] An important concept to understand is that during IONM, disappearance of SSEP responses (electrical failure) occurs before the "ion pump failure" or cellular death.[8] Thus, real-time continuous SSEP collection and interpretation during EEA can present situations where the decrease in SSEP amplitude secondary to cerebral ischemia can be reversed by restoration of perfusion prior to the development of significant perioperative neurological injury.[2]

To our knowledge, the utility of SSEP recording in pediatric EEA is limited to just one study performed by our group. We have reported the use of SSEP monitoring in 129 pediatric patients who underwent EEA for resection of skull base tumors.[3] SSEP monitoring was conducted as described earlier. ▶ Fig. 6.2 shows example SSEPs obtained from a pediatric patient undergoing EEA skull base surgery. While changes in SSEPs due to anesthesia and changes in MAP were noted preoperatively, no intraoperative SSEP changes were observed in any of the patients. These correlated with absence of postoperative neurological deficits.[3]

Given the demonstrated efficacy of SSEPs in adult skull base surgery and its successful execution in the aforementioned pediatric study, SSEPs are likely valuable in pediatric EEA as well. As a method of continuous neurophysiological monitoring, a significant decrease in amplitude and increase in latency can be particularly useful for identifying ischemia-induced damage in somatosensory pathways. However, SSEPs provide no information regarding motor pathways, requiring the need for a multimodality approach to protect descending brainstem pathways from ischemic damage.

6.2 Brainstem Auditory Evoked Potentials

Brainstem auditory evoked potentials (BAEPs) have become a routine component of IONM during skull base surgeries

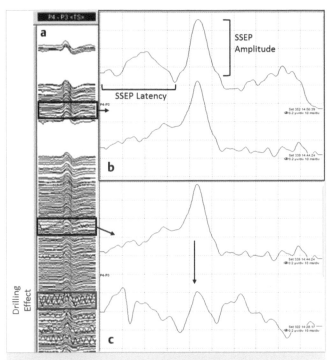

Fig. 6.2 (a) Intraoperative somatosensory evoked potential (SSEP) monitoring in a pediatric patient undergoing endoscopic endonasal approach (EEA) surgery with effect of drilling illustrated in red rectangle. **(b)** Normal SSEP waveforms illustrating amplitude and latency measurements. **(c)** Change in SSEP amplitude during EEA surgery.

involving manipulation of the brainstem, cochlear nerve, and vertebrobasilar vasculature. BAEPs are recorded from the scalp following the unilateral delivery of auditory stimuli (clicks consisting of 100-μs-long pulses of an 85- to 99-dB intensity delivered at a frequency range of 9.1–17.5 Hz via foam earbuds placed in the external auditory canal). BAEPs monitor the functional integrity of ascending auditory pathways beginning at the distal aspect of the vestibulocochlear nerve, progressing to cochlear nuclei, superior olivary nuclei, the lateral lemniscus, and ending at the inferior colliculi in the midbrain.[9] In addition to assessing cochlear nerve conduction, BAEPs are also sensitive to ischemic changes in component structures along these pathways. Further, BAEPs are used to assess the degree of cerebellar retraction and its effects on cochlear nerve function as well as cochlea and brainstem perfusion in the auditory pathways during EEA procedures.

JNAs and clival tumors, which increase susceptibility to vascular injury, warrant the addition of BAEPs during EEA procedures. BAEP monitoring can help identify intraoperative vascular compression and injury by detecting impaired propagation of auditory signals to and through the brainstem. The use of SSEPs and BAEPs together provides a multimodality approach with the monitoring of auditory tracts (by BAEPs) in the brainstem in addition to somatosensory pathways utilizing SSEPs.

Baseline BAEPs should be obtained following the initiation of anesthesia and positioning of the patient but before surgically accessing brainstem structures. The resultant waveform

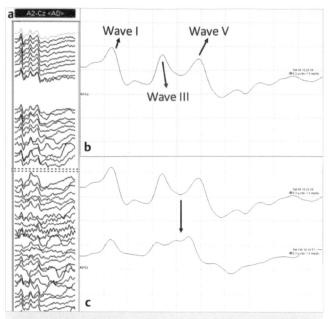

Fig. 6.3 **(a)** Intraoperative brainstem auditory evoked potential (BAEP) monitoring in a pediatric patient undergoing endoscopic endonasal approach (EEA) surgery. **(b)** Example of BAEP waveform with waves I, III, and V. **(c)** Change in amplitude of wave V during EEA surgery.

typically consists of five peaks, each corresponding to the distal auditory nerve, proximal auditory nerve, cochlear nucleus, superior olivary complex, and inferior colliculus, respectively.[9] Each of these anatomical structures serves as a generator of neuronal activity and allows for localization of ischemia. ▶ Fig. 6.3 shows example BAEP waveforms obtained from a pediatric patient undergoing EEA.

The amplitudes of each peak and the latencies from one peak to the next (interpeak latency) are used in evaluation of BAEP responses. Given that most EEA procedures involve the brainstem at or above the level of the superior olivary sulcus, alterations in amplitude and latency of peak V represent the majority of changes observed.[9] In general, surgeons should be informed of changes in BAEP following a consistent decrease in amplitude or increase in latency, as these indicate impaired impulse transmission along auditory neurons. The American Society of Neurophysiological Monitoring (ASNM) recommend alerting the surgeon of a 10% (1-ms) increase in latency and/or a 50% decrease in the amplitude of peak V compared to baseline.[4] However, these guidelines are not specific to the pediatric population, and a controlled study is required to establish alarm criteria for pediatric patients.

Similar to SSEPs, vascular compromise is expected to cause alterations in BAEP waveforms. A more distal vascular occlusion in the posterior circulation (e.g., posterior cerebral artery) could result in disappearance of later BAEP peaks, while a proximal vascular occlusion would prevent the auditory stimulus from propagating to the cochlea or cochlear nucleus, resulting in disappearance of all BAEP peaks. Studies in primates have shown that brainstem ischemia, due to reduced brainstem blood flow (12–15 mL/100 g/min), increases the latency of BAEP waveforms.[10] Similarly, reversible changes in BAEPs correlating with reduction in MAP have also been observed in humans during

EEA procedures.[1] Significant changes in the peak V response during EEA procedures are indicative of neurological compromise due to reduced perfusion or compressive forces.[9]

Reported use of BAEPs in pediatric EEA procedures is very limited. Our group[3] has described BAEP monitoring in 16 pediatric patients. We noted transient wave V amplitude changes that improved with increases in MAP in two patients, neither of whom developed postoperative deficits. The two cases with changes in BAEPs were both in patients with JNAs.[3] As such, BAEPs can be useful in evaluating the cerebellopontine angle (CPA) structures and brainstem perfusion during EEA.

6.3 Motor Evoked Potentials

Motor evoked potentials (MEPs) have traditionally been used during spine surgery but are now commonly utilized during supra- and infratentorial procedures. Transcranial MEPs are generated by stimulating the primary motor cortex via scalp electrodes using a train of square wave constant voltage stimuli of 50- to 75-μs duration. Recordings are made in the form of compound muscle action potentials (CMAP) from the contralateral upper and lower extremity skeletal musculature.[11] Hence, MEPs evaluate the functional integrity of motor neurons of the corticospinal tract as well as the descending cortical and spinal cord pathways. Each stimulation/response cycle provides an immediate evaluation of the corticospinal tract. As such, it is not a continuous method of IONM.

During EEA procedures, MEPs can be helpful in assessing the function of pyramidal corticospinal tracts. A consistent amplitude reduction of 50% is considered significant, although no consensus regarding alarm criteria has been established.[12] To our knowledge, there are no studies to date describing the use of MEPs during pediatric or adult EEA. Cranial nerve (CN) MEPs in response to transcranial electrical stimulation have also been recorded but have not become a mainstay of IONM due to electrical spread from transcranial stimulation and poor correlation between MEP results and postoperative neurological outcomes.

6.4 Electromyogram

Electromyogram (EMG) is a commonly utilized technique to monitor the function of individual CN during adult skull base surgical procedures and has shown efficacy in detecting and preventing CN injury.[13] CN vary in size, follow a circuitous course, and have a structurally delicate epineurium, making them more susceptible to injury in the setting of tumor compression and resection. Nerve injury can result from mechanical trauma from the surgical instruments, unintended manipulation, and ischemia during surgery. Surgical removal of tumors in close proximity to the CN can result in spontaneous EMG activity due to unintended mechanical activation, causing CN depolarization and resultant motor unit action potentials. Surgically exposed CN can also be electrically triggered, which will generate a CMAP from target, innervated musculature. The nature of EEA surgery often makes it difficult to clearly identify a CN from the pathology without the use of electrical stimulation and triggered EMG (t-EMG) techniques.

While many CN have motor and sensory components, EMG monitoring only evaluates the motor function of these nerves.

Our monitoring protocol includes EMG recording from the extraocular muscles including medial rectus, superior oblique, and lateral rectus muscles. These recordings allow for the evaluation of the integrity of CN III, IV, and VI, respectively, during tumor resection.[13] The masseter muscle is used to evaluate the motor component of CN V, whereas the orbicularis oculi, orbicularis oris, and mentalis muscles allow for evaluation of CN VII.[14] Bipolar recording electrodes are placed in or on the soft palate, vocal cords, trapezius, and tongue for monitoring of CN IX, X, XI, or XII, respectively.[15]

Numerous studies describing EMG evaluation of facial nerve function in the setting of acoustic neuroma resection at the CPA suggest improved postoperative facial nerve function with the use of EMG.[14] The use of EMG monitoring of CN also has been utilized in adult EEA procedures for localizing and preventing CN deficits.[13,15] EMG can be monitored in two forms, free-running or triggered.

6.4.1 Free-Running Electromyogram

Free-running EMG (f-EMG) is the real-time continuous recording of muscle activity in the form of spikes, bursts, and neurotonic discharges that can occur secondary to unintended mechanical stimulation by surgical instruments or irrigation of the surgical field.[15] We utilize two standard 13-mm needle electrodes, placed in muscle groups corresponding to particular CN, for monitoring of f-EMG activity. At baseline, f-EMG shows no activity. When CN are activated via surgical manipulation during EEA, short-duration monophasic or polyphasic spike and bursts with low frequencies of 10 to 30 Hz with amplitudes ranging from 50 to 2,000 µV can be recorded. These discharges are typically benign. Conversely, neurotonic discharges, characterized by high frequency (>100 Hz), prolonged duration (>100 ms), and high amplitudes have been shown to indicate nerve injury. Our team, with the understanding of limitations provides real-time audio feedback of f-EMG activity to the surgical team, which serves as an alarm for altering surgical technique.

Though f-EMG has significant utility during EEA, diagnostic accuracy has been evaluated only for CN VII during skull base surgery. In our experience, we have observed neurotonic discharges from CN XII during adult EEA procedures. However, transection of nerves results in no f-EMG activity, highlighting a major limitation of this technique. Analyses conducted by our group have shown high sensitivity of f-EMG in locating CN but limited value in identifying CN deficits.[13,15]

To our knowledge, the study by Elangovan et al from our group is the only report that describes the use of f-EMG for CN IONM in pediatric EEA procedures. F-EMG was performed in 62 pediatric EEA patients with 321 monitored nerves.[3] Significant f-EMG activity was observed in 55 nerves and no activity in 266 nerves. The incidence of CN deficits was 9% and 1.5% in the significant f-EMG and no significant f-EMG activity groups, respectively.[3] f-EMG monitoring was found to have a low sensitivity (55%) but high specificity (83%) and negative predictive value (98%) in identifying CN deficits.[3] The higher rate of deficits in the significant f-EMG activity group is reflective of greater intraoperative manipulation of CN, increasing the likelihood of injury. The low sensitivity of f-EMG can be improved by employing t-EMG techniques along with the f-EMG.

6.4.2 Triggered Electromyogram

t-EMG is recorded in the form of CMAP from the muscles supplied by CN secondary to discrete electrical stimulation. Unlike f-EMG, this is not a continuous method of CN monitoring. Electrical current is delivered using a monopolar stimulator introduced into the surgical field with a return electrode placed on the forehead or shoulder of the patient when desired during the surgical procedure. In our experience, a dissecting monopolar stimulator can also be utilized to perform microsurgical manipulation while delivering electrical stimulation. We utilize constant voltage stimulation for our CN t-EMG monitoring, as the consistency of current delivery is less susceptible to changes in resistivity. Our neurophysiology staff provide real-time audio feedback of t-EMG activity to the surgical team.

Given that f-EMG often does not provide indication of nerve transection, supplementation with t-EMG has been used extensively for finer localization and more precise measurements of facial nerve function during acoustic neuroma resection procedures.[14] t-EMG waveforms can be evaluated using the stimulation thresholds (mV), onset latency (ms), and CMAP amplitude (µV) of recorded waveforms. Stimulation threshold is defined as the minimum current needed to elicit a CMAP from the target musculature and can indicate proximity to neural structures or the degree to which nerve function is preserved. Studies have shown CN injury with changes in stimulation thresholds[14]; therefore, we routinely obtain a threshold response before and after resection if possible during our EEAs. CMAP amplitude is directly proportional to the number of stimulated muscle fibers and therefore reflects the number of intact axons in the target CN. The response is generally measured as the peak-to-peak amplitude of the largest polyphasic waveform (▶ Fig. 6.4B). Finally, onset latency is the time from stimulation to the CMAP onset (▶ Fig. 6.4B). Latency may be increased in the setting of nerve damage but is also influenced by the distance of the stimulation electrode from the CN.

Unfortunately, there is a paucity of data on the use of t-EMG during pediatric EEA procedures. However, our group has implemented t-EMG as a routine component of our pediatric EEA IONM protocol.[3] Examples of t-EMG responses recorded from a pediatric patient are provided in ▶ Fig. 6.4. To our knowledge, there have been no reports documenting the efficacy of t-EMG in preventing CN injury or affecting outcomes in the pediatric or adult EEA procedures. However, based on experience with conventional skull base surgery approaches, we believe t-EMG IONM is likely to be beneficial for pediatric EEA procedures.

6.5 Conclusion

Various methods of IONM that have been utilized during conventional skull base surgery procedures have also shown to be efficacious in pediatric EEA procedures. However, there have been relatively few studies evaluating these techniques in the pediatric population. More studies will be needed to standardize IONM techniques and alarm criteria to further solidify the aforementioned IONM techniques for pediatric EEA.

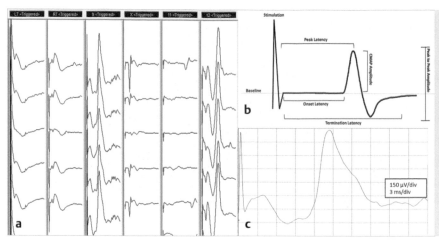

Fig. 6.4 **(a)** Triggered electromyogram (EMG) responses from cranial nerves (CN) VII, IX, X, XI, and XII following 2,000-mV stimulation in a 10-year-old pediatric patient undergoing EEA tumor resection. **(b)** Parameters of interest in a typical t-EMG waveform. **(c)** Example response following 2,000-mV stimulation of CN IX of patient depicted in **(a)**.

References

[1] Thirumala P, Lai D, Engh J, Habeych M, Crammond D, Balzer J. Predictive value of somatosensory evoked potential monitoring during resection of intraparenchymal and intraventricular tumors using an endoscopic port. J Clin Neurol. 2013; 9(4):244–251

[2] Thirumala PD, Kassam AB, Habeych M, et al. Somatosensory evoked potential monitoring during endoscopic endonasal approach to skull base surgery: analysis of observed changes. Neurosurgery. 2011; 69(1) Suppl operative:64–76, discussion ons76

[3] Elangovan C, Singh SP, Gardner P, et al. Intraoperative neurophysiological monitoring during endoscopic endonasal surgery for pediatric skull base tumors. J Neurosurg Pediatr. 2015:1–9

[4] American Electroencephalographic Society. Guideline eleven: guidelines for intraoperative monitoring of sensory evoked potentials. J Clin Neurophysiol. 1994; 11(1):77–87

[5] Gilmore R. The use of somatosensory evoked potentials in infants and children. J Child Neurol. 1989; 4(1):3–19

[6] Symon L. The relationship between CBF, evoked potentials and the clinical features in cerebral ischaemia. Acta Neurol Scand Suppl. 1980; 78:175–190

[7] Lopez JR. Intraoperative neurophysiological monitoring. Int Anesthesiol Clin. 1996; 34(4):33–54

[8] Astrup J, Symon L, Branston NM, Lassen NA. Cortical evoked potential and extracellular K + and H + at critical levels of brain ischemia. Stroke. 1977; 8(1):51–57

[9] Thirumala PD, Kodavatiganti HS, Habeych M, et al. Value of multimodality monitoring using brainstem auditory evoked potentials and somatosensory evoked potentials in endoscopic endonasal surgery. Neurol Res. 2013; 35(6):622–630

[10] Baik MW, Branston NM, Bentivoglio P, Symon L. The effects of experimental brain-stem ischaemia on brain-stem auditory evoked potentials in primates. Electroencephalogr Clin Neurophysiol. 1990; 75(5):433–443

[11] Macdonald DB. Intraoperative motor evoked potential monitoring: overview and update. J Clin Monit Comput. 2006; 20(5):347–377

[12] Singh H, Vogel RW, Lober RM, et al. Intraoperative neurophysiological monitoring for endoscopic endonasal approaches to the skull base: a technical guide. Scientifica (Cairo). 2016; 2016:1751245

[13] Thirumala PD, Mohanraj SK, Habeych M, et al. Value of free-run electromyographic monitoring of extraocular cranial nerves during expanded endonasal surgery (EES) of the skull base. J Neurol Surg Rep. 2013; 74(1):43–50

[14] Acioly MA, Liebsch M, de Aguiar PH, Tatagiba M. Facial nerve monitoring during cerebellopontine angle and skull base tumor surgery: a systematic review from description to current success on function prediction. World Neurosurg. 2013; 80(6):e271–e300

[15] Thirumala PD, Mohanraj SK, Habeych M, et al. Value of free-run electromyographic monitoring of lower cranial nerves in endoscopic endonasal approach to skull base surgeries. J Neurol Surg B Skull Base. 2012; 73(4):236–244

7 Endonasal Corridors and Approaches

Harminder Singh, Jeffrey P. Greenfield, Gustavo J. Almodóvar-Mercado, Vijay K. Anand, and Theodore H. Schwartz

Abstract

Numerous endonasal surgical approaches to the anterior skull base have been described in the literature. These utilize a variety of terminologies and trajectories, which can sometimes be difficult to comprehend for the novice practitioner. In this chapter, we present a straightforward algorithm to conceptualize these approaches. It is based upon five different nasal corridors that must be transgressed to reach various anterior skull base targets.

Keywords: transsphenoidal corridor, transethmoidal corridor, transpterygoid/transmaxillary corridor, transnasal corridor, transfrontal corridor

7.1 Transsphenoidal Corridor

The sphenoid sinus has been called the "gateway to the anterior skull base." Via the transsphenoidal corridor, one can access the sella, tuberculum, planum, upper clivus, and the medial cavernous sinus (CS; ▶ Fig. 7.1).

The transsphenoidal approach begins by lateralizing the middle (▶ Fig. 7.2) and superior turbinates and identifying the sphenoid ostium, which is located in the sphenoethmoid recess posterior to the superior turbinate (▶ Fig. 7.3).

The sphenoid ostium can be enlarged with a mushroom punch to gain entry into the sphenoid sinus, either unilaterally or bilaterally, depending on the pathology. Care must be taken not to punch inferolaterally into the territory of the sphenopalatine artery (SPA), which can cause unwanted bleeding. The SPA provides blood supply to the nasoseptal mucosa. In cases where a nasoseptal flap (NSF) must be harvested for skull base repair, it is critical to preserve this blood supply (▶ Fig. 7.4).

The anterior wall of the sphenoid sinus is removed for a panoramic view of the sphenoid sinus region (▶ Fig. 7.5). The posterior one-third of the nasal septum (consisting of the perpendicular plate of the ethmoid bone superiorly and the vomer inferiorly) can be removed for a binarial approach to the sphenoid. The posterior inferior portion of the vomer (the "Keel") should also be removed if an NSF is used to reconstruct the skull base. This maneuver prevents kinking of the vascular

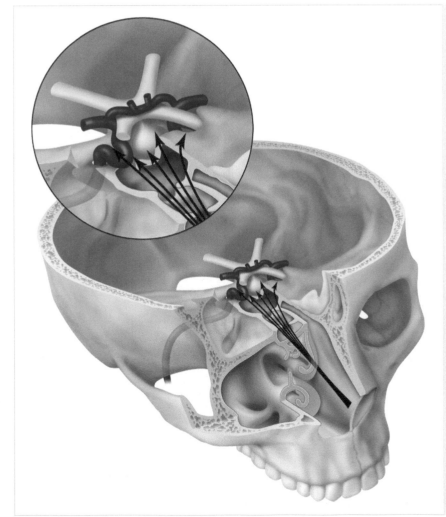

Fig. 7.1 The transsphenoidal corridor is the most commonly used corridor and permits approaches to the sella, suprasellar cistern, medial cavernous sinus, and superior clivus.

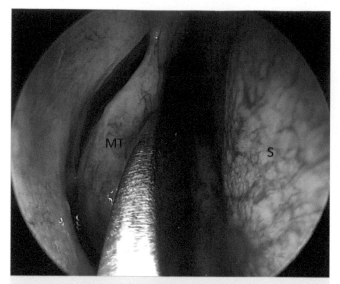

Fig. 7.2 Right nostril. The middle turbinate (MT) is lateralized to gain access to the superior turbinate. The septum (S) is seen on the right.

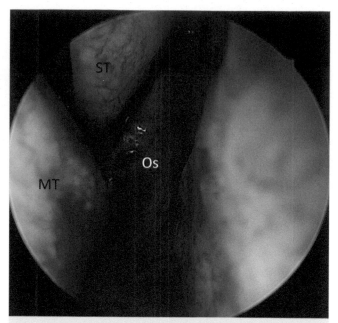

Fig. 7.3 The ostium (Os) of the sphenoid sinus is seen in the sphenoethmoid recess, posterior to the superior turbinate (ST).

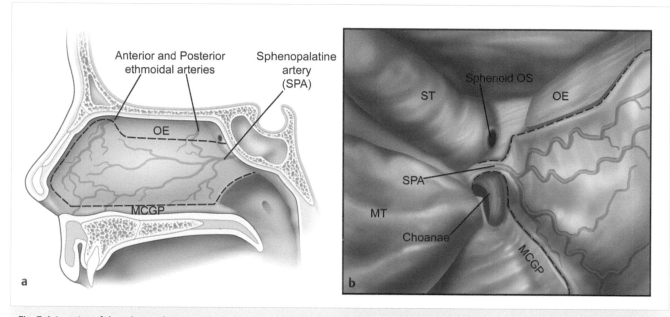

Fig. 7.4 Location of the sphenopalatine artery (SPA) in relation to the sphenoid ostium and choanae, and the surgical cuts (dotted line) that need to be made to harvest the nasoseptal flap (NSF). In pediatric patients, the olfactory epithelium (OE) and the maxillary crest growth plate (MCGP) need to be preserved. (a) Sagittal view. (b) Coronal view.

pedicle of the NSF and allows the flap to sit flush with the skull base, promoting healing[1].

In the pediatric population, there can be incomplete pneumatization of the sphenoid sinus. In the sagittal plane, five different pneumatization patterns have been described[2] (▶ Fig. 7.6):

- Type 1: conchal (completely missing or minimal sphenoid sinus).
- Type 2: presellar (posterior wall of sphenoid sinus is in front of the anterior wall of the sella).
- Type 3: sellar (posterior wall of sphenoid sinus is between anterior and posterior wall of sella).
- Type 4A: postsellar (posterior wall of sphenoid sinus is behind the posterior wall of sella).
- Type 4B: postsellar (posterior wall of sphenoid sinus is behind the posterior wall of sella, with air dorsal to the sella).

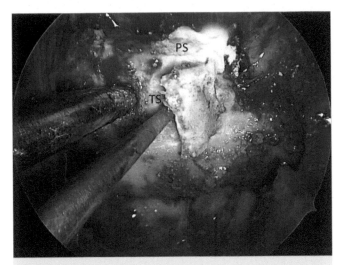

Fig. 7.5 View inside the sphenoid sinus. From superior to inferior, the following structures are identified: S, sella; TS, tuberculum sella; PS, planum sella; C, clivus.

Conchal pneumatization patterns are a *relative* limitation in pediatric endoscopic endonasal surgery, because the cancellous bone can be easily drilled down to approach the sella (▶ Fig. 7.7).

Laterally, the bone between the optic nerve and the carotid artery, or medial opticocarotid (mOCR) recess can be removed to expose the superomedial aspect of the CS. This opening can be extended inferolaterally to expose the carotid siphon in the medial CS. In order to access the lateral inferior portion of the CS, the medial pterygoid plate (mPP) will have to be removed for better exposure (▶ Fig. 7.8).

7.2 Transethmoidal Corridor

The transethmoidal corridor allows access to the lateral anterior skull base, from the frontal sinus anteriorly to the sphenoid sinus posteriorly. The orbital apex, the lateral CS, and the anterior fossa (though the fovea ethmoidalis) can be reached through this corridor. The anterior and posterior ethmoidal arteries are important landmarks, which must be cauterized and transected (▶ Fig. 7.9a; ▶ Fig. 7.9b).

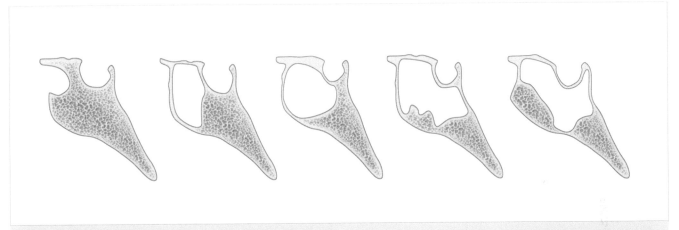

Fig. 7.6 Sphenoid sinus pneumatization patterns in the sagittal plane. From left to right: type 1, conchal; type 2, presellar; type 3, sellar; type 4A, postsellar; type 4B, postsellar, with air dorsal to the sella.

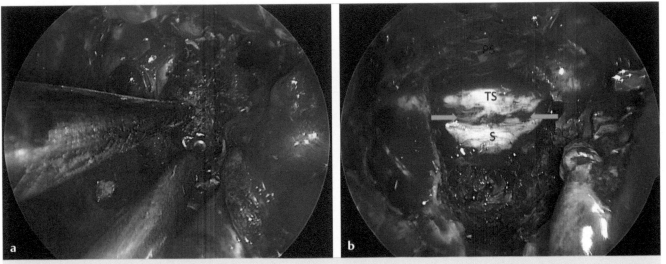

Fig. 7.7 (a) Type 1: conchal pneumatization of the sphenoid sinus. The cancellous bone can be easily drilled to reach the sella. (b) The cancellous bone in the sphenoid sinus has been removed with a high-speed drill to reveal the PS (planum sphenoidale), TS (tuberculum sphenoidale), and the S (sella).

A total ethmoidectomy is performed in an anterior to posterior fashion, lateral to the superior turbinate after first removing the uncinate process (UP) to expose the bulla ethmoidalis (▶ Fig. 7.10). This will lead to the exposure of the fovea ethmoidalis superiorly (roof of the ethmoid cells, which leads into the anterior cranial fossa) and the lamina papyracea laterally (leading into the medial orbit; ▶ Fig. 7.11; ▶ Fig. 7.12).

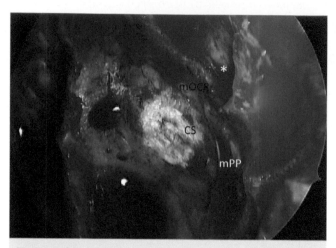

Fig. 7.8 Endoscopic view of the left lateral aspect of the sphenoid sinus, showing the medial opticocarotid recess (mOCR) and the medial pterygoid plate (mPP). The bone over the medial aspect of the cavernous sinus has been scored with a drill (CS). In order to access the lateral superior aspect of the cavernous sinus (*), the ethmoid air cells lateral and anterior to the sphenoid sinus have been removed. In order to access the lateral inferior aspect of the cavernous sinus, the superior portion of the medial pterygoid plate (mPP) has to be removed.

The lateral superior aspect of the CS can be accessed via the transethmoidal corridor, in conjunction with the transsphenoidal corridor. In order to access the lateral inferior aspect of the CS, the superior portion of the mPP has to be removed (▶ Fig. 7.8).

Individual variations in the posterior ethmoidal sinus anatomy must be studied prior to utilizing this approach corridor. Onodi cells are posterior ethmoidal cells extending into the sphenoid bone, abutting the optic nerves (▶ Fig. 7.13). There might be variations in the course of the carotid artery in the lateral wall of the sphenoid sinus, as well as pneumatization variations of the sphenoid sinus,[3] placing the neurovascular structures at risk (▶ Fig. 7.14).

7.3 Transpterygoid/Transmaxillary Corridor

The transpterygoid/transmaxillary corridor allows access to the pterygopalatine fossa, infratemporal fossa, Meckel's cave, and lateral petrous apex (▶ Fig. 7.15).

The approach begins by medializing the middle turbinate and identifying the UP and ethmoidal bulla (EB; ▶ Fig. 7.16). The maxillary sinus ostium (in the semilunar hiatus) is obscured by the UP.

The UP is removed and a wide maxillary sinus antrostomy is performed. The EB and surrounding ethmoid cells are opened and removed (▶ Fig. 7.17). The ethmoidal crest, or crista ethmoidalis (CE), is a good localizer for the SPA emanating from the sphenopalatine foramen. Removing the perpendicular plate of the palatine bone and the posterior wall of the maxillary

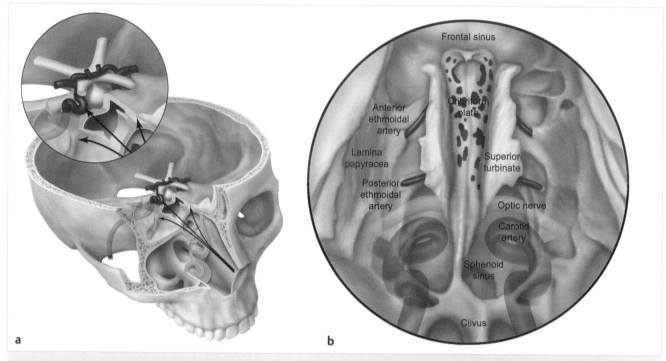

Fig. 7.9 (a) The transethmoidal corridor exposes the orbital apex, the lateral cavernous sinus, and the anterior fossa though the fovea ethmoidalis. (b) Complete ethmoidectomy is performed on both sides of the superior turbinate. Note the location of the anterior and posterior ethmoidal arteries.

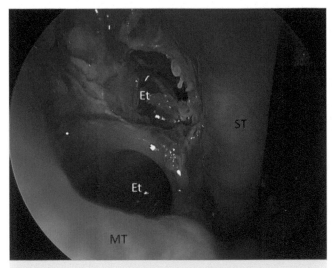

Fig. 7.10 A total ethmoidectomy is performed, lateral to the superior turbinate (ST) and cephalad to the middle turbinate (MT). Et, ethmoid cells

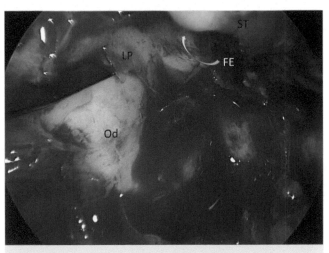

Fig. 7.12 The lamina papyracea (LP) is removed revealing the medial orbital dura (Od). The fovea ethmoidalis (FE) superiorly is being obscured by the superior turbinate (ST).

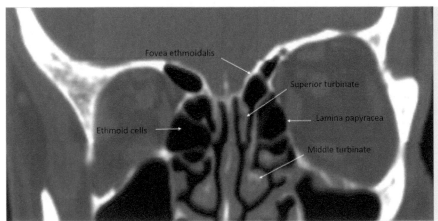

Fig. 7.11 A coronal CT scan showing the relationship of the ethmoid air cells to the turbinates, the fovea ethmoidalis superiorly, and the lamina papyracea laterally.

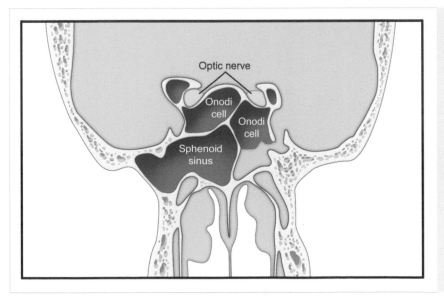

Fig. 7.13 Onodi cells. Posterior ethmoid cells, extending into the sphenoid bone superior to the sphenoid sinus, abutting the optic nerves superolaterally.

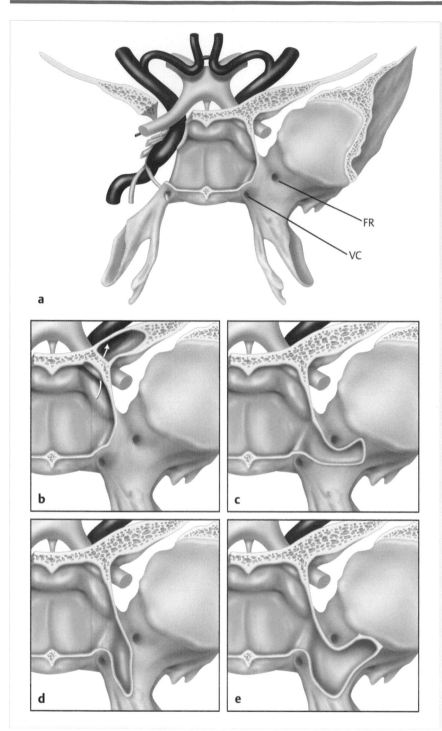

Fig. 7.14 Pneumatization variations of the sphenoid sinus in the coronal plane. **(a)** Body type: the pneumatization is confined to the body of the sphenoid sinus. **(b)** Lesser wing type: the sinus pneumatizes through the optic strut (*arrow*) and into the anterior clinoid process. **(c)** Greater wing type: the pneumatization extends laterally between the foramen rotundum (FR) and vidian canal (VC) into the greater wing. **(d)** Pterygoid type: the pneumatization extends laterally between the FR and VC and inferiorly into the pterygoid process. **(e)** Full lateral type: the sinus extends laterally into both the greater wing and the pterygoid process.

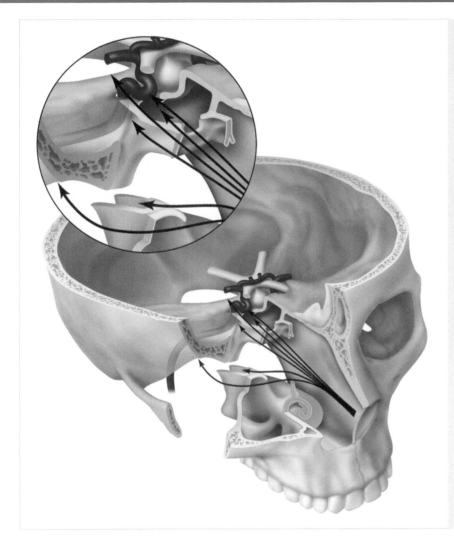

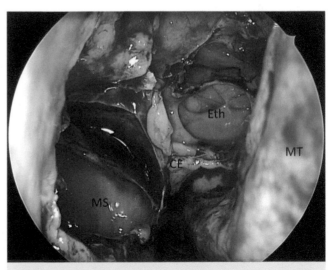

Fig. 7.15 The transpterygoid/transmaxillary corridor facilitates approaches to the pterygopalatine fossa, infratemporal fossa, Meckel's cave, and petrous apex.

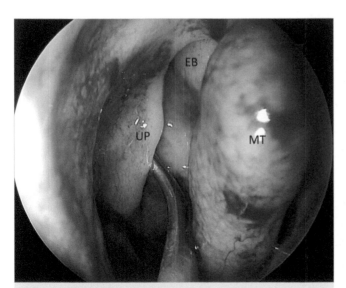

Fig. 7.16 Right nostril. The medial turbinate (MT) is medialized to reveal the uncinate process (UP) and the ethmoidal bulla (EB). The maxillary sinus ostium is obscured by the uncinate process. Probe tip is in the maxillary sinus ostium.

Fig. 7.17 The uncinate process is removed, and a maxillary sinus (MS) antrostomy is performed. The ethmoid (Eth) air cells are exposed after opening the ethmoidal bulla. The crista ethmoidalis (CE) localizes the sphenopalatine artery as it emanates from the sphenopalatine foramen. MT, middle turbinate.

sinus exposes the pterygopalatine fossa (▶ Fig. 7.18; ▶ Fig. 7.19). The perpendicular plate of the palatine bone forms the medial wall of the pterygopalatine fossa. The posterior wall of the maxillary sinus forms the anterior wall of the pterygopalatine fossa.

An artist depiction of the neurovascular anatomy of the pterygopalatine fossa is shown in ▶ Fig. 7.20.

The SPA, which is a branch of the internal maxillary artery (IMA), exits at the sphenopalatine foramen. The SPA is

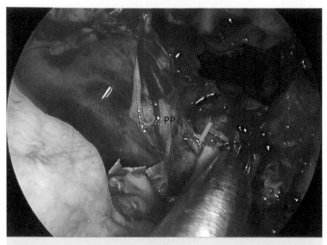

Fig. 7.18 Sphenopalatine artery (SPA; *blue arrow*), emerging from pterygopalatine fossa. Removing the perpendicular plate (PP) of the palatine bone exposes the pterygopalatine fossa.

coagulated and cut, and the contents of the pterygopalatine fossa are pushed laterally, to reveal the vidian nerve (VN; ▶ Fig. 7.21). The VN enters the pterygoid canal, which is located at the junction of the sphenoid sinus floor and mPP, and travels along the floor of the sphenoid sinus. Following the VN into the pterygoid canal will lead us to the petrous carotid, and is an important landmark in endoscopic endonasal surgery.

Further drilling laterally through the pterygomaxillary fissure (PMF) will expose the infratemporal fossa, with branches of the mandibular nerve (V3; ▶ Fig. 7.22). The roof of the infratemporal fossa is the inferior surface of the greater wing of the sphenoid, and contains two foramina: foramen ovale (V3) and foramen spinosum (middle meningeal artery).

Drilling the medial pterygoid bone medially and posteriorly exposes the lateral recess of the sphenoid sinus and the CS dura. Encephaloceles can sometimes originate within the lateral recess of the sphenoid sinus, in Sternberg's canal, which is a lateral craniopharyngeal canal resulting from incomplete fusion of the greater wings of the sphenoid bone with the basisphenoid.

Drilling the medial pterygoid bone posteriorly along the vidian (pterygoid) canal will lead to the junction of the paraclival and lacerum segment of the ICA. The carotid canal can then be drilled from medial to lateral using a standard egg shelling technique, freeing up the carotid. The carotid can then be mobilized as needed to reach lesions of the lateral petrous apex (▶ Fig. 7.23).

Drilling between the vidian canal and foramen rotundum (V2) will help in exposure of the *quadrangular space*, which can be used to reach lesions in the inferior CS and Meckel's cave. Once again, the vidian canal is followed back to the carotid

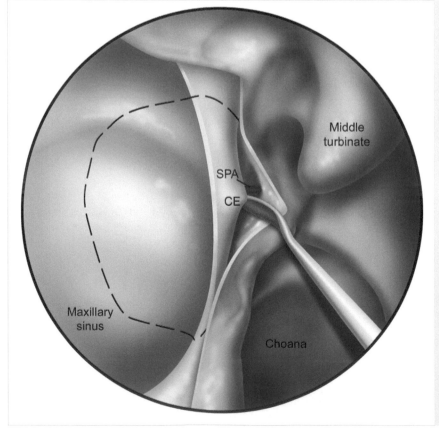

Fig. 7.19 The perpendicular plate of the palatine bone and the posterior wall of the maxillary sinus need to be removed to access the pterygopalatine fossa.

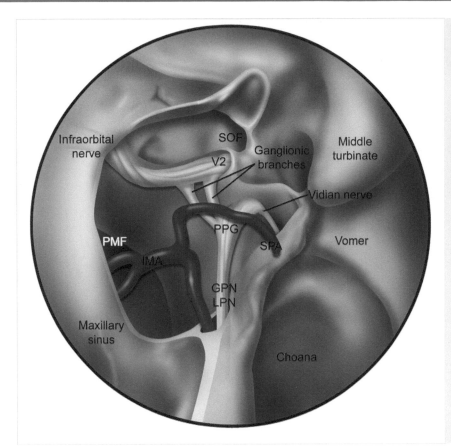

Fig. 7.20 The neurovascular anatomy of the pterygopalatine fossa is shown. The sphenopalatine artery (SPA), which is a branch of the IMA, exits at the sphenopalatine foramen. The SPA is coagulated and cut, and the contents of the pterygopalatine fossa are pushed laterally, to reveal the VN going into the vidian (pterygoid) canal. V2, maxillary nerve at foramen rotundum; PPG, pterygopalatine ganglion; GPN and LPN, greater and lesser palatine nerves; PMF, pterygomaxillary fissure.

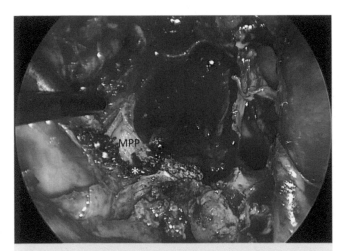

Fig. 7.21 The sphenopalatine artery (SPA) is coagulated and cut (*). The contents of the pterygopalatine fossa are pushed laterally to reveal the vidian nerve (VN; *blue arrow*) entering the pterygoid canal. MPP, medial pterygoid plate.

artery. The quadrangular space is bound by the paraclival carotid medially and the lacerum carotid inferiorly, by the maxillary nerve (V2) laterally and by the abducens nerve (CN 6) and ophthalmic nerve (V1) superiorly. The dura of the quadrangular space can be opened along V2 to access lesions in Meckel's cave (▶ Fig. 7.23).

7.4 Transnasal Corridor

All endoscopic endonasal approaches utilize the nostrils as entry portals. The transnasal corridor is defined as one in which no sinus cavities need to be transgressed to reach the target. From cephalad to caudal, these targets are the cribriform plate, medial petrous apex, jugular foramen, lower two-thirds of the clivus, craniovertebral junction, and the odontoid (▶ Fig. 7.24).

The cribriform plate can be visualized by working lateral to the septum but medial to the middle turbinate, and is a narrow channel, usually medial to the superior turbinates (▶ Fig. 7.9a). The cribriform plate can frequently be the source of encephaloceles and must be removed along with the fovea ethmoidalis when reaching the anterior fossa for esthesioneuroblastomas and olfactory groove meningiomas (▶ Fig. 7.25).

Working parallel to the hard palate along the nasal floor, one can reach the clivus and the odontoid. In children, prominent adenoids can occasionally obscure the posterior nasopharynx and choana (▶ Fig. 7.26). The adenoids can be resected and the lower clivus and anterior arch of C1 can be reached after making a vertical incision in the posterior pharyngeal musculature using Bovie cautery (▶ Fig. 7.27). The C1 arch can be drilled away to reach the odontoid tip.

The paraclival (C3 lacerum segment) and petrous (C2) segments of the internal carotid artery are the lateral limits of the exposure, and can be avoided by staying medial to the VN at C3, and the eustachian tube at C2 inferiorly (▶ Fig. 7.28). The medial

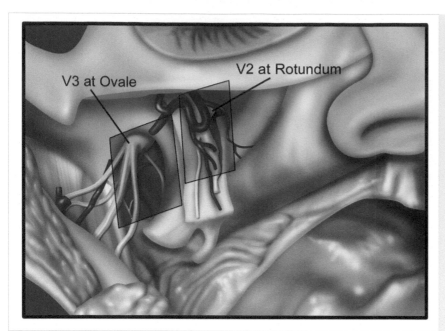

Fig. 7.22 Relationship between the pterygopalatine fossa (*yellow shading*) and the infratemporal fossa (*red shading*).

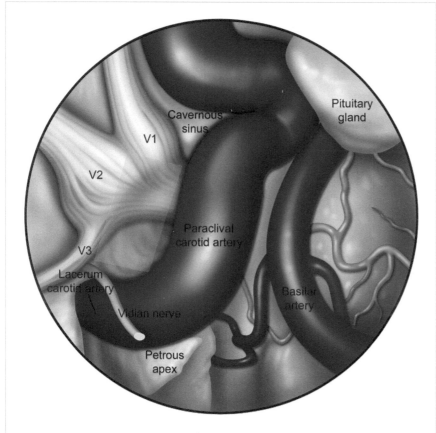

Fig. 7.23 The *quadrangular space* (*blue shading*) is bound by the paraclival carotid medially and the lacerum carotid inferiorly, by the maxillary nerve (V2) laterally and by the abducens nerve (CN 6) and ophthalmic nerve (V1) superiorly. The dura of the quadrangular space can be opened along V2 to access lesions in Meckel's cave.

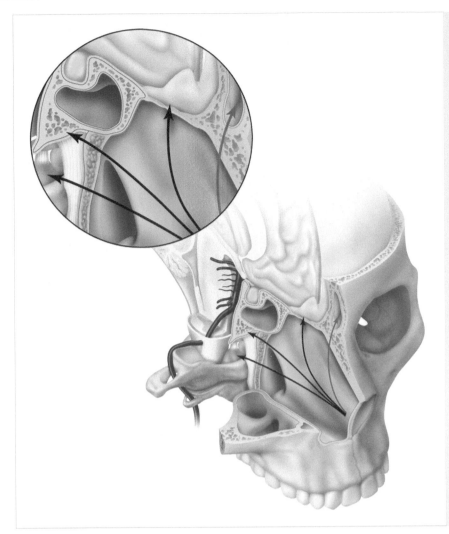

Fig. 7.24 The transnasal corridor does not involve any breach of the paranasal sinuses. Approaches to the cribriform plate, the inferior two-thirds of the clivus and odontoid are feasible through this surgical corridor. The frontal sinus can be reached via the transfrontal corridor (*purple arrow*).

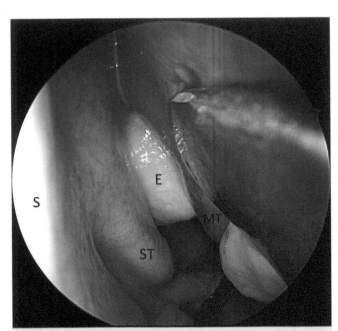

Fig. 7.25 An encephalocele (E) is visualized in the left nostril, lateral to the septum (S). The middle turbinate (MT) is displaced laterally by the instrument. ST, superior turbinate.

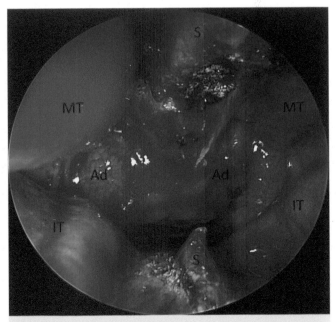

Fig. 7.26 A posterior septectomy is performed and the nasopharynx approached using a binarial approach. In pediatric patients, large adenoids (Ad) can occasionally obscure the choana. S, septum; MT, middle turbinate; IT, inferior turbinate.

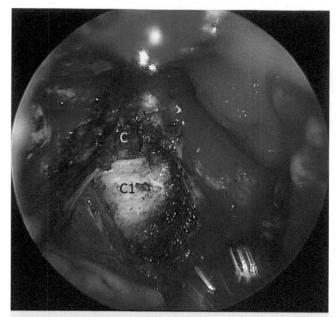

Fig. 7.27 The adenoids are resected and a vertical incision made in the posterior pharyngeal musculature using Bovie electrocautery. The anterior arch of the C1 ring can be seen underneath. The clival mucosa can also be cauterized to expose the clivus (C) above.

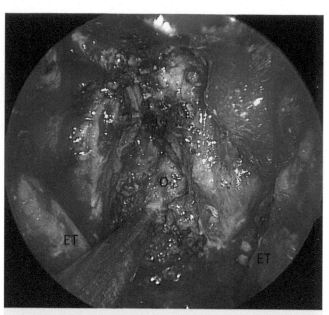

Fig. 7.28 The anterior arch of C1 is drilled off to expose the odontoid peg. The Eustachian tubes (ET) mark the lateral borders of the dissection.

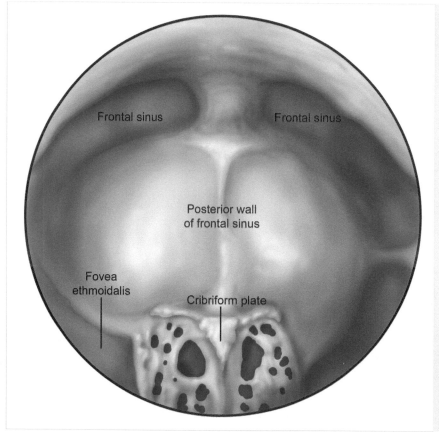

Fig. 7.29 The frontal sinus ostia can be opened bilaterally for a panoramic view into the frontal sinus.

petrous apex can also be reached medial to the Eustachian tube; however, reaching the jugular foramen may require mobilization of the Eustachian tube.

7.5 Transfrontal Corridor

The transfrontal corridor can be used to access the frontal sinus and the anterior frontal fossa (▶ Fig. 7.24). A 30- or 45-degree angled scope is usually needed to visualize the frontal recess (frontal sinus opening into the nasal cavity), lateral to the middle turbinate and medial to the ethmoid sinus air cells. The frontal sinus ostia (recess) can be widely opened by performing a Draf III to achieve a panoramic view into the frontal sinus bilaterally. The posterior wall of the frontal sinus can be opened to enter the anterior cranial fossa to provide access to the crista galli (▶ Fig. 7.29).

In some patients, frontal bullar cells might be present, which can masquerade as the posterior wall of the frontal sinus. These additional air cells must be removed to reach the posterior wall of the frontal sinus. Review of preoperative CT imaging should alert the surgeon of the presence and location of these additional air cells in the anterior skull base.

7.6 Conclusion

In section 2 of this book, the readers will find one or a combination of these approach corridors being utilized to surgically treat pathology at the anterior pediatric skull base. Having an anatomic understanding of these surgical corridors, along with their limitations and inherent pitfalls, will prepare the surgeon to safely and successfully treat pathology in this location via the endonasal approach.

References

[1] Schwartz TH, Fraser JF, Brown S, Tabaee A, Kacker A, Anand VK. Endoscopic cranial base surgery: classification of operative approaches. Neurosurgery. 2008; 62(5):991–1002, discussion 1002–1005

[2] Güldner C, Pistorius SM, Diogo I, Bien S, Sesterhenn A, Werner JA. Analysis of pneumatization and neurovascular structures of the sphenoid sinus using cone-beam tomography (CBT). Acta Radiol. 2012; 53(2):214–219

[3] Wang J, Bidari S, Inoue K, Yang H, Rhoton A, Jr. Extensions of the sphenoid sinus: a new classification. Neurosurgery. 2010; 66(4):797–816

7.7 Additional Resources

Online anatomical videos to gain a comprehensive understanding of the anterior skull base anatomy via the endonasal approach:

* The Rhoton Collection: Anterior Skull Base—Part 1 and 2, 2D video, AANSNeurosurgery. YouTube Channel.
* The Rhoton Collection: The Nose for Neurosurgeons, 2D video, AANSNeurosurgery. YouTube Channel.

8 Combined Transcranial and Endonasal Approaches

Jennifer L. Quon, Gerald A. Grant, Peter H. Hwang, Griffith R. Harsh IV, and Michael S.B. Edwards

Abstract

Combined approaches can be used to treat a number of different skull base lesions. In adults, they have been applied to a wide variety of skull base pathology. In the pediatric population, purely endonasal approaches are limited by the small anatomic dimensions and limited aeration of sinuses. Transcranial approaches alone may be sufficient for extensive supratentorial lesions, but more challenging tumors with extension along the skull base or into the nasal cavity may require a combined approach for optimal access to the necessary corridors. Collaboration with otolaryngology colleagues is crucial to this approach.

Keywords: combined approach, skull base tumor, pediatric skull base

8.1 Patient Selection

Patients with anterior skull base lesions may present with a variety of symptoms, including endocrine dysfunction and cranial nerve compression due to tumor invasion into the periorbita, optic canal, superior orbital fissure, sella, or cavernous sinus.[1] Further supratentorial extension may lead to compression of the optic chiasm or obstruction of the third ventricle and hydrocephalus.

8.1.1 Transcranial

Favorable Anatomy

For tumors larger than 4 cm in diameter and 80 cm³, gross total resection is feasible using a transcranial approach.[2]

Limitations

Transcranial approaches may require significant brain retraction to reach the sella. Tumors that extend into the sphenoid sinus and nasal cavity may be more challenging from this approach.

8.1.2 Endonasal

Favorable Anatomy

A purely endoscopic endonasal approach is favorable for tumors with extracranial extension into the paranasal sinuses and can be used to access the transsphenoidal, transethmoidal, and transpterygoid compartments. When tumors have significant extension into the third and lateral ventricle, adequate visualization can be challenging with just the endoscope.[3] Removal of the tuberculum sellae and planum sphenoidale in an extended transsphenoidal approach allows access to the suprasellar cistern and third ventricle using angled endoscopes.[3]

Limitations

Tumors that extend into the lateral ventricle are difficult to access from a purely endoscopic endonasal approach. Lateral extension beyond the internal carotid arteries prohibits gross total resection using a purely endoscopic endonasal approach.[4] A craniotomy may be required for tumors with lateral extension beyond the lamina papyracea, especially those requiring an orbital extenteration.[5] For very small children, in particular, an endoscopic endonasal approach may be limited by the small intercarotid distance and lack of a pneumatized sella. Pneumatization of the sella begins as early as 2 months of age but may not be complete until about 9 years.[6]

8.1.3 Combined Approach

Favorable Anatomy

Combined approaches allow a more extensive resection while limiting damage to surrounding anatomy. They should be used for extensive tumor growth, either infrasellar or suprasellar.[4] For tumors invading the orbital or periorbital regions, optic canal, cavernous sinus, or anterior and middle fossae, a combined approach may expand access into different corridors. If a single approach does not allow safe resection, and the goal is gross total resection, then a planned combined approach may be indicated. Combined approaches may benefit from the advantages while reducing the disadvantages of each approach used separately.

Endoscopic approaches can access skull base lesions from the posterior table of the frontal sinus to the foramen magnum. The transcranial portion of a combined procedure typically adds a subfrontal, a pterional, or an orbitozygomatic craniotomy.[3] An endoscopic endonasal approach can even be combined with a retrosigmoid approach.[4] Endoscopic approaches may be limited laterally at the frontal sinus and in the anterior cranial fossa; exposure lateral to the midpupillary line is limited. In the parasellar region, extension of tumors lateral to the internal carotid artery is a relative contraindication to an endoscopic approach. In transpterygoid approaches to the pterygopalatine fossa and infratemporal fossa, extensive tumor involvement of the middle fossa dura or temporal lobe may contraindicate a solely endoscopic approach. A combined approach can be also used after a failed single approach, either in the near term if one approach has been unsuccessful or later, when recurrent growth favors one approach over another. Combined approaches are most often undertaken in attempt to achieve gross total resection.

Tumor Pathology

Certain tumor subtypes may have consistencies more favorable for one approach over another. Combined approaches are particularly useful for malignant skull base tumors such as esthesioneuroblastomas and clival chordomas, and for frontoethmoidal osteomas and giant pituitary adenomas. Combined approaches may be favored for highly vascular lesions, such as intradural juvenile nasopharyngeal angiofibromas (JNA), where an endoscopic-only approach may compromise the surgeon's ability to control surgical bleeding.[1,2,3,4,5,7] For malignant tumors, in particular, achieving negative tumor margins is crucial for disease control.[5] Sinonasal carcinomas widely invading brain may be more

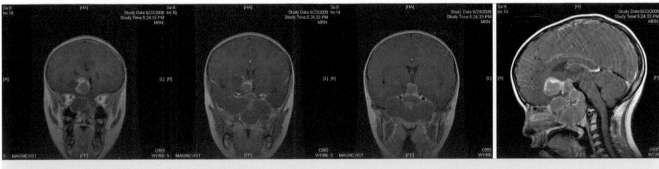

Fig. 8.1 Case 1: Preoperative coronal and sagittal MRI.

safely managed with a combined approach. Combined approaches have also been used for sphenoid wing meningiomas with inferior and lateral invasion of the paranasal sinuses; these tumors can widely involve dura, the transcranial resection can result in a high rate of cerebrospinal fluid (CSF) leakage.[1] Although most anterior skull meningoencephaloceles can be managed through a purely endoscopic approach, a combined approach may be needed for massive encephaloceles or if sinonasal anatomy has been significantly altered.[8]

Special Considerations

Most combined approaches are performed collaboratively by neurosurgeons and otolaryngologists. Preoperatively, a balloon-occlusion test can be used to assess the safety of sacrifice of the internal carotid artery. Preoperative tumor embolization can reduce blood loss during resection of some JNA and meningiomas.[9]

More extensive tumor resection can increase the risk of CSF leak.[4] A multilayer closure including a vascularized nasoseptal flap is extremely important in preventing CSF leakage. In cases of extensive resection, collaboration with plastic surgery may improve reconstruction of the orbit and skull base. As combined approaches performed in tandem can be lengthy, some surgeons prefer to stage them.

8.2 Case Examples

At our institution, planned combined approaches have been reserved for cases of tumor extension beyond regions accessible with one approach alone. There is a paucity of data on the use of combined approaches in the pediatric population. Although endoscopic endonasal approaches are becoming more common in the pediatric population, reported experience with combined approaches is very limited. In children, we have used combined approaches for craniopharyngioma, Rathke's cleft cyst, JNA, esthesioneuroblastoma, alveolar rhabdomyosarcoma, and melanotic neuroectodermal tumor of infancy. We will discuss several technical case examples below.

8.2.1 Case 1: Craniopharyngioma

Clinical Presentation

The patient is a 10-year-old boy who presented with a several year history of intermittent headaches but was otherwise neurologically intact. He later began to have vomiting and lethargy, prompting his physicians to obtain a head CT, which demonstrated a skull base lesion that was faintly calcified with approximately 4 mm of midline shift. An MRI better characterized the lesion as a 4.7 × 6.9 × 7.6 cm multiloculated cystic skull base originating from the sella turcica (▶ Fig. 8.1). Notably, the lesion obliterated the sphenoid and posterior ethmoid sinus and invaded bilateral cavernous sinuses. In addition, the lesion extended superiorly, displacing the optic chiasm superiorly and compressing the frontal lobe. The patient did not have any visual field deficits or gross endocrine abnormalities but had no have short stature and obesity, which are classic features of a child with a craniopharyngioma. Although diabetes insipidus can occur with craniopharyngiomas and even more so with germ cell tumors, the patient did have symptoms of DI. To confirm the diagnosis of craniopharyngioma, and rule out other lesions such as a sarcoma, the child underwent an endoscopic transnasal biopsy.

Surgical Approach

A combined approach from above and below was planned because of the superior to inferior extent of the lesion and goal for an aggressive resection of the benign pathology. The tumor was initially debulked from above through a bifrontal craniotomy. At the end of the resection, an endoscope was inserted endonasally to ensure that there was no residual tumor.

At the beginning of the procedure, the patient was given preoperative steroids and antibiotics. A lumbar drain was placed for brain relaxation and postoperative diversion of CSF to prevent CSF leak. The patient was placed supine and the head was fixed in three-pin Mayfield head holder in a neutral position. Even a little head extension is preferred to flexion. Neuronavigation was used for the procedure to help identify proximity to critical structures. The patient was prepped for a bicoronal incision with the nose covered with a sterile towel. A large pericranial flap was dissected and left attached posteriorly to keep it vascularized. Subgaleal dissection was performed down to the level of both orbital rims with special care not to injure the supraorbital nerve artery and vein. The supraorbital foramen was opened with a small chisel to free the nerve and subperiosteal dissection was carried out bilaterally into the orbit and in the midline to the level of the nasofrontal suture. The orbitofrontal craniotomy consisted of a bifrontal bone flap and resection of the orbital rim with an orbital bandeau bilaterally. Small burr holes were placed on either side of the sagittal sinus and at the keyholes laterally in the pterion underneath the temporalis muscle. The bifrontal craniotomy was then performed using a craniotome. The frontal lobe dura was freed from the orbital roof and partially freed from the crista galli anteriorly. The supraorbital osteotomies were then performed from an intracranial approach using the reciprocating saw and small chisels and a mallet. The removal of the supraorbital bar was critical to extend the subfrontal access, which opens up the anterior corridor to allow the surgeon to look up with minimal to no retraction on the frontal lobe. The dura was then opened, and the sagittal sinus was isolated and ligated with two 2–0 silk sutures and transected along with the falx. CSF was drained off through the lumbar drain for better frontal lobe relaxation. Greenberg 3/8 inch retractors were used to gently elevate the frontal lobe over wet Telfa to keep the brain moist. Using neuronavigation, we localized the intracranial portion of the tumor and its frontal extent. The olfactory nerve and olfactory bulbs were identified and transected, as planned, on the right side. The gyrus rectus on the right side was also partially resected subpially to avoid further retraction on the frontal lobe while exposing the large multilobulated cystic tumor. The operative microscope was then brought in for closer microdissection.

A firm capsule of the tumor was dissected from the surrounding frontal lobe white matter. After the dissection along the lateral margin of the tumor, the dissection was carried out along the inferior and medial aspects of the tumor. Birefringent calcium specks could be visualized inside of the capsule, which is classic for craniopharyngioma. The takeoff of the R A1 off the supraclinoid carotid and optic nerve was dissected free of the tumor capsule and we then followed the A1 medially to the anterior communicating (ACom) complex. We dissected the tumor capsule on either side of the A2 segments as well as optic nerves between both carotid arteries. It was also important to open up the Sylvian fissure to identify the M1 perforators, which were adherent to the tumor capsule. This dissection is much higher risk at the time of reoperation or post radiation since the adventitia around the vessel wall is often violated. A CT angiogram can be helpful prior to reoperation to rule out a pseudoaneurysm or vasculopathy due to the craniopharyngioma in particular. After a significant portion of the tumor was debulked, the tumor capsule was gently pulled down and dissected from the overlying frontal lobe white matter and hypothalamus. A tumor capsule that is markedly adherent to the hypothalamus and basal ganglia might be better left due to the high risk for hypothalamic dysfunction. The tumor extended into the sellar region, although the pituitary could not clearly

be identified as separate from the tumor. In the end, approximately 90% of the intracranial tumor mass was debulked from above. Our otolaryngology colleagues then began their portion of the operation endonasally. This second surgery could be staged if needed in a very young child or if there was any frontal lobe swelling or coagulopathy.

The enlarged sella was further opened with an ethmoidectomy, allowing access to the anteromedial and posterior aspect of the skull base. The eroded bone structures within the sphenoid and ethmoid sinuses were identified and a remnant of a midline bony septum was removed. We then performed a radical resection of the remaining intracranial tumor mass and tumor capsule guided by neuronavigation. Along the soft palate, the tumor capsule was very adherent to the mucosa as well as the basilar artery.

For closure, the pericranial flap was divided and first used to line the subcranial resection cavity as a free graft. The endoscope was introduced through the right nostril and the resection cavity was inspected, with any visible residual tumor resected. The endoscope was also introduced through the widened sella from above to inspect all angles of the tumor resection. Gross total removal, apart from the adherent capsule as mentioned earlier along the A2 s, was confirmed using the endoscope. Two Merocel nasal packings were introduced through both nostrils to support the cranial base reconstruction from below. The vascularized pericranial flap was then used to line the anterior cranial fossa. To reconstruct the bony defect, a split bone graft from the calvarium was obtained in the right frontal area. The calvarium was split using the oscillating saw and chisels. A 2 × 1.5 cm piece of calvarium was now placed in the bony defect of the skull base. Tissue glue was put on top of the pericranial flap to hold it in place. The dura was then closed primarily except in the areas where the dura was detached from the crista galli where a dural matrix graft was used with Tisseel. Tack-off sutures were performed in the frontal craniotomy area. The orbitofrontal bone flap including the frontal bone and orbital bandeau was now reconstructed using resorbable fixation. We left the lumbar drain in place but clamped until a postoperative scan was obtained and we had a postoperative examination to follow. The lumbar drain was then opened at a drain rate of 10 mL/h. Special attention was paid in the pediatric intensive care unit (ICU) to the occurrence of syndrome of inappropriate antidiuretic hormone (SIADH) and diabetes insipidus (DI) with frequent serum sodium checks. Final diagnosis was a craniopharyngioma and the patient has not had any recurrence of his tumor over a the 10-year follow-up (▶ Fig. 8.2).

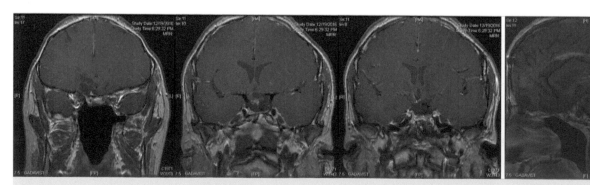

Fig. 8.2 Case 1: Postoperative coronal and sagittal MRI.

Rationale

Intercarotid distance, suprasellar extent.

8.2.2 Case 2: Juvenile Nasopharyngeal Angiofibromas

Clinical Presentation

A combined approach was used for three patients with JNA. Presenting symptoms included a remote history of nosebleeds, snoring, nasal congestion, facial numbness, and hearing loss. In all three cases, there was significant tumor involvement along the skull base from the nasal cavity, ethmoid and maxillary sinuses, the orbital apex, sphenoid sinus, clivus and infratemporal fossa to the cavernous sinus, and middle cranial fossa. Bony dehiscence was noted in several cases. In each case, the decision was made to use a combined open and endoscopic approach because of extensive disease across several corridors. Given the impressive vascular network, these patients also went for preoperative embolization. A representative preoperative MRI from one of these cases is shown in ▶ Fig. 8.3.

Surgical Approach

A curvilinear incision beginning in the preauricular area was carried superiorly just posteriorly behind the ear, across the superior temporal line, toward the anterolateral hairline. It was injected with 5 mL of local anesthetic and carried through skin, subcutaneous tissue, galea, and pericranium. The soft-tissue flap was mobilized anteriorly over the orbital rim. The anterior temporal fat pad was elevated to preserve the facial nerve branches. The orbital rim was exposed from external orbital angle down to its junction with the zygomatic arch. The zygomatic arch was cleared of attachments anteriorly and posteriorly and divided at the zygomatic–maxillary junction and posteriorly at its root. It was left attached to underlying muscle. The temporalis muscle was incised to the superior temporal line and mobilized from its fossa down through the zygomatic arch opening, providing exposure of the inferior and anterior aspect of the middle cranial fossa floor. Three trephinations were used to elevate a free bone flap, extending the craniotomy to the floor. Additional subtemporal bone was removed, working posterior to anterior beneath the temporal pole. Tumor had penetrated through the outer table of the bone and any tumor-involved bone was removed with a rongeur. Working in concert with the otolaryngology team, tumor was removed from the infratemporal space by centrally debulking and resecting from regions of bony expansion in the greater sphenoid wing pterygoid structures and surrounding soft tissues. The tumor was accessed endoscopically via a transmaxillary, transpterygoid approach to the pterygopalatine fossa and infratemporal fossa components of the tumor, and a transsphenoidal approach was used for the sphenoid and nasopharyngeal components of the tumor. Further dissection simultaneously with the otolaryngology team from below identified the inferolateral aspect of the cavernous sinus. The internal carotid artery and the cavernous sinus were identified by Doppler ultrasonography and confirmed by StealthStation navigation. Tumor was stripped away from this region and simultaneously removed from the upper reaches of the pterygopalatine fossa, and tumor extending underneath the greater wing of the sphenoid into the sphenoid sinus cavity was also removed. Communication of the two approaches facilitated this dissection. At this point, we further resected the tumor from the intranasal cavity into the sphenoid sinus. The tumor seemed invested along the sphenopalatine foramen and extending posteriorly along the path of the vidian nerve. Using a combined external and endoscopic approach, the remaining tumor was removed from the pterygopalatine fossa, lateral extension along temporal lobe and infratemporal fossa. Inspection of all tumor surfaces suggested a gross total resection. Hemostasis was achieved and cavities were irrigated with antibiotic solution. Gelfoam was used to plug the communication in the middle cranial fossa floor with the nasal cavities. The dura was confirmed to be intact and covered with a single layer of Surgicel. The bone plate was fixed with titanium mini plates. Temporalis muscle was sewn back to its fascia superiorly and posteriorly. The zygomatic arch was fixed with titanium mini screws and linear strips. The wound was closed in layers with 2–0 Vicryl in galea and staples on skin. The upper aspect of the transnasal exposure was packed with Gelfoam as well. The patient was allowed to awaken, extubated, and taken to the ICU in stable condition.

A representative postoperative MRI from one of these cases is shown in ▶ Fig. 8.4.

Rationale

Tumor extension lateral to the carotid arteries, tumor vascularity.

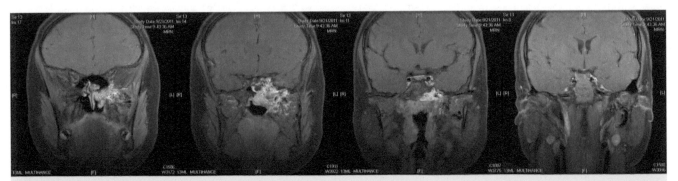

Fig. 8.3 Case 2: Preoperative coronal MRI.

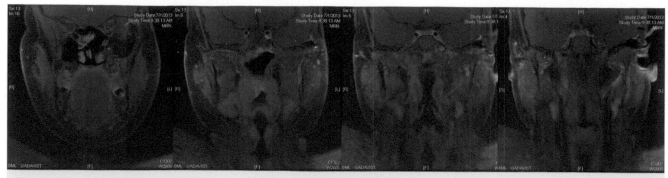

Fig. 8.4 Case 2: Postoperative coronal MRI.

8.3 Adjuvant Therapy

8.3.1 Radiation Therapy

Postoperative radiotherapy is commonly administered for control of microscopic disease after combined skull base resection of sinonasal carcinomas. Other tumors whose gross total resection may be precluded by tumor invasion of the superior orbital fissure or cavernous sinus may require postoperative radiotherapy for control of residual disease.[1] Adjuvant stereotactic radiotherapy, radiosurgery, or proton beam therapy is routinely employed after surgical resection of clival chordomas.[4] Neoadjuvant radiation may also be considered for certain sinonasal malignancies, such as sinonasal undifferentiated carcinoma and esthesioneuroblastoma.[5]

8.3.2 Chemotherapy

For some advanced Kadish stages/Hyams grades of esthesioneuroblastoma, adjuvant chemotherapy is added to surgery and radiation.[5] Neoadjuvant chemotherapy has also been used for advanced stage esthesioneuroblastoma and sinonasal undifferentiated carcinoma (neoadjuvant chemoradiation), with combined surgical approaches reserved for surgical salvage.[10,11]

8.4 Conclusion

Combined transcranial endonasal approaches are performed collaboratively by neurosurgeons and otolaryngologists. They are most valuable and even necessary for anterior skull base lesions with extensive growth into the surrounding anatomy. These approaches are particularly useful for achieving gross total resection in malignant pathologies, but when necessary can be combined with adjuvant radiation or chemotherapy.

References

[1] Attia M, Patel KS, Kandasamy J, et al. Combined cranionasal surgery for spheno-orbital meningiomas invading the paranasal sinuses, pterygopalatine, and infratemporal fossa. World Neurosurg. 2013; 80(6):e367–e373

[2] Fraser JF, Nyquist GG, Moore N, Anand VK, Schwartz TH. Endoscopic endonasal transclival resection of chordomas: operative technique, clinical outcome, and review of the literature. J Neurosurg. 2010; 112(5):1061–1069

[3] Greenfield JP, Leng LZ, Chaudhry U, et al. Combined simultaneous endoscopic transsphenoidal and endoscopic transventricular resection of a giant pituitary macroadenoma. Minim Invasive Neurosurg. 2008; 51(5):306–309

[4] Koechlin NO, Simmen D, Briner HR, Reisch R. Combined transnasal and transcranial removal of a giant clival chordoma. J Neurol Surg Rep. 2014; 75(1):e98–e102

[5] Komotar RJ, Starke RM, Raper DM, Anand VK, Schwartz TH. Endoscopic endonasal compared with anterior craniofacial and combined cranionasal resection of esthesioneuroblastomas. World Neurosurg. 2013; 80(1–2):148–159

[6] Jang YJ, Kim SC. Pneumatization of the sphenoid sinus in children evaluated by magnetic resonance imaging. Am J Rhinol. 2000; 14(3):181–185

[7] Park MC, Goldman MA, Donahue JE, Tung GA, Goel R, Sampath P. Endonasal ethmoidectomy and bifrontal craniotomy with craniofacial approach for resection of frontoethmoidal osteoma causing tension pneumocephalus. Skull Base. 2008; 18(1):67–72

[8] Schaberg M, Murchison AP, Rosen MR, Evans JJ, Bilyk JR. Transorbital and transnasal endoscopic repair of a meningoencephalocele. Orbit. 2011; 30(5):221–225

[9] Naraghi M, Saberi H, Mirmohseni AS, Nikdad MS, Afarideh M. Management of advanced intracranial intradural juvenile nasopharyngeal angiofibroma: combined single-stage rhinosurgical and neurosurgical approach. Int Forum Allergy Rhinol. 2015; 5(7):650–658

[10] Patil VM, Joshi A, Noronha V, et al. Neoadjuvant chemotherapy in locally advanced and borderline resectable nonsquamous sinonasal tumors (esthesioneuroblastoma and sinonasal tumor with neuroendocrine differentiation). Int J Surg Oncol. 2016; 2016:6923730

[11] Su SY, Bell D, Ferrarotto R, et al. Outcomes for olfactory neuroblastoma treated with induction chemotherapy. Head Neck. 2017; 39(8):1671–1679

9 Transorbital and Multiportal Approaches

Kris S. Moe, Randall A. Bly, and Jeremy N. Ciporen

Abstract

Endoscopic endonasal corridors have significantly improved our ability to safely access challenging lesions of the mid-line anterior skull base. Transorbital endoscopic approaches have further expanded surgical access to the anterior and middle cranial fossae, particularly those lesions that are obstructed by the orbits, or may involve the orbital bone and contents. We describe our four quadrant approach whereby the orbit is used as a pathway to access lesions of the anterior and middle cranial fossa.

The surgical outcomes with transorbital procedures have been highly favorable, including in the pediatric population. Our experience with transorbital and multiportal approaches including transnasal, transmaxillary, and infratemporal fossa portals provides excellent visualization, as well as superior dimensions and angles for safe and successful treatment of skull base pathology.

Keywords: transnasal, transorbital, multiportal approach, endoscopic corridors

9.1 Introduction

Transnasal endoscopic approaches have added tremendously to our ability to treat midline skull base lesions in the pediatric population. From the crista galli to the upper cervical spine, we are now able to address many lesions that until recently would have required an open surgical approach. Though often effective, traditional open approaches create a significant amount of collateral damage and morbidity that should be avoided if possible.

While transnasal corridors are highly effective to approach the majority of midline skull base lesions, in some cases the pathology is obstructed by the orbits or may actually involve the orbital bone or contents. Given their position occupying much of the anterior cranial fossa (ACF) and anterior aspect of the middle cranial fossa (MCF), the orbits block much of the transnasal corridor to these regions.

Rather than being considered an obstacle to be avoided, the orbits might be looked at as large potential portals to the ACF, MCF, and adjacent structures. With this possibility in mind, over a decade ago we began looking into whether endoscopic pathways within and through the orbit could serve as alternative or adjunct routes to targets that were challenging to reach through nasal portals.[1] We found that through four transorbital endoscopic approaches that can be used in monoportal or multiportal technique,[2,3,4,5] we can expand our endoscopic armamentarium to access the majority of skull base pathology involving or adjacent to the orbit.[6,7] This chapter will describe our current concept of a quadrant-centered model of transorbital endoscopic skull base surgery.

9.2 Terminology

Endoscopic surgery of the orbit can be divided into two primary types: **transorbital** and **transnasal**. The former includes transcutaneous and transconjunctival portals that provide direct entrance into the orbit. The latter refers to corridors that proceed through a naris, the ethmoid sinuses and lamina papyracea to enter the medial orbit, or through the maxillary sinus to enter the medial orbital floor. It is also possible to enter the orbit using a portal in the face of the maxillary sinus, traveling through the maxillary sinus to enter the floor of the orbit, though monoportal transmaxillary orbital approaches are uncommonly used for tumor surgery.

Within the realm of transorbital approaches, there are four primary portals, one for each quadrant (superior, medial, inferior, and lateral). These approaches can be used for surgery within the orbit (**endoscopic orbital surgery**); for pathways through the orbit to adjacent targets (**transorbital endoscopic surgery**); or for pathways through the orbit to neurologic targets (**transorbital neuroendoscopic surgery [TONES]**). For these procedures, we use the term "**pathway**" to connote a surgical route through a volume that is created by dissection, in distinction to "**corridor**," which suggests a preexisting space such as the nasal cavity through which access is achieved. We do not consider these procedures to be "**minimally invasive**," as invasiveness is dictated by the nature and location of the pathology rather than the approach. However, these procedures are "**minimally disruptive**," in that they minimize collateral damage to tissue that is not involved in the disease process, thereby creating the least possible morbidity and allowing the swiftest possible return to previous lifestyle.

9.3 Experience and Outcomes in Transorbital Surgery

There have been multiple reports on experience with transorbital surgery, and these are appearing with increasing frequency and with perspectives from international sources. These approaches have been described for the treatment of skull base tumors,[8,9,10] infectious processes such as epidural abscess and sinogenic pathology,[11] cerebrospinal fluid (CSF) leak repair,[12] cavernous sinus pathology,[13] seizure disorders,[14] ethmoid artery ligation for control of epistaxis, and trauma surgery[15] through endoscopic and robotic techniques.[4]

The surgical outcomes with transorbital procedures have been highly favorable. In an early report of our initial outcomes with transorbital endoscopic procedures on over 100 patients, we found no complications due to the surgical approach, and had a high success rate in achieving the surgical goals. Our results in the 5 years since that publication have been similarly favorable.

The morbidity that patients experience postoperatively depends on the orbital quadrant involved, as well as the extent of the pathology and duration of surgery. Temporary ptosis is expected with superior quadrant pathology due to retraction of the levator muscle, as is forehead numbness from retraction of the supraorbital and supratrochlear nerves. If these nerves are preserved, sensation is expected to return. Likewise, temporary diplopia is not uncommon after surgery in any of the four quadrants, due to retraction of the extraocular muscles that is required to access and treat the surgical target. Postoperative pain from the surgical approach is typically minimal: when a transorbital portal is combined with a transnasal approach, in our experience, patients typically report less pain from the orbital component of the surgery. Given that the alternative to these approaches is in many instances bifrontal or other open craniotomy, we believe that these techniques constitute truly minimally disruptive surgery.

Our experience with pediatric applications of these procedures has also been excellent. Pathology, including trauma (brain, dural, orbital, and frontal sinus injury), tumors (esthesioneuroblastoma, juvenile nasopharyngeal angiofibroma [JNA], neuroma, orbital osteoma with extension into the brain), orbital lymphatic malformation, and complications of sinogenic pathology involving the orbit and skull base have been favorably addressed in the pediatric population. We have performed tumor excisions, including resectioning of the skull base and orbital bone in patients as young as 18 months of age without adverse outcomes. Though there remain few reports in the literature of the use of these procedures in the pediatric population, based on our favorable experience to date we believe that cautious use of transorbital surgery in the pediatric population is safe when used appropriately, particularly when faced with the alternative of open craniotomy.

9.4 Indications and Contraindications

Transorbital endoscopic approaches are indicated for benign or malignant lesions of similar pathology and extent to those that are treated with a transnasal approach. The decision to use a transorbital endoscopic approach must be based on the location, extent, and characteristics of the pathology. Major considerations are whether the pathology could be treated by an endoscopic approach, and whether the safety of adjacent critical neurovascular structures can be ensured. For larger tumors invading the orbital contents that require exenteration, transorbital endoscopic technique can be quite useful. Endoscopic enucleation can be performed, after which there is a wide field for any further endoscopic resection that might be required, such as a tumor invading the frontal lobe of the brain. For appropriate defects, transorbital endoscopy can be combined with endoscopic brow lift portals for multiportal harvest of a vascularized pericranial flap.

Transorbital procedures are contraindicated in patients who have had recent orbital trauma with hyphema or globe rupture. These procedures should be undertaken with caution in patients who have had ocular surgery within the last 6 months, recent orbital infection, significant inflammatory disease, or loss of corneal sensation.[7]

9.5 Issues Peculiar to Pediatric versus Adult Skull Base Surgery

Endoscopic skull base surgery in pediatrics deserves special attention due to the age and stages of craniofacial development of the patients. Preoperative planning is essential in both the pediatric and adult populations. The limited volume of the nasal cavity and under-pneumatized sphenoid sinus in younger children impairs the use of the four-handed endoscopic and microsurgical technique used for endoscopic endonasal approach (EEA) to skull base pathology. In addition, the intercarotid distance (ICD) has been shown to be significantly more narrow in the 2- to 4-year-old range and progressively widens with age as the sphenoid becomes pneumatized.[16] This pneumatization is usually completed by the age of 16 years. However, most pediatric patients are divided into the less-than - 11-year-old and the greater-than - 11-year-old categories when addressing the access of the EEA. A conchal sphenoid is associated with a narrow ICD and therefore should be strongly considered prior to EEA. An ICD of 10 mm is recommended prior to considering an EEA for intradural pathology.

The delayed pneumatization of the frontal sinus, however, expands the opportunities for the supraorbital keyhole craniotomy via an eyebrow incision as either a single approach or used as an operative and endoscopic port.

The volume of the nasal cavity in the pediatric patient is a significant concern when addressing complex and highly vascular lesions of the skull base. The smaller working area causes the "coning down" of instruments and more instrument "sword fighting" (▶ Fig. 9.11). This is most apparent as surgeons address clival and more lateral pathology. The pediatric population has a decreased blood volume as compared to an adult and therefore the minimization of blood loss is even more crucial, thereby raising the importance of a four-handed endoscopic and microsurgical technique. The dual-portal approach, TONES combined with an EEA, affords improved visualization and increased degrees of instrument working room when an endoscopic transsphenoidal or transclival approach is utilized.[17] While the utilization of this approach is too limited to quote outcome data, it has been studied in a simulated real-time adult cadaver vascular perfusion model. Utilizing a dual or multiportal approach may be considered to address these complex lesions.

The growth centers or suture lines along these portal pathways should be evaluated prior to surgery. The avoidance of suture line disruption should be considered. A medial TONES approach via a pre-or transcaruncular approach to the central skull base may be safer, as the surgeon remains below the frontoethmoidal suture. Similarly, the same approach to the subfrontal region can be achieved by staying above the frontoethmoidal suture. There are not enough outcome data at this time to further assist in the decision-making process; however, this may serve as a guide. Delaying surgery until the patient matures should be considered to avoid the risks of growth-plate disruption. However, this may not be feasible, given that most pathology needs to be addressed. There are potential advantages to adding a port, and therefore it should not be dismissed but rather considered carefully.

A special consideration in the pediatric population is the effect of surgery on the developing craniofacial skeleton. Specific to the maxillary sinus, the biggest risk is a hypoplastic maxillary sinus. This does not typically result in maxillary retrusion or maxillary deficiency as seen in certain craniofacial syndromes with midface deficiency (e.g., Crouzon's syndrome), but it may have long-term implications if the patient develops chronic sinusitis. Indeed, studies have shown that the most consistent factor to alter the maxillary sinus volume is prior Caldwell–Luc procedure.[18] However, many of the alternative surgical approach options for surgical targets in these regions incur even more morbidity, such as a

Le Fort I osteotomy or a craniotomy. Thus, despite the risk for decreased maxillary sinus volume, if it permits adequate access to a lesion that would otherwise require an approach with more morbidity, it should be strongly considered with adequate patient and patient-family counseling.

A child's ability to cooperate and follow guidance is also important postoperatively. Cases of children with hyperactivity disorders can at times make their care highly challenging.

9.6 Anatomy

The anatomy of the eyelids and their support structures dictates the location and geometry of the portals that are created for transorbital endoscopy; deeper anatomy of the orbital bone and adjacent orbital structures influences the pathways and optical chambers that are created.

The eyelids consist of skin, orbicularis oculi muscle, and, deep to that, the orbital septum. The septum is a continuation of the periosteum of the orbital rim. Deep to the septum is located the eyelid support system (▶ Fig. 9.1).

The primary support consists of the superior tarsus and inferior tarsus, the superior tarsus being supported by the levator muscle and aponeurosis, and the inferior tarsus being stabilized by the lower lid retractors. A critical difference between the upper and lower lids is that the lower lid retractors can be transected without deleterious effect, while the upper lid levator system must be preserved to prevent severe ptosis. As a result, we can perform a transconjunctival lower lid approach, but the upper lid approach must be transcutaneous. Also important in eyelid support are the medial canthus, which surrounds the lacrimal system, and the lateral canthus. The lateral canthus can be separated and detached from the orbital rim (canthotomy and cantholysis) as long as it is reconstructed at the end of the procedure. The medial canthal tendon cannot be transected without damage to the lacrimal system, and must therefore be preserved. The medial canthal tendon attaches to the anterior and posterior limbs of the lacrimal crest, enveloping the lacrimal sac. The lateral canthal tendon attaches 1 to 2 mm posterior to the anterior aspect of the orbital rim, inferior to the frontozygomatic suture.

For endoscopic surgery, the orbit is divided conceptually into superior, medial, inferior, and lateral quadrants by intervening structures that must be preserved. Each quadrant is entered through a unique portal (orbitotomy). The trochlea of the superior oblique muscle separates the superior from the medial quadrant; the insertion of the inferior oblique muscle demarcates the medial and inferior quadrants. The inferior and lateral quadrants are separated by the contents of the inferior fissure, while the superior fissure separates the lateral and the superior quadrants (▶ Fig. 9.1; ▶ Fig. 9.2).

Once the orbitotomy is created and the pathway is established, the subperiosteal dissection within the orbit can be widened to cross quadrants. This is not the case with all portals, however; the superior transcutaneous portal cannot be connected with the transconjunctival medial portal.

The key anatomic structures of the superior approach include the lacrimal gland laterally, and the trochlea medially. These structures can be elevated off the orbital bone in the subperiosteal plane. Dissecting posteriorly along the roof, there are no obstacles until the orbital apex is reached. Medially, the optic nerve is approached where it enters the orbit through the posterior medial wall. Laterally, the anterior aspect of the superior fissure is encountered.

For the medial dissection, key structures to be aware of include the posterior limb of the medial canthal tendon, which is visualized immediately deep to the incision. This structure is followed posteriorly to the posterior lacrimal crest, where the subperiosteal plane is entered. Dissecting posteriorly, the ethmoid arteries are encountered at the junction of the orbital roof and medial wall. These (typically three or more) are cauterized with bipolar forceps sequentially, dissecting posteriorly until the optic nerve is encountered.[19] The bone of the medial wall, the lamina papyracea, is extremely thin and must be handled delicately if it is to be preserved. Inadvertent fracture of the bone can cause minor bleeding from the underlying mucosa, which subsides spontaneously.

The inferior approach proceeds directly through the conjunctiva of the inferior fornix, through a small amount of fat, and then to the subperiosteal plane at the inferior orbital rim. Further posteriorly, the inferior fissure is located at the lateral floor. Some fibrous tissue, small vessels, and the zygomatic (sensory) nerve traverse the inferior fissure, and can be transected without notable deficits. The inferior fissure courses posteriorly and medially, where deep to the periosteum it joins the superior fissure (▶ Fig. 9.2).

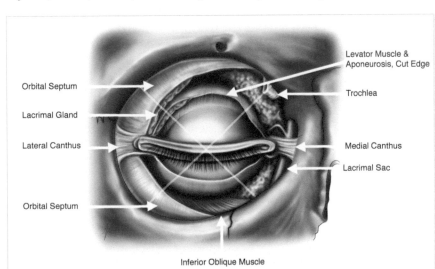

Orbital Septum
Lacrimal Gland
Lateral Canthus
Orbital Septum
Levator Muscle & Aponeurosis, Cut Edge
Trochlea
Medial Canthus
Lacrimal Sac
Inferior Oblique Muscle

Fig. 9.1 Orbital anatomy, skin and orbicularis muscle removed. Crossed lines demonstrate division of the orbit into four quadrants, each with a unique surgical approach.

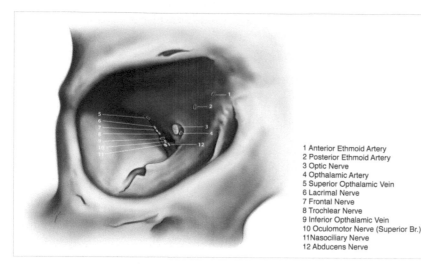

Fig. 9.2 Anatomy of the orbital bone and fissures. Note that the superior fissure contains multiple cranial nerves and must be protected, while the structures of the inferior fissure can be transected as needed.

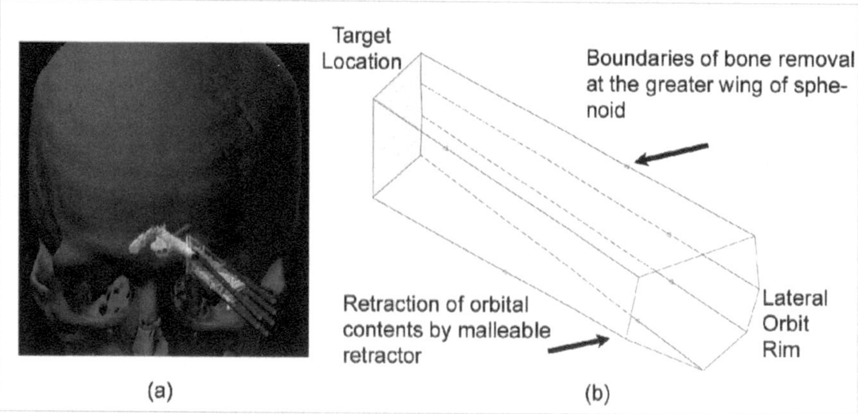

1 Anterior Ethmoid Artery
2 Posterior Ethmoid Artery
3 Optic Nerve
4 Opthalamic Artery
5 Superior Opthalamic Vein
6 Lacrimal Nerve
7 Frontal Nerve
8 Trochlear Nerve
9 Inferior Opthalamic Vein
10 Oculomotor Nerve (Superior Br.)
11 Nasociliary Nerve
12 Abducens Nerve

Target Location

Boundaries of bone removal at the greater wing of sphenoid

Retraction of orbital contents by malleable retractor

Lateral Orbit Rim

(a)　　　　(b)

Fig. 9.3 A surgical pathway to provide access to the lateral cavernous sinus through a lateral retrocanthal transorbital approach. Note this is a simplified pathway design with simply connecting an entrance polygon to a target polygon. The intersection of the pathway with the middle fossa is indicated and this represents the size of the craniotomy required (see ▶ Fig. 9.4). (Adapted from Bly et al.[13])

The lateral approach can be accessed through a retrocanthal transconjunctival portal, or a canthotomy and cantholysis can be added to the dissection. The subperiosteal plane is entered, and dissection continues posteriorly. In the anterior orbit, the dissection can be extended to the orbital roof or floor. More posteriorly, however, the fascia of the superior and inferior fissures become the boundaries of the dissection, converging to meet at the posterior orbit. As noted, the contents of the superior fissure must be preserved, while the structures of the inferior fissure can be cauterized and divided. Meticulous hemostasis in this region is critical.

9.7 Choice of Approach

Accurate surgical approach selection for access to skull base pathology is critical for successful outcomes. The approach (or approaches) dictates the incurred morbidity and collateral tissue damage, and the ability to perform the surgical task required at the target site, whether that be obtaining a tissue sample for biopsy or complete resection and reconstruction. The optimal surgical approach maximizes visualization and instrumentation at the target site, yet minimizes collateral tissue damage. As mentioned earlier, the term "minimally invasive" is a misnomer as the degree of "invasive" is determined by the pathology, and it is our job to determine an approach that offers adequate access to pathology while minimizing damage to collateral tissue in the process. We promote the term "minimally disruptive."

In an ideal case, the surgical pathway is direct, short, and has geometric boundaries that are just large enough to permit adequate instrumentation. Depending on the surgical task, fundamental minimum dimensions of the surgical pathway are required. For example, if endoscopic visualization with a 4-mm endoscope, plus one instrument (pituitary forceps) is required to perform a biopsy at a skull base location, then the initial surgical pathway shape must meet the minimum dimensions to permit the 4-mm-diameter endoscope working in concert with pituitary forceps. In this instance, the dimension at the midpoint (center of instrument angulation) must be 9 mm in the typical biconical shape (4-mm diameter of endoscope + 4-mm diameter of pituitary forceps + 1-mm clearance). The biconical shape is hypothesized to be the ideal endoscopic surgical pathway because it permits adequate instrument angulation. This was demonstrated in an engineering optimization study gaining access to the lateral cavernous sinus through a lateral retrocanthal approach. Prior to iterative computer analysis, the proposed surgical pathway was the same width throughout the length, but with computer planning and dimension optimization at the center point of instrument angulation, the volume of the pathway reduced by 27% without compromising visualization and instrumentation at the target site. The size of the craniotomy in the MCF (middle cranial fossa) was also reduced by 48%, and thus the collateral tissue damage was reduced (▶ Fig. 9.3; ▶ Fig. 9.4).[13]

In addition to instrument range of motion within the pathway, the angle of approach to a given pathology significantly

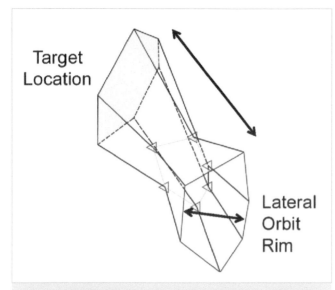

Target Location

Lateral Orbit Rim

Fig. 9.4 A surgical pathway to the lateral cavernous sinus, now after iterative computer planning to optimize the shape. The biconical configuration does not affect instrumentation at the target site, yet permits a significant reduction in the size of the craniotomy at the greater wing of the sphenoid compared to initial pathway design seen in ► Fig. 9.3. (Adapted from Bly et al.[13])

impacts the ability to safely perform surgical tasks at the target site. Indeed, with greater than 20 endoscopic surgical approaches described through the craniofacial skeleton to access the skull base, there is a wide range of approach angles available to the surgeon. One specific example where approach angle becomes critical is in the region of the optic canal. In this instance, dissection from a perspective that is near parallel to the nerve has distinct advantages over an approach that is near-perpendicular. A near-parallel approach offers the surgeon an optimal endoscopic view to remove thinned bone along the optic nerve because the nerve is visualized along its length during bone removal. Thus, selecting the surgical approach angle may have a high priority for addressing specific pathology, and it may be that a surgical pathway that is longer, but has a better approach angle, provides the best overall access.

In the multiportal approach, the angle of the two (or more) portals relative to each other is important. These angles determine how two or more instruments will work in concert, and it determines the viewing angle. In endoscopic sinus surgery, it is routine that a single instrument works through the same portal as endoscope, and the two are nearly parallel. These are advantageous in the ability to instrument at the target site when the angulation is widened. It allows for reproduction of standard microsurgical techniques where multiple instruments are working in concert providing retraction and maintaining tension on the tissue that is being dissected or divided. Current surgical robotic platforms have limitations on the angle, and most require at least 20° between them to work effectively without collision.

Finally, a major factor to consider in the selection of a surgical approach is the degree of instrumentation required at the target site, and the number of simultaneous instruments required in addition to an endoscope. In the literature, the optimal endoscopic skull base surgery is done in a "four-handed" technique with two surgeons working together, each with two instruments.

Perhaps a more accurate determination to make is not the number of instruments or hands required, but rather the number of functions needed, such as ablation, irrigation, suction, cautery, and navigation. The number of functions is a more relevant number because an increase in the functions may not result in an increase in the number of surgical portals. It is acceptable, and in fact better if the same surgical effect can be achieved with fewer instruments. Many advanced instruments now have multiple functions. For example, an ultrasonic bone aspirator provides multiple functions, including ablation, irrigation, and suction. A Coblator provides suction, irrigation, and radiofrequency ablation and hemostasis. As technology emerges that continues to combine functions, it may reduce the need for either additional surgical pathways or wider dimensions for any given pathway.

The selection of a pathway requires many considerations, including visualization, instrumentation, pathology type and location, and individual anatomy, but selected pathways should be as close to ideal as possible in order to maximize the surgical effect while minimizing collateral tissue damage.

9.8 Transorbital Approaches

The approach is determined by the quadrant of the orbit that is occupied by the pathology or that the path to the pathology will traverse (► Fig. 9.5).

Once the quadrant of the orbit is noted that involves or provides access to the pathology, the type of incision to enter that quadrant is decided upon. While there are some variations in the exact placement of the incision, the primary incisions and access techniques used for each quadrant will be described below.

Before making the incision, the patient is given appropriate antibiotics and, unless contraindicated, 8 to 10 mg of dexamethasone. The size and shape of the pupils at the beginning of the case is noted. If desired, exophthalmometry can be performed with the patient asleep to aid in deciding on reconstructive options at the end of the procedure. A temporary tarsorrhaphy is typically placed at the lateral limbus bilaterally, allowing the lids to be opened to monitor the shape and size of the pupils. Ophthalmic lubricant is placed and maintained throughout the case. During the operation, the ipsilateral pupil is regularly checked for any change in shape or size, either of which can indicate excessive pressure on the globe or other orbital contents. This is particularly important when dissecting behind the equator of the globe toward the orbital apex. If this occurs, retractors and instruments are removed from the globe until the pupils become symmetric. While a corneal protector may give the surgeon added comfort, if one is used it needs to be removed frequently to check the pupils.

Retraction of the orbital contents is performed with malleable brain retractors. Care is taken not to angle the distal end of the retractor into the orbital contents, but rather to gently distract the contents with even pressure along the retractor. A thin sheet of Silastic can be placed between the orbital contents and retractor to aid in both retraction and maintaining a patent optical cavity.

9.8.1 Superior Quadrant

The superior quadrant lies between the lacrimal gland laterally and the trochlea of the superior oblique muscle medially. A

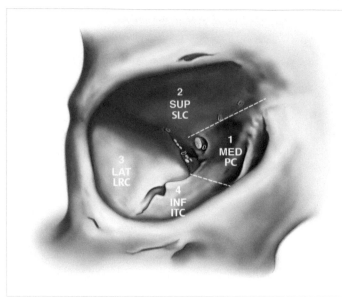

Fig. 9.5 Region of the orbit that is accessed by each approach. PC, precaruncular; SLC, superior lid crease; LRC, lateral retrocanthal; ITC, inferior transconjunctival.

2 SUP SLC

1 MED PC

3 LAT LRC

4 INF ITC

1 Medial wall
2 Orbital roof
3 Lateral wall
4 Floor

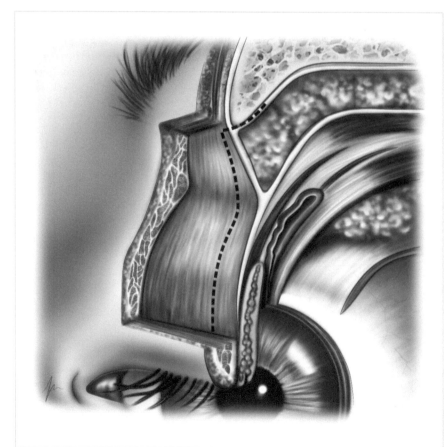

Fig. 9.6 Superior lid crease approach. Skin and orbicularis muscle removed. Arrow shows dissection superficial to orbital septum, and thence to the superior orbit.

transcutaneous blepharoplasty incision is used for this approach (▶ Fig. 9.6), placed in a dominant crease of the upper eyelid skin. The incision is typically 3 to 4 cm wide, and extends through the orbicularis oculi muscle. Dissection continues toward the superior orbital rim following the undersurface of the muscle, superficial to the orbital septum. This plane lies superficial to the prelevator fat. Once the orbital rim is encountered, the supraorbital and supratrochlear neurovascular bundles are located and preserved. In some cases, these run through a palpable notch in the orbital rim which can aid in their location. The periosteum of the superior orbital rim is then incised and lifted off the bone with a periosteal elevator, creating a plane into which the orbit is entered inferior to the bone of the orbital roof and superior to the orbital periosteum (periorbital). The plane is developed posteriorly to a depth of approximately 1 cm, at which time a 0-degree endoscope is introduced and dissection continues under endoscopic visualization. A suction Freer elevator is useful for the dissection that, though largely bloodless, is helpful when a small amount of bleeding is encountered. Any blood vessels extending through the periorbital into the bone can be ligated with bipolar cautery. Dissection then continues, exposing the region of the orbit or adjacent orbital roof that is needed. If a craniotomy is performed for transorbital access to the frontal lobe, this is done with a diamond burr or ultrasonic bone aspirator. If entry into the frontal sinus is desired, the entry point is determined by navigation guidance, and the bone is taken down in a similar fashion. If dissection to the orbital apex is required, as the posterior limit of the orbital roof is encountered, navigation is checked to ascertain the exact position of the optic nerve and superior orbital fissure, both of which are bounded by periosteum. If access to the brain is desired, the position of the dural opening is confirmed by navigation, and the incision in the dura is made in standard fashion. Once the procedure is completed, the reconstruction is completed as noted below.

9.8.2 Medial Quadrant

The medial quadrant of the orbit extends from the trochlea of the superior oblique muscle to the origin of the inferior oblique muscle (▶ Fig. 9.1). These structures are located on the orbital side of the periosteum, and are not seen during the dissection unless intentionally sought. The medial orbit is opened using a precaruncular transconjunctival approach (▶ Fig. 9.7).[1,20] This approach is created posterior to the lacrimal canaliculi and sac. Until the approach is mastered, it may be helpful to place lacrimal probes in the canaliculi and tape them to the adjacent skin

until the dissection is well within the orbit. It is critical not to use monopolar cautery adjacent to the canaliculi to prevent stenosis.

A small, sharp scissor is used to incise the conjunctiva medial to the caruncle. The incision is extended superiorly as needed, taking care not to damage the levator aponeurosis. Dissection continues inferiorly as far as desired, extending the incision into the fornix of the lower eyelid if needed. It is important to place the incision at least 3 mm inferior to the lower eyelid tarsus if the approach is extended, to prevent postoperative lid retraction.

Once the plane between the caruncle the medial canthus is opened, the caruncle is retracted laterally with a forceps and dissection continues toward the posterior lacrimal crest, on the deep side of the medial canthal tendon (the Horner muscle). When the posterior lacrimal crest is reached, the periosteum of the lamina papyracea posterior to this can be sharply incised, and the plane between the lamina and the periosteum is entered with endoscopic visualization. Dissection continues using a Freer elevator in the planned surgical route. At the superior aspect of the exposure, the ethmoid arteries are located and transected with bipolar cautery. It is important to realize that more often than not there are three or more ethmoid arteries[19] located at the junction of the lamina and the skull base, and by projecting the plane of these vessels posteriorly, the location of the optic nerve can be determined. Dissecting posteriorly, the curvature of the medial orbit becomes more pronounced as the location of the optic nerve at the posterior superior aspect of the medial orbital wall is approached. Navigation is used to confirm location of the nerve as this region is approached.

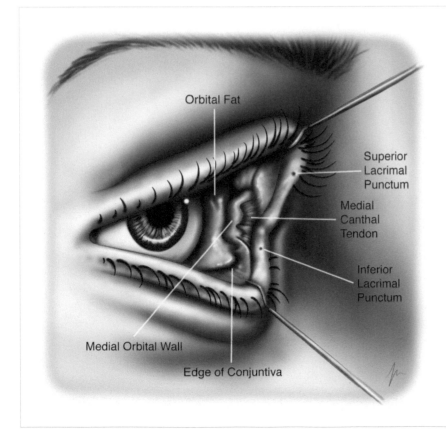

Fig. 9.7 Precaruncular approach. Note the pathway follows the posterior limb of the medial canthal tendon to lamina papyracea.

Orbital Fat

Superior Lacrimal Punctum

Medial Canthal Tendon

Inferior Lacrimal Punctum

Medial Orbital Wall

Edge of Conjuntiva

Depending on the goal of the surgery, the lamina papyracea may be partially or completely removed. This can be done as noted for the superior quadrant approach. Bleeding will be encountered if the sinus mucosa is disturbed on the deep side of the bone. Once the goal of the procedure has been fulfilled, bone that has been removed from the medial wall of the orbit is reconstructed as noted below.

9.8.3 Inferior Quadrant

The inferior quadrant extends from the origin of the inferior oblique on the periosteum of the medial floor of the orbit laterally to the junction of the floor with the lateral wall (▶ Fig. 9.1; ▶ Fig. 9.5). The portal to this quadrant can be transcutaneous through the skin and muscle of the lower eyelid, or transconjunctival through a preseptal or inferior fornix incision. We prefer the transconjunctival inferior fornix result because it is scarless, provides direct access to the inferior orbital rim, and can be extended contiguously into the transconjunctival precaruncular or lateral retrocanthal approaches (▶ Fig. 9.8).[1] A canthotomy and cantholysis can also be performed to allow increased lower eyelid retraction if desired.

A lubricated corneal protector can be used as desired. The incision is made 3 to 4 mm inferior to the tarsus using a number 15 scalpel, or needle-tip monopolar cautery on low power, taking care to maintain a safe distance from the lacrimal system as noted earlier. Dissection continues directly through the orbital fat onto the inferior orbital rim. A malleable retractor is used to protect the orbital contents, and a small retractor is used to distend the lower eyelid. The periosteum of the inferior orbital rim is then incised and raised, dissecting posteriorly onto the orbital floor. Once several millimeters of periosteum have been elevated, the dissection continues posteriorly under endoscopic guidance using a suction Freer elevator. The dissection contin-

ues laterally and posteriorly until the fibrovascular contents of the inferior orbital fissure are encountered. If access to the bone of the lateral wall is required, or if the inferior fissure is involved with the pathology, it is cauterized with some bipolar forceps and divided. The canal of the infraorbital nerve can often be seen in the bone of the orbital floor, and posteriorly the nerve may become dehiscent within the orbit on its course from the foramen rotundum. The nerve can be dissected to access and open foramen rotundum as needed, for example, in following tumor metastases within the nerve. The periosteum is elevated from the orbital floor as needed, and any necessary bone resection from the floor can be performed with a drill or ultrasonic bone aspirator. The optic nerve, entering the orbit high on the posterior aspect of the medial wall, is generally not at risk during this dissection. However, excessive retraction in the posterior orbit can cause venous congestion, and pupil response should be closely monitored when operating in this region.

9.8.4 Lateral Quadrant

The lateral quadrant of the orbit extends from the lacrimal gland superiorly to the orbital floor inferiorly (▶ Fig. 9.1). We generally prefer to access the region from a lateral retrocanthal transconjunctival approach (▶ Fig. 9.9).[1,21] This can be extended superiorly, or inferiorly into an inferior fornix incision as needed. For added room, a canthotomy and cantholysis can also be performed as needed. The periosteum of the lateral wall is incised, the subperiosteal plane is developed, and endoscopic dissection continues toward the orbital apex. As noted earlier, the contents of the inferior fissure can be cauterized and divided if the orbital floor is to be included into the pathway. To access the infratemporal fossa, the bone of the lateral wall is removed beginning posterior to the orbital rim. Dissecting

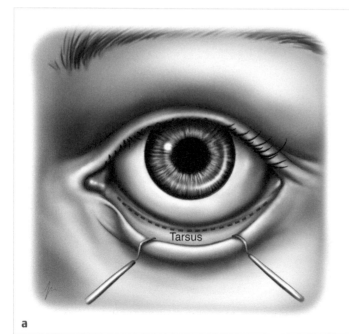

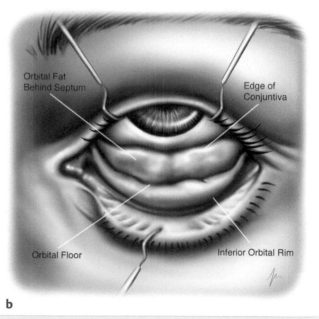

a   b

Fig. 9.8 Inferior transconjunctival approach. **(a)** Incision, at least 3 mm inferior to tarsus. **(b)** Bone of inferior rim exposed prior to entering orbit.

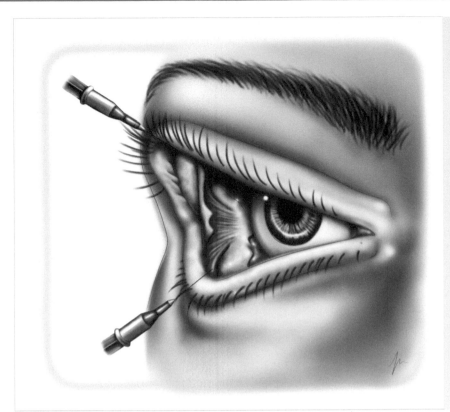

Fig. 9.9 Lateral retrocanthal approach. The conjunctival incision is placed posterior to the attachment of the lateral canthal tendon.

further posteriorly within the orbit, the approach is narrowed by the confluence of the superior and inferior orbital fissures (▶ Fig. 9.5). While the inferior fissure can be transected as noted earlier without functional compromise, this is not the case with the superior orbital fissure due to the course of components of the third, fourth, fifth, and sixth cranial nerves that pass through. The periosteum adherent to these structures at the fissure generally protects the contents from inadvertent transection. A pathway to the Meckel cave and lateral aspect of the cavernous sinus can be developed dissecting lateral to the superior orbital fissure through the greater wing of the sphenoid bone to reach the dura of the MCF.[1,13] For cases with an extensive lateral recess of the sphenoid sinus, the sphenoid sinus can also be reached through this lateral approach to treat, for example, meningoceles or other CSF leaks. The bone of the greater wing of the sphenoid can be resected as needed to access the temporal lobe of the brain or floor of the MCF.

9.9 Reconstruction of Transorbital Approaches and Postoperative Care

In general, we do not close the transconjunctival incisions at the end of the procedure; they heal well without suturing, and this allows ready egress for any residual bleeding that may occur. If a precaruncular incision is used and the caruncle does not readily return to its original position due to swelling, a single resorbable 6–0 suture is placed at the apex of the medial canthus. Cutaneous incisions are closed in a two-layer fashion with 5–0 resorbable sutures through the orbicularis oculi muscle, and 6–0 resorbable or permanent sutures through the skin. If a superior quadrant approach is undertaken and there is a CSF leak, a watertight running permanent suture is used and left in place for 7 days.

The decision whether or not to reconstruct the orbital bone depends on the location and amount, if any, of bone that was removed during the procedure. We routinely perform exophthalmometry at the beginning and end of the procedure. Two to 3 mm of proptosis is expected from the procedure due to edema in a typical procedure lasting 2 to 3 hours. For longer procedures, or if the dissection is more extensive than usual, a small degree of additional proptosis may occur. When possible, we prefer to use "preconstruction before deconstruction" of bone defects. At the beginning of the procedure when the bone has been exposed, as long as it is not obscured by tumor, we place the reconstruction material and "preconstruct" it to conform exactly to the native contouring before the bone is removed. We then remove the implant and replace it at the end of the case. If the orbital bone is already absent or involved with the disease process, "preconstruction" is not possible, and we use computer-guided mirror-image overlay of the contralateral orbit as a template for implant placement and in situ shaping at the end of the procedure.[22]

Except in unusual cases of complete removal, reconstruction of the bone of the orbital roof is unnecessary; the periorbita will seal against the bone margins and dura. The patient may have pulsatile exophthalmos in the immediate postoperative period, but this typically resolves within 1 to 2 weeks after surgery. This is also true when the frontal sinus is opened. If there is concern for herniation of orbital contents into the frontal sinus, particularly in the region of the frontal outflow tract, or if there is herniation of orbital fat, we place a resorbable layer of

0.25-mm-thick polydioxanone foil to maintain anatomic partitioning. If dura is resected, small defects can be reconstructed with allogenic dermis or other dural substitutes when the periorbital is intact. For larger dural defects, particularly if orbital exenteration has been performed, we recommend reconstruction with a layer of vascularized tissue. Pericranium is excellent for this, and it can be harvested endoscopically, pedicled laterally, and delivered over the superior orbital rim into the dural defect.

Reconstruction of the lateral orbital wall depends on the extent of bone removal. If much of the greater wing of the sphenoid is removed, failure to replace the volume will lead to postoperative enophthalmos. This can be analyzed by exophthalmometry at the end of the procedure as noted earlier. In the case of a small bone defect, we often place a layer of thin polydioxanone foil to prevent herniation of the lateral rectus muscle into the defect. This is particularly true if the lateral rectus muscle is exposed during the dissection and tethering of the muscle to the bone of the lateral wall is a risk. Polydioxanone provides an excellent glide layer during healing. If reconstruction is desired for volumetric indications, a fat graft can be used with the expectation of partial resorption of the graft postoperatively. We generally fill the bone defect with fat and then line the lateral wall with polydioxanone foil.

Reconstruction of the bone of the medial wall and floor of the orbit is more critical. For small defects of the medial wall,

we typically use thin polydioxanone to prevent herniation or adherence of the medial rectus muscle. If a larger bone defect is present, we prefer to use a preformed thin titanium mesh orbital implant, bending the implant in situ to conform to the patient's anatomy. We line this with thin polydioxanone foil to prevent adherence of orbital contents. The same is true for orbital floor defects; the majority of these are reconstructed with titanium mesh implants and the implant is shaped in situ. If preconstruction was not possible, we perform mirror-image overlay of the contralateral orbit onto the ipsilateral CT scan (▶ Fig. 9.10), using navigation software as previously described.[22] Preoperatively, the navigation CT scan is uploaded and prepared for standard navigation. The scan is then reimported in reversed, mirror-image position. The image is segmented, colored, and fused with the standard CT so that a template of the opposite (normal) side is placed over the anatomically altered orbit. The implant is then positioned at the end of the case, and its position is checked against the template by navigating over the bone contours under endoscopic visualization. The implant is then adjusted in situ to conform to the surgical plan. We then perform exophthalmometry as a confirmation of the expected globe position.

Postoperatively, the visual acuity and pupils are checked to confirm baseline function. Lubricating ointment is used twice daily for the first week after surgery. A light ice pack or iced saline sponge is applied 20 minutes per hour while awake for the

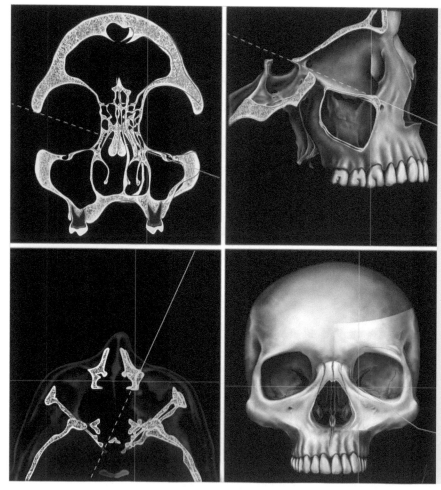

Fig. 9.10 Computer planning in orbital reconstruction. The CT of the contralateral (normal) orbit is colored green, mirrored, and superimposed on the abnormal orbit CT. This creates a reconstruction template. After placement of the implant, the construct is navigated and adjusted in position and shape to conform to the template.

first 48 hours after surgery. If significant edema is expected, intravenous steroid can be used for 24 to 48 hours after surgery, and the temporary tarsorrhaphy stitch can be left in place for several days.

With any orbital surgery, it is important to warn the patient regarding symptoms of retrobulbar hematoma (increased retrobulbar pain, proptosis, visual loss) and the need for emergent canthotomy and cantholysis should this rare event occur. We have not had this occur with transorbital endoscopic procedures, probably due to the excellent ability to visualize and treat any areas of bleeding. The primary regions where bleeding tends to occur are the inferior orbital fissure and the ethmoid arteries if bipolar cautery is not used when dividing these structures.[23]

9.10 Multiportal Surgery

9.10.1 Logic and Rationale

Multiportal skull base surgery affords surgeons the opportunity to optimize the visualization gained by endoscopy while performing two-handed microsurgical dissection. The optimal direct pathway to a lesion and its main vascular supply are determined by its site of origin and preoperative imaging characteristics. Preoperative planning is the key to successful resection and reconstruction of complex lesions involving the skull base. Complimentary studies such as MRI with and without contrast and CT angiogram identify both the important soft-tissue bone involvement and vascular supply. The use of 3D stereotactic navigation is valuable both preoperatively and intraoperatively. Vascular lesions, highly vascular tumors, and large lesions involving multiple compartments are those in which a multiportal technique should be considered. The risks and benefits of each port selected need to be assessed carefully, given each have their potential benefits and risks. These ports can be utilized interchangeably by the endoscope and instruments to optimize visualization and microsurgical dissection.

9.10.2 Combinations Utilized

The bi-nares endoscopic ports, EEA, are the "work horse" for central and anterior endoscopic skull base surgeries. The complementary ports include the transorbital (or TONES approaches), caldwell–Luc (maxillary antrostomy) and supraorbital craniotomy. These ports maybe utilized for complex pathology involving the sellar, parasellar, cavernous sinus, clivus, middle fossa, infratemporal fossa, pterygopalatine fossa, and petrous apex regions.

In two recent publications, we demonstrated that optimal aneurysm clip application and visualization of the cavernous carotid artery and vessels of the posterior circulation are achieved when the TONES port was added to the endoscopic endonasal transsphenoidal or transclival approach, respectively. The addition of the TONES port minimized the risk of passpointing of the clip tines beyond the vessel being clipped. In the case of the transclival approach and clipping of the posterior circulation vessels in a real-time cadaveric bleeding simulation model, this dual-portal approach minimized incorporating the brainstem tissue in the clip tines when the TONES port was added. On the other hand, the endoscopic transclival approach alone is a more inline view of the clip tines decreasing the perspective of the clip tines to the vessel being clipped and the brainstem. Pass pointing was more common using this approach. The use of angled endoscopes (30° and 45°) improved the perspective of the clip tines, yet the working area was significantly more limited when the EEA to the cavernous sinus and the transclival approach to the posterior circulation was utilized alone. The addition of TONES to the EEA improved the degrees of working freedom and visualization by minimizing the "coning down effect" and the "sword fighting" between the endoscope and instruments. ▶ Fig. 9.11 and ▶ Fig. 9.12 illustrate the advantages of utilizing a dual transsphenoidal or transclival and precaruncular transorbital approaches to address complex pathology of these regions. The dual approach and four-handed technique provided improved working area, degrees of freedom and accurate clip placement.[17]

Another port to consider utilizing is the supraorbital port. The supra orbital port is created via an eyebrow incision and a keyhole supraorbital craniotomy.[24] Dr. Axel Perneczky popularized this approach to address neoplasms and aneurysms. When modified and utilized as a port, it provides improved visualization and access of instrumentation to the suprasellar, parasellar and subfrontal regions when combined with the EEA.[2]

The Caldwell–Luc (maxillary antrostomy) approach has been beneficial in addressing lesions of the infratemporal and

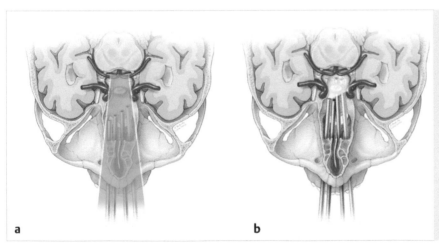

Fig. 9.11 Schematic showing the endoscopic transclival approach alone is limited by **(a)** coning down effect and **(b)** instrument sword fighting.

a   b

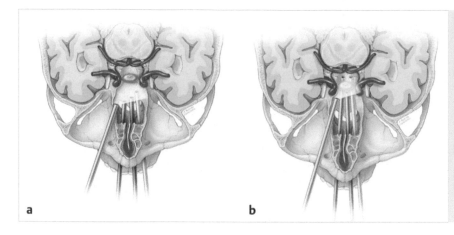

Fig. 9.12 Schematics showing that the right transorbital view of the combined endoscopic multiportal transorbital and endonasal approaches increases (a) visualization and (b) working area for instrumentation.

pterygopalatine fossae. This port is utilized for tumor resection as well as visualization and obtaining improved vascular control of the sphenopalatine vessels. Endovascular embolization of the sphenopalatine vessels is recommended prior to the resection of lesions. However, significant bleeding may still occur and this additional port has low morbidity and had been commonly used for sinus surgery for decades prior to its utilization as a port for endoscopic skull base surgery. Given the laterality of lesions extending into or from infratemporal and pterygopalatine fossae, the Caldwell–Luc port when combined with an EEA allows both the visualization and instrumentation access needed to safely resect these lesions, thereby, in many cases, obviating the need for the more potentially disfiguring open approaches.

9.11 Outcomes and Complications

We described our early outcomes with transorbital endoscopic procedures,[15] and our more recent results performing transorbital endoscopic skull base lesions.[8] This demonstrated that transorbital approaches are safe and allow rapid recovery. The experience of others has been similar.[9,10]

Our experience with pediatric applications of these procedures has mirrored our adult experience; we have had no complications due to the surgical approach, and none of our procedures required conversion to an open approach due to endoscopic failure. In particular, we have had no instances of visual loss, persistent diplopia or ptosis, corneal damage, or globe malposition after these procedures. The following discussion presents several unique applications of these procedures, as well as challenges that have been encountered with their use.

9.11.1 Case 1

A 13-year-old girl developed epiphora and nasal congestion for which she was treated with allergy medicine. She eventually developed hypertropia and received a CT scan, shown in ▶ Fig. 9.13. She was referred for evaluation and a transnasal biopsy demonstrated esthesioneuroblastoma, Kadish stage C. A navigation-guided multiportal approach was undertaken. The procedure began with an extended medial, inferior, and lateral quadrant transorbital approach (a single transconjunctival

incision) for examination of the frontal lobe dura and orbital contents. Surveillance of the dura demonstrated that it was not involved with tumor (▶ Fig. 9.13d). Tumor was then excised from the orbit. A sublabial approach was used for a transmaxillary approach, and a transnasal approach was also undertaken to resect the remaining tumor from the nose. Her surgical margins were negative. Reconstruction was performed with porous polyethylene-covered titanium mesh. Postoperatively she had no diplopia, but had epiphora as expected, given resection of her lacrimal sac. She was noted to have mild enophthalmos. She underwent proton radiation and chemotherapy.

Two years later, she developed progressive enophthalmos and an implant infection. Three years later, the implant began to extrude and was replaced. Still free of disease 9 years postoperatively (▶ Fig. 9.13), she again developed partial extrusion of the implant, which was treated by trimming and closure of the defect with adjacent tissue. She also had progressive enophthalmos, despite symmetric implant position, and diffuse soft-tissue retraction in the area with lower lid retraction.

This case illustrates several important points. The triportal surgical access allowed excellent visualization and access to the surgical field. Because we were able to ascertain the status of the dura at the beginning of the operation, we could operate outward from the brain, ensuring its safety. Likewise, we could determine that the orbital contents were not invaded with tumor, and operated from the orbital contents outward into the nasal cavity and maxilla. Triportal surgery allowed us to have clear visualization and instrumentation from various trajectories.

Her postoperative recovery was rapid, and despite the extent of her surgery and adjuvant treatment, she did well for several years. She then developed an infection of her polyethylene implant as well as progressive enophthalmos, forcing removal and replacement of the implant. We have encountered a number of similar infections of this type of implant, and thus now use only thin titanium mesh with a liner of polydioxanone. This has decreased our implant infection rate. She also developed progressive loss of volume of the orbital contents, most likely due to atrophy and scarring of the orbital and periorbital soft tissue from the proton radiation. While these complications would most likely have risen with any surgical approach given the extent of the tumor, they represent significant long-term issues that arise in the management of pediatric patients who undergo multimodality therapy.

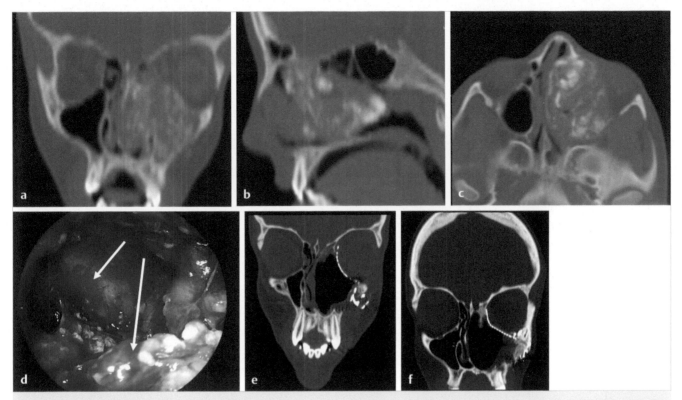

Fig. 9.13 Case 1. **(a–c)** Preoperative coronal, sagittal, and axial CT scans. **(d)** Intraoperative view inspecting dura through L orbit. **(e)** Postoperative CT scan demonstrating reconstructed orbit. **(f)** CT 9 years later after replacement of orbital implant.

9.11.2 Case 2

This 10-year-old boy presented with a history of worsening nasal obstruction and decreased sense of smell and taste, and worsening vision. He was undergoing orthognathic surgery, when his family inquired about changes in the position of his left eye and worsening facial asymmetry. Imaging was obtained and a large mass was noted disrupting his maxilla, invading the orbit and infratemporal fossa on the left. High on the initial diagnosis was JNA. Complete imaging was obtained, and angiography with selective embolization was performed. A multiportal transnasal, transmaxillary, infratemporal fossa, and transorbital procedure was planned. The tumor resection went very well, and because it was fairly soft, the majority of it could be removed from the three inferior portals without a transorbital approach. Frozen section diagnosis was consistent with JNA. At the conclusion of the procedure while still on the operating table Hertel's exophthalmometry demonstrated that the left globe was 2-mm proptotic relative to the normal side, having been 3 mm proptotic before resection of the mass. Given that the orbital volume was largely unchanged and the periorbita had been preserved intact, the decision was made not to reconstruct the orbital bone that had been destroyed by the tumor. The final pathologic diagnosis was schwannoma. Postoperative CT scan demonstrated complete tumor resection. His recovery was uneventful; on outpatient visit 5 days after surgery, his vision was subjectively improving before he returned to his home state and the care of his referring surgeon where he has continued to do well. We will follow the position of his globe and the orbital volume as his face continues to grow (▶ Fig. 9.14).

9.11.3 Case 3

A 15-year-old adolescent boy with a history of amblyopia and visual acuity of 20/400 presented with orbital cellulitis. Imaging demonstrated a large osteoma extending from the skull base superiorly into the left frontal lobe, and inferiorly into the left frontal sinus and orbit, extending between the superior oblique and medial rectus muscles. He had no history of sinus symptoms or facial pain. He was referred for excision.

He underwent a biportal approach to the mass. A left superior quadrant transorbital approach was undertaken through a blepharoplasty incision, and dissection continued posteriorly around the orbital component of the osteoma. The mass was amputated at the floor of the frontal sinus and orbital roof using an ultrasonic bone aspirator and removed. A transorbital frontal sinusotomy was performed, removing the bone adjacent to the osteoma. The osteoma was then resected in a similar fashion leaving the intradural component intact, removing all the tumor in the frontal sinus and skull base, taking down the intersinus septum. A left transnasal frontal sinusotomy was performed. The tumor extending into the frontal lobe of the brain was then dissected free and removed. The frontal lobe dura was reconstructed with inlay and onlay technique using allogenic dermis. The frontal sinus was filled with fibrin sealant. The orbital roof was reconstructed with a thin layer of polydioxanone foil. Postoperatively, he did well. His vision returned to baseline, and he had normal globe and eyelid position (▶ Fig. 9.15).

We have not yet followed small children for a period long enough to rule out the possibility of any future craniofacial growth disturbances due to conservative resection of orbital

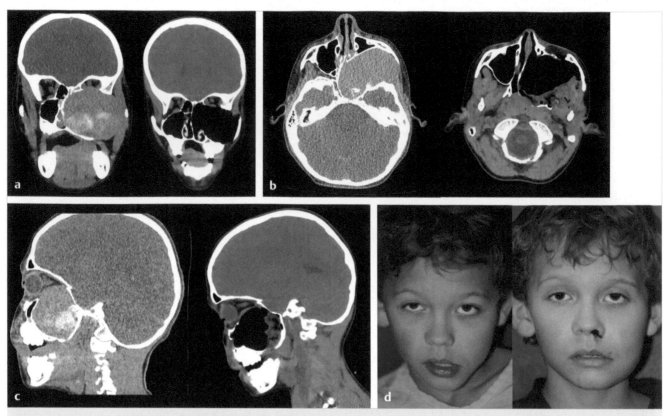

Fig. 9.14 Case 2. (a) Coronal CT pre- and postoperative. (b) Axial CT pre- and postoperative. (c) Sagittal CT pre- and postoperative. (d) Photograph of facial appearance preoperative and 5 days after surgery.

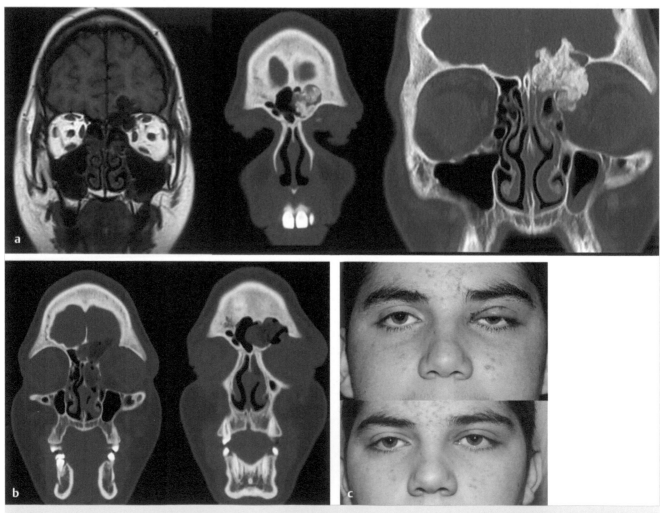

Fig. 9.15 (a) Preoperative coronal MRI and CT scans. Note invasion of osteoma into frontal lobe of brain. (b) Postoperative coronal CT scans. (c) Photographs 5 and 21 days after surgery.

bone. However, given the location of the pathology and the extensive nature of the alternative surgical approaches, we believe that the use of these minimally disruptive transorbital pathways is justified. Our experience with transorbital and multiportal approaches, including transnasal, transmaxillary, and infratemporal fossa portals provides excellent visualization, as well as superior dimensions and angles for safe and successful treatment of skull base pathology.

9.12 Future Directions

As flexible, digital, and 3D endoscopy develop, dual- and multiportal endoscopic techniques to the skull base will become more widely utilized. Multiportal approaches to the skull base have expanded our capabilities when addressing complex pathology of these regions. The improved degrees of instrument working room and visualization gained from the endoscopic multiportal approaches expand the role of endoscopic endonasal clipping of cerebral aneurysms. Likewise, the lateral TONES approach to the supraorbital fissure expands the role of resecting temporal lobe lesions.

Skull base surgery has a rich multidisciplinary history. The collaborative efforts between neurosurgeons, otorhinolaryngologists, oculoplastic, and plastic surgeons will lead to further innovations.

References

[1] Moe KS, Bergeron CM, Ellenbogen RG. Transorbital neuroendoscopic surgery. Neurosurgery. 2010; 67(3) Suppl operative:16–28

[2] Ciporen JN, Moe KS, Ramanathan D, et al. Multiportal endoscopic approaches to the central skull base: a cadaveric study. World Neurosurg. 2010; 73(6): 705–712

[3] Bly RA, Su D, Hannaford B, Ferreira M, Jr, Moe KS. Computer modeled multiportal approaches to the skull base. J Neurol Surg B Skull Base. 2012; 73(6) B6:415–423

[4] Bly RA, Su D, Lendvay TS, et al. Multiportal robotic access to the anterior cranial fossa: a surgical and engineering feasibility study. Otolaryngol Head Neck Surg. 2013; 149(6):940–946

[5] Alqahtani A, Padoan G, Segnini G, et al. Transorbital transnasal endoscopic combined approach to the anterior and middle skull base: a laboratory investigation. Acta Otorhinolaryngol Ital. 2015; 35(3):173–179

[6] Moe KS, Ellenbogen RG. Transorbital neuroendoscopic approaches to the middle cranial fossa. In: Snyderman C, Gardner P, eds. Master Techniques in Otolaryngology: Head and Neck Surgery—Skull Base Surgery. Philadelphia, PA: Wolters Kluwer; 2014

[7] Ellenbogen RG, Moe KS. Transorbital Neuroendoscopic Approaches to the Anterior Cranial Fossa. In: Snyderman C, Gardner P, eds. Master Techniques in Otolaryngology: Head and Neck Surgery—Skull Base Surgery. Philadelphia, PA: Wolters Kluwer, 2014

[8] Ramakrishna R, Kim LJ, Bly RA, Moe K, Ferreira M, Jr. Transorbital neuroendoscopic surgery for the treatment of skull base lesions. J Clin Neurosci. 2016; 24:99–104

[9] Dallan I, Castelnuovo P, Locatelli D, et al. Multiportal combined transorbital transnasal endoscopic approach for the management of selected skull base lesions: preliminary experience. World Neurosurg. 2015; 84(1):97–107

[10] Lubbe D, Mustak H, Taylor A, Fagan J. Minimally invasive endo-orbital approach to sphenoid wing meningiomas improves visual outcomes - our experience with the first seven cases. Clin Otolaryngol. 2017; 42(4): 876–880

[11] Lim JH, Sardesai MG, Ferreira M, Jr, Moe KS. Transorbital neuroendoscopic management of sinogenic complications involving the frontal sinus, orbit, and anterior cranial fossa. J Neurol Surg B Skull Base. 2012; 73(6):394–400

[12] Moe KS, Kim LJ, Bergeron CM. Transorbital endoscopic repair of cerebrospinal fluid leaks. Laryngoscope. 2011; 121(1):13–30

[13] Bly RA, Ramakrishna R, Ferreira M, Moe KS. Lateral transorbital neuroendoscopic approach to the lateral cavernous sinus. J Neurol Surg B Skull Base. 2014; 75(1):11–17

[14] Chen HI, Bohman LE, Loevner LA, Lucas TH. Transorbital endoscopic amygdalohippocampectomy: a feasibility investigation. J Neurosurg. 2014; 120(6): 1428–1436

[15] Balakrishnan K, Moe KS. Applications and outcomes of orbital and transorbital endoscopic surgery. Otolaryngol Head Neck Surg. 2011; 144(5):815–820

[16] Banu MA, Guerrero-Maldonado A, McCrea HJ, Garcia-Navarro V, Souweidane MM, Anand VK, Heier L, Schwartz TH, Greenfield JP. Impact of skull base development on endonasal endoscopic surgical corridors. Journal of Neurosurgery: Pediatrics. 2014 Feb;13(2):155-69.

[17] Ciporen J, Lucke-Wold B, Dogan A, Cetas J, Cameron W. Endoscopic endonasal transclival approach versus dual transorbital port technique for clip application to the posterior circulation: a cadaveric anatomical and cerebral circulation simulation study. J Neurol Surg B Skull Base. 2017; 78(3): 235–244

[18] Lawson W, Patel ZM, Lin FY. The development and pathologic processes that influence maxillary sinus pneumatization. Anat Rec (Hoboken). 2008; 291 (11):1554–1563

[19] Berens AM, Davis GE, Moe KS. Transorbital endoscopic identification of supernumerary ethmoid arteries. Allergy Rhinol (Providence). 2016; 7(3):144–146

[20] Moe KS. The precaruncular approach to the medial orbit. Arch Facial Plast Surg. 2003; 5(6):483–487

[21] Moe KS, Jothi S, Stern R, Gassner HG. Lateral retrocanthal orbitotomy: a minimally invasive, canthus-sparing approach. Arch Facial Plast Surg. 2007; 9(6): 419–426

[22] Bly RA, Chang SH, Cudejkova M, Liu JJ, Moe KS. Computer-guided orbital reconstruction to improve outcomes. JAMA Facial Plast Surg. 2013; 15(2): 113–120

[23] Shaftel SS, Chang SH, Moe KS. Hemostasis in orbital surgery. Otolaryngol Clin North Am. 2016; 49(3):763–775

[24] Reisch R, Perneczky A, Filippi R. Surgical technique of the supraorbital keyhole craniotomy. Surg Neurol. 2003; 59(3):223–227

10 Endonasal versus Supraorbital Eyebrow Approaches: Decision-Making in the Pediatric Population

Reid Hoshide, Richard Harvey, and Charles Teo

Abstract

The eyebrow/transcranial and the endonasal approaches are very versatile, and can successful address most pathology in the anterior skull base. Specific pediatric anatomical variations, such as the size of the nose, both soft tissue and bony apertures, morphology of the skull base and the size, extent, long axis and shape of the lesion itself need to be closely and comprehensively studied pre-operatively to decide on the correct approach.

In this chapter, through case examples, we discuss the nuances of both approaches, as they pertain to the developing pediatric skull base.

Keywords: pediatric, transcranial, endonasal keyhole, suborbital eyebrow approach, parasellar, sella, two-point rule

10.1 Introduction

The development of minimally invasive transcranial and endonasal keyhole approaches to the skull base has progressed significantly over the past few decades. These developments have made the approaches to the parasellar region safer and less invasive. Two approaches, specifically, have risen with the popularity of minimally invasive techniques. The approaches are the endonasal transsphenoidal approach and the subfrontal approach through an eyebrow incision. Here, we dissect the factors that help decide which approach is appropriate for varying pathologies in the pediatric population.

10.2 Specific Pediatric Considerations

The three factors that deserve special attention in the pediatric population are the concerns with the growing skull, the pyriform aperture width, and the development of the paranasal sinuses. Any cranial opening that bridges a skull suture has the potential to alter growth patterns. Done properly, the eyebrow craniotomy should not transgress any calvarial suture and, therefore, should not alter any of the normal growth patterns of the pediatric skull.

Many of the instruments designed for extended endonasal surgery are either larger or the same diameter as the endoscope and when the surgery requires more than one instrument, cluttering will occur and may impede the natural fluidity of surgery. One has to imagine a scenario where the carotid artery is injured and several suction instruments and endoscopes are urgently needed through two extremely small apertures. If the size of the pyriform aperture is limiting the rapid and unimpeded passage of instruments to the skull base, the result could be disastrous. Consequently, our recommendation is that the endonasal approach to the parasellar region should be reserved for children with pyriform apertures greater than 6 mm in diameter.

The sphenoid sinus normally reaches half of its adult size by the age of 7 years, reaching its maximal size at the end of the adolescent growth spurt (▶ Fig. 10.1).[1] It goes without saying that the pneumatization of the sphenoid sinus provides an ideal, though not absolutely necessary, operative corridor to

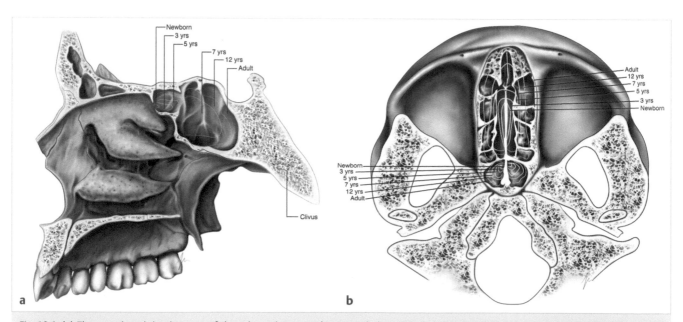

Fig. 10.1 (a) The growth and development of the sphenoid sinus in the saggital plane. **(b)** The growth and development of the sphenoid sinus and nasal cavity in the axial plane.

perform a routine transsphenoidal approach to the sellar region. Many times, however, the sellar region can still be approached through a variant of the presellar or conchal sphenoid sinus. In direct correlation with the sphenoid sinus pneumatization is the development of the bony impressions of the internal carotid artery and the optic nerves in the sphenoid bone. These protuberances provide helpful landmarks for the surgeon and are useful in the anatomical orientation necessary to avoid neurovascular injuries. When absent in an underdeveloped sphenoid sinus, there is added risk of disorientation and subsequent injury. Other anatomical, perhaps more reliable, landmarks such as the Vidian canal, orbital apex, medial orbital wall, sphenoid roof, and paraclival carotid may mitigate this risk. As the sphenoid sinus grows, it also expands the intercaro-

tid distance—the horizontal distance between each of the internal carotid arteries. An average adult's intercarotid distance is between 12 and 18 mm (▶ Fig. 10.2).[2] It has been studied that an intercarotid distance less than 10 mm would make transsphenoidal surgery more difficult, which is approximately the size of a normal 3- to 4-year-old child's intercarotid distance.[2,3] A narrow intercarotid corridor is not unique to the pediatric population but certainly encountered more often in the diminutive pediatric skull base. For pathology that extends above the diaphragma sellae, an intercarotid distance greater than 15 mm is mandatory for facile and safe instrument manipulation.

When one combines all these pediatric requirements, a suitable candidate for the endonasal approach to the parasellar region is a patient older than 7 years of age. This will vary by the size of the child and the size of the nose, but as a general rule, any complex parasellar pathology in a child younger than 7 years should be approached transcranially.

10.3 The Two-Point Rule

As a general rule, most tumors have a long axis. In other words, tumors are rarely perfectly round and more often than not are oval or even cylindrical. If you mark both extreme ends of the tumor and draw a line between the points and then carry that line to the surface, it will give some indication as to the best approach. In ▶ Fig. 10.3, the long axis of the tumor projects to the coronal suture. The best trajectory for this craniopharyngioma is a transcallosal, transforaminal approach. Conversely, the long axis of the tumor in ▶ Fig. 10.4, as seen best on the axial images, when carried to the surface, projects to the eyebrow. Finally, the long axis of the tumor in ▶ Fig. 10.5 projects to the tip of the nose and hence should be removed by an endonasal approach. When a tumor has several axes, the endoscope

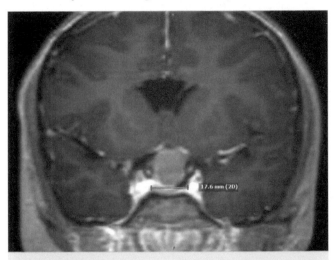

Fig. 10.2 Coronal MRI showing the normal intercarotid distance within the pituitary fossa.

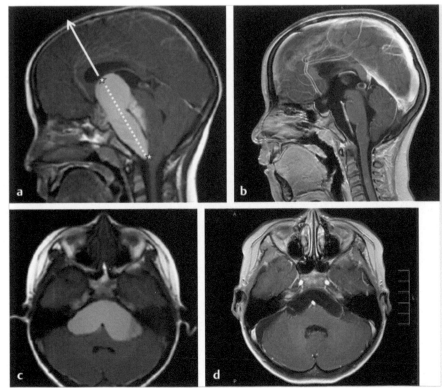

Fig. 10.3 (a) The long axis of this craniopharyngioma projects to the coronal suture and hence was removed through a transcallosal/transforaminal approach. (c) It also extended into both cerebellopontine angles and required extensive endoscopic-assisted surgical dissection to achieve (b,d) a complete and radical resection.

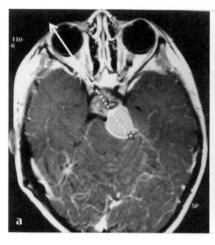

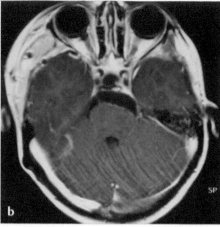

Fig. 10.4 (a) The long axis of this craniopharyngioma projects to the subfrontal space and the sphenoid sinus is poorly pneumatized and hence, it was completely removed through an eyebrow craniotomy (b).

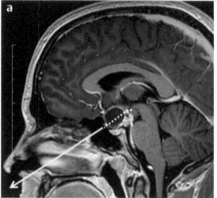

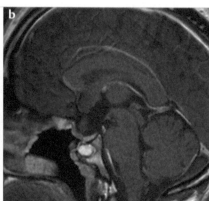

Fig. 10.5 (a) The long axis of this craniopharyngioma projects to the tip of the nose and the sphenoid sinus is well pneumatized; and hence was completely removed using an extended endonasal approach (b).

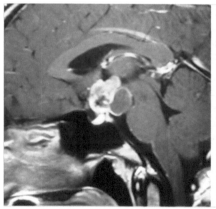

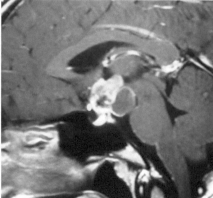

Fig. 10.6 (a) This patient has a well-aerated sphenoid sinus and a prefixed optic chiasm as shown by the yellow dot in (b). Furthermore, the pituitary gland is well positioned for an endonasal approach.

is invaluable in assisting the surgeon to look around corners and remove those parts of the tumor that are hidden from the limited line of view afforded by the microscope (▶ Fig. 10.3c, d).

10.4 The Optic Chiasm

A high-resolution midsagittal MRI image may show the position of the optic chiasm. When the chiasm is prefixed, it diminishes the prechiasmatic space and thereby limits the corridors

by which one reaches a suprasellar lesion transcranially. ▶ Fig. 10.6 shows a tumor that would be ideal for an endonasal approach. The chiasm is prefixed, the sphenoid sinus is well aerated, and the long axis of the tumor projects to the tip of the nose. Conversely, the tumor in ▶ Fig. 10.7 would be ideally approached through an eyebrow incision and a subfrontal trajectory because the optic chiasm is in the normal position, the sphenoid sinus is poorly aerated, and the long axis of the tumor is in the anteroposterior plane.

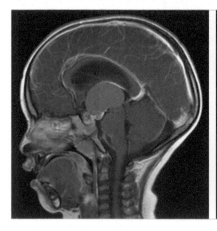 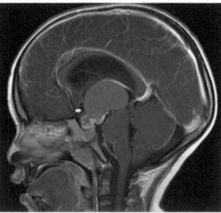

Fig. 10.7 **(a)**This patient has a poorly aerated sphenoid sinus and a normally positioned optic chiasm as shown by the yellow dot in **(b)**. Hence, this craniopharyngioma was completely removed through an eyebrow approach.

10.5 Endonasal Transsphenoidal Approach: Special Considerations in the Pediatric Population

From the moment the patient is draped, every effort should be made to reduce the impediments to unconstrained movement of instruments and scopes through the nostrils. This means judicious placement of drapes, limited use of adhesive drapes, and minimal submucosal infiltration of vasoconstricting agents. We prefer the use of a combination of topical (1:1,000–1:2,000) and injectable (1:100,000) epinephrine for local vasoconstriction, which has been demonstrated to be safe from untoward cardiovascular events.[4] If one has a selection of scopes to choose from, we would prefer to use a smaller diameter endoscope to reduce cluttering down the nose. Of course, if the endoscope is too small, it will not be adequately rigid enough to withstand the force applied within the intranasal structures, thus risking damage to the endoscope. We normally recommend a standard 4-mm rigid scope used without a sheath or attached irrigating device. We will select a 3-mm scope only if absolutely necessary. Although the 3 mm endoscope offer a similar range of view, they carry less capacity to illuminate the skull base, and this hinders their use.

We normally do not recommend extreme lateral dissection of the nares off the edges of the pyriform aperture. Craniofacial maldevelopment and disfiguring cosmetic sequelae have been documented.[1] Furthermore, lateral rhinotomies produce very significant cosmetic defects due to destruction of the alar attachments. The bone supporting the ala is often removed, and this leads to collapse and retraction of the ala. This collapse produces both cosmetic and functional deformities. For these reasons, lateral rhinotomies are rarely practiced in our institution. While there is no debate with lateralizing the inferior or medial turbinates, there is ongoing argument on the necessity of resecting these turbinates for the approach. The middle turbinate does not constrict at either the anterior (pyriform aperture) or the posterior (sphenoid aperture) access points. Thus, we rarely ever find an indication to resect the middle turbinate at our institution. However, in the unusual situation of a small nose with limited access, whether pediatric or adult, resection of the lower half of the middle turbinate and even part of the inferior turbinate will further expand the corridor to the skull base.

It is mandatory that a bilateral sphenoidal approach incorporates at least one posterior ethmoid cavity. This incorporation of the posterior ethmoid cavity is normally on the side of the endoscope. This allows the endoscope to park in a location whereby bimanual instrumentation can be performed in an unencumbered manner. Incorporating a full sphenoethmoidectomy on one or both sides allows the entire orbit to be identified and the surgeon can work medial and inferior to the orbital apex. Drilling of a poorly aerated or nonaerated sphenoid is dangerous without a comprehensive knowledge of the anatomy of the carotid artery and the optic nerves. Frameless stereotactic guidance is helpful but not essential.

It is important to note that the endonasal approach is not ideal for tumors of the planum sphenoidale at the posterior edge of the olfactory groove. Not only are these tumors better accessed via an eyebrow approach, but an endonasal approach will likely require the destruction of the posterior olfactory mucosa. This destruction will invariably cause a significant loss of olfaction. Worse, the posterior olfactory mucosa is involved in retronasal smell that senses the "flavor" of food; thus, any loss of this sensory function will greatly frustrate patients.

Despite the significant sinus drilling and mucosal manipulation, patients generally are able to have a preservation of quality of life following this procedure. If done correctly, studies have shown that there is no added morbidity from this procedure itself, where the primary pathology of the sellar lesion is the better predictor of morbidity.[5] Although postoperative meningitis has been a serious concern for this type of procedure, a large analysis of the literature has shown the relative rarity of this complication in the setting of advanced techniques to prevent leaking of cerebrospinal fluid and subsequent meningitis.[6]

10.6 Eyebrow Approach

The eyebrow approach to the parasellar anatomy is a very versatile one. With endoscopic assistance, almost all parasellar tumors can be accessed through this approach, with few exceptions. This approach, unlike the endonasal approach, is not affected by pediatric sinus limitations. In fact, the underdevelopment of the pediatric frontal sinus is convenient in eyebrow approaches. At birth, the frontal sinus is rudimentary and exists only as a small pouch at the superior end of the nasofrontal duct (► Fig. 10.8).[1] The expansion of the frontal sinus continues in a superolateral fashion, reaching half its adult size by the

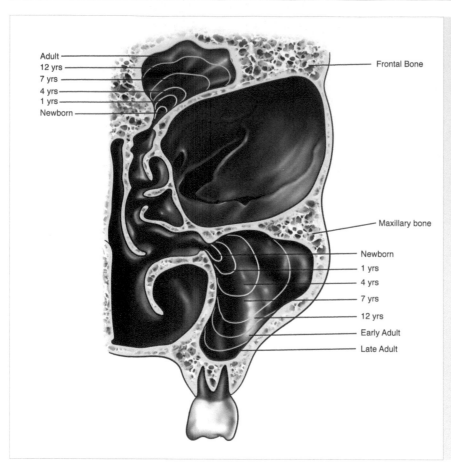

Adult
12 yrs
7 yrs
4 yrs
1 yrs
Newborn

Frontal Bone

Maxillary bone

Newborn
1 yrs
4 yrs
7 yrs
12 yrs
Early Adult
Late Adult

Fig. 10.8 The growth and development of the frontal maxillary sinus.

age of 4 years, and completing its pneumatization by midado-lescence.[1]

When compared to the endonasal approach, the eyebrow approach does create an externally visible surgical scar, but it is still a very cosmetically pleasing technique. Aside from the rare problem of keloid formation, surgical scars through an eyebrow incision are hardly noticeable once healed over. Injury to the nearby supraorbital nerve can cause temporary numbness on the forehead above the eyebrow, but this is rarely permanent.[7,8,9] Injury to the frontalis branch can occur less commonly, but this is also rarely permanent.[7,8,9] In patients with a developed frontal sinus, a frontal sinus breach can cause postoperative cerebrospinal fluid (CSF) leaks, and so liberal waxing of the medial edges of the craniotomy should be undertaken to seal off any occult entry into the frontal sinus. The use of a pericranial, muscle, or fat graft can also be used to seal off larger entries into the frontal sinus. While the endoscope can be used to access areas of the sella, parasellar and suprasellar regions, there are anatomic regions in which the eyebrow approach cannot access, even with the endoscope. In adults, a tumor that extends superficially into the temporal fossa may sometimes be accessible from a subfrontal trajectory. This is a consequence of "flattening" of the alar wing with skull base development. Of course, a tumor that extends deep into the temporal fossa should be approached through a temporal or a mini-pterional approach. In children, the immature skull base accentuates the alar wing and access to any part of the temporal fossa is near impossible from an eyebrow approach. This is the same

morphology that accounts for retroalar herniation and middle cerebral artery compression seen in children with swelling and contusions of the frontal lobe but almost never seen in the adult patient. Close examination of the preoperative parasagittal MRI may give a better idea of the suitability of the eyebrow approach (▶ Fig. 10.9a, b). Tumors that are suprasellar and retrochiasmatic would be better addressed by an endonasal approach. Uncommonly, sellar lesions can extend into the olfactory grooves. The olfactory grooves are midline structures that are similar to the valley between two hills. The hills, in the anterior cranial fossa, are the orbits that, when prominent, will obstruct access to the valley when coming from an anterolateral approach, which is the eyebrow approach. Lesions of this area might be better accessed through an endonasal or a larger, subfrontal approach, depending on the size and extent of the tumor. The ipsilateral inferomedial aspect of the optic canal and the lateral sphenoid wall are also very difficult regions to reach through a supraorbital craniotomy. These are better accessed through an endonasal approach.

There are very few specific considerations for the pediatric population. The eyebrow itself may be extremely thin, so it is important to keep the incision within the hair-bearing area. The burr hole must be placed below the temporal line and within the temporal fossa to achieve a good cosmetic outcome. The dura in the very young is thin and stuck to the inner surface of the cranial vault, so care must be taken when creating the bony free flap. Tearing the dura may be inconsequential with craniotomies anywhere else on the calvarium, but on the

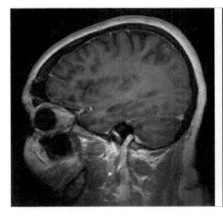
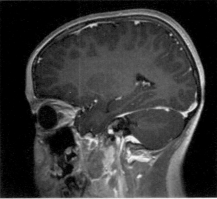

Fig. 10.9 **(a)** This parasagittal slice of a 58-year-old woman shows a relatively shallow angle between the anterior cranial fossa and the middle cranial fossa created by a "flattened" sphenoid wing. **(b)** A very acute angle created by a prominent sphenoid wing in a 7-year-old boy.

forehead, a dural tear results in a poor dural closure, which results in a large CSF subgaleal and periorbital fluid collection.

Once the operation is completed, the dura should be closed in a watertight fashion. The bone flap should be replaced and secured with absorbable plates, and the plates should not bridge a normal skull suture. They should also be very low profile. The skin incision is closed with a nonabsorbable nylon suture that is removed at postoperative day 5. We prefer a running 4.0, subcuticular stitch that is brought out beyond the apices of the incision and tied over with a nonstick dressing beneath it to prevent the stitch from being buried in the healing wound.

10.7 Conclusion

Surgical approaches to sella and parasellar tumors in the pediatric population must be carefully considered. Specific pediatric anatomical variations, such as the size of the nose, both soft-tissue and bony apertures, morphology of the skull base and the size, extent, long axis, and shape of the lesion itself need to be closely and comprehensively studied preoperatively. When all these factors are taken into consideration, the eyebrow/transcranial and the endonasal approaches are so versatile that almost all pathology in this area can be adequately addressed.

References

[1] Scuderi AJ, Harnsberger HR, Boyer RS. Pneumatization of the paranasal sinuses: normal features of importance to the accurate interpretation of CT scans and MR images. AJR Am J Roentgenol. 1993; 160(5):1101–1104

[2] Tatreau JR, Patel MR, Shah RN, et al. Anatomical considerations for endoscopic endonasal skull base surgery in pediatric patients. Laryngoscope. 2010; 120 (9):1730–1737

[3] Renn WH, Rhoton AL, Jr. Microsurgical anatomy of the sellar region. J Neurosurg. 1975; 43(3):288–298

[4] Gunaratne DA, Barham HP, Christensen JM, Bhatia DD, Stamm AC, Harvey RJ. Topical concentrated epinephrine (1:1000) does not cause acute cardiovascular changes during endoscopic sinus surgery. Int Forum Allergy Rhinol. 2016; 6(2):135–139

[5] Harvey RJ, Malek J, Winder M, et al. Sinonasal morbidity following tumour resection with and without nasoseptal flap reconstruction. Rhinology. 2015; 53(2):122–128

[6] Lai LT, Trooboff S, Morgan MK, Harvey RJ. The risk of meningitis following expanded endoscopic endonasal skull base surgery: a systematic review. J Neurol Surg B Skull Base. 2014; 75(1):18–26

[7] Dlouhy BJ, Chae MP, Teo C. The supraorbital eyebrow approach in children: clinical outcomes, cosmetic results, and complications. J Neurosurg Pediatr. 2015; 15(1):12–19

[8] Teo C. Application of endoscopy to the surgical management of craniopharyngiomas. Childs Nerv Syst. 2005; 21(8–9):696–700

[9] Wilson DA, Duong H, Teo C, Kelly DF. The supraorbital endoscopic approach for tumors. World Neurosurg. 2014; 82(6) Suppl:S72–S80

11 Ventral Approaches to Intraparenchymal Tumors of the Skull Base and Brainstem

Harminder Singh, Allen Ho, Lily Kim, Walid I. Essayed, and Theodore H. Schwartz

Abstract

Endonasal surgery to address intraparenchymal pathology at the skull base and brainstem, although challenging, is feasible in the pediatric population in appropriately selected cases. A thorough understanding of brainstem nuclei and tracts is required to operate successfully in this region. Classic anterolateral safe entry zones, such as peritrigeminal zone in the pons and olivary zone in the medulla, are not easily accessible when using the anterior endoscopic trajectory. This endoscopic window is safe only for approaching midline exophytic pontine lesions, but might also be extended to nonexophytic lesions strictly anterior to cortico-spinal tracts. Neuromonitoring and image guidance are valuable tools that can be utilized during the endoscopic resection of intraparenchymal oncologic pathology. Since the pathology is intradural, accessing it requires a durotomy and creation of a high-flow cerebrospinal fluid (CSF) leak. A multilayered skull base reconstruction strategy must be used to prevent post-op CSF leaks.

Keywords: endoscopic endonasal surgery, ventral approach, brainstem anatomy, fibertracts, nuclei, safe-entry zones

11.1 Introduction

Endonasal surgery to address intradural pathology at the skull base and brainstem presents its own set of challenges. Since the pathology is intradural, accessing it requires a durotomy and the creation of a high-flow cerebrospinal fluid (CSF) leak. This creates unique challenges in reconstructing the skull base after removal of the lesion. While numerous "safe zones" have been described in the transcranial literature to approach intra-axial brainstem pathology, only a few of these are accessible from a ventral endonasal route. Removal of intradural, intra-axial pathology also puts various cranial nerves, fiber tracts, and brainstem nuclei at risk, necessitating deployment of a neuromonitoring montage, as well as image guidance, to guide the surgeon. These intradural oncologic considerations during endonasal surgery will be the focus of this chapter.

11.2 Considerations

11.2.1 Approach Selection

There are numerous endonasal approaches to intradural skull base pathology, and choice of approach will depend largely on the anatomic area of interest, as well as the planned extent of resection of lesions and strategies for dural and skull base repair. These approaches can be categorized into five different endonasal corridors (transsphenoidal, transethmoidal, transmaxillary, transnasal, and transfrontal) to reach specific skull base and brainstem targets, as has been described in Chapter 7.

11.2.2 Neuromonitoring

When considering endoscopic endonasal approach (EEA) for intradural lesions of the skull base and brainstem, the region of interest and the anticipated neurovascular structures to be encountered should determine which neuromonitoring modalities should be utilized. For skull base approaches involving the parasellar region and cavernous sinus, in the vicinity of the internal carotid artery and its branches, global cortical mapping with electroencephalogram (EEG) and somatosensory evoked potentials (SSEPs) should be employed to monitor for global and brainstem ischemia. The same is true for transclival approaches involving the vertebrobasilar junction.[1,2,3,4] Both of these modalities have been validated in EEA surgeries to account for both cortical ischemia, which would be captured on EEG, and the subcortical ischemia that can be better monitored with SSEPs.[1,2] The addition of motor evoked potentials (MEPs) can be useful in certain suprasellar or petroclival lesions, given the false-negative rates of EEG/SSEPs.[5]

EMG has been utilized successfully in EEA surgery to provide real-time feedback for cranial nerve (CN) irritation and probe the functional integrity of a mixed or motor CN. The oculomotor, trochlear, and abducens nerves can be monitored with needle electrodes placed in the inferior rectus, superior oblique, and lateral rectus muscles, respectively. These CNs are most at risk during intradural EEA procedures,[6,7,8] even in cases where the cavernous sinus is *not* accessed. The oculomotor nerve, for example, is vulnerable in the interpeduncular cistern via the transsphenoidal and transplanum routes, with vascular compromise possible from injury to the inferolateral trunk of the cavernous carotid or its branches. The trochlear nerve may be exposed at the ambient cisternal segment through the transsellar transtuberculum route, and ischemic injury may occur with injury to the superior cerebellar artery. The abducens nerve, being the longest and most ventrally located CN at the level of the clivus and cavernous sinus, is particularly at risk during approaches to petroclival lesions via the midline transclival, paramedian suprapetrous, and medial petrous apex approaches. In these cases, the risk may be increased by abnormal anatomy (e.g., medial displacement of the nerve by a petroclival tumor or upward displacement by a cisternal mass). Like the oculomotor nerve, the abducens nerve may also suffer vascular compromise by injury to the inferolateral trunk from the cavernous segment of the internal carotid artery. The trigeminal nerve may be violated in Meckel's cave via the transpterygoid corridor. As EEAs are extended to the inferior clivus, as well as through the transcondylar and transjugular corridors, attention must be paid to lower CN monitoring, including the glossopharyngeal, vagus, accessory, and hypoglossal nerves[5] (▶ Table 11.1).

For endonasal endoscopic removal of tumors involving the brainstem, brainstem auditory evoked potentials (BAEPs) can be beneficial for detecting brainstem ischemia during surgery at

Table 11.1 Surgical approaches using the endoscopic, endonasal route, and recommended IONM modalities based on pathologies commonly encountered via that approach[5]

Surgical approach	IONM montage	Common pathology
Transsphenoidal to sella	None	Adenoma, Rathke's cleft cyst
Transsphenoidal, transplanum, transtuberculum to suprasellar region	EEG, SSEPs, MEPs	Meningioma, craniopharyngioma, giant pituitary adenomas
To orbital apex	EEG, SSEPs, MEPs, EMG (CN III, IV, VI)	Hemangioma, meningioma, neoplasm
Transethmoidal, transcribriform to anterior cranial fossa	EEG, SSEPs, MEPs	Meningioma, esthesioneuroblastoma, meningocele
Transclival/transpetrous to brainstem and posterior fossa	EEG, SSEPs, MEPs, EMG (CN VI, VII), BAEPs	Chordoma, chondrosarcoma
Transpterygoid	EEG, SSEPs, MEPs, EMG (CN V)	Meningocele, meningoencephalocele, schwannoma
To cavernous sinus	EEG, SSEPs, MEPs, EMG (CN III, IV, VI)	Adenoma, meningioma
Transcondylar/transjugular	EEG, SSEPs, MEPs, EMG (CN IX, X, XI, XII)	Chordoma, chondrosarcoma

Abbreviations: BAEPs, brainstem auditory evoked potentials; CN, cranial nerve; EEG, electroencephalogram; EMG, electromyogram; IONM, intraoperative neuromonitoring; MEPs, motor evoked potentials; SSEPs, somatosensory evoked potentials.

or around the vertebrobasilar junction, as is the case for transclival approaches.

As shown in ▶ Table 11.1, multimodal neuromonitoring, tailored to approach and specific intradural pathology, endeavors not only to detect and identify iatrogenic nervous system dysfunction but also to guide the use of surgical interventions and monitor their efficacy.

For an in-depth analysis of how intraoperative neuromonitoring is applicable to pediatric endoscopic endonasal skull base surgery, please refer to Chapter 6.

11.2.3 Image Guidance

Intraoperative image guidance is especially useful in endoscopic surgeries because of the distorted depth perception inherent in 2D endoscopes, which are still more commonly used than newly developed 3D endoscopes. The utility of image guidance has been well described in the literature for adult endonasal approaches but not for pediatric cases. The few studies in the pediatric population suggest that the benefits of having enhanced localization and immediate feedback through image guidance can optimize pediatric endonasal endoscopic skull base surgery as well.[9,10,11] The small corridor, incomplete pneumatization of the sphenoid sinus, and crowding of the neurovascular structures make image guidance even more critical for pediatric patients.

In a traditional setting, image guidance in the operating room relies on the scans taken *preoperatively*. These images are then utilized for image guidance intraoperatively, but this method has limited ability to offer accurate anatomical information due to changes from patient positioning or the anatomical shifts during surgery. Intraoperative use of live CT or MR eliminates this problem, as the imaging accurately reflects patient positioning at the time of operation.[12] With live intraoperative imaging, surgeons can guide their resections for optimal safety around critical structures and minimize the risk of incomplete resection and prevent reoperation due to residual pathology.[13,14]

The additional arrangement needs for an intraoperative scanner and image guidance system lengthens operation time due

to setup and registration. Moreover, intraoperative CT may expose pediatric patients to excessive radiation, which should be avoided. Despite these inconveniences, real-time image guidance may still be desirable in certain *extended* endonasal cases, considering the extra time and cost incurred, as well as the increased morbidity, from a repeat surgery in the case of incomplete resection. For a thorough understanding of the variations in the operating room setup with and without intraoperative imaging, please refer to Chapter 4.

11.2.4 Ventral Safe Entry Zones into Brainstem

Brainstem lesions represent a challenge to both the surgeon and the patient. The dense concentration of critical nuclei and fibers located in a region roughly the size of the human thumb underlies the morbidity and mortality associated with brainstem pathology. To minimize disruption of eloquent tissue in this region, microsurgical approaches in conjunction with safe entry zones have been developed to optimize safe exposure and resection in different portions of the brainstem.[15,16,17,18,19,20] These safe entry zones and trajectories represent areas where eloquent structures and perforators are sparse, thus minimizing possible damage with a neurotomy.

As endoscopic endonasal surgery has continued to evolve beyond straightforward approaches to the sellar and suprasellar regions, extended endoscopic approaches have allowed for access to ventral brainstem lesions with good results.[21,22,23,24] In particular, the EEA allows for safe midline, ventral exposure of the clivus down to the craniovertebral junction.[25,26] This allows for endoscopic access to three classic ventral safe entry zones: anterior mesencephalic zone (AMZ) in the midbrain, the peritrigeminal zone (PTZ) in the pons, and the olivary zone in the medulla.[19,27]

Anterior Mesencephalic Zone

The AMZ may be accessed via a standard endoscopic endonasal approach to the sella. However, unilateral transposition of the pituitary gland is necessary to obtain more direct access to the midbrain and anterior mesencephalic sulcus. While complete transposition often causes hypopituitarism,[28] unilateral or extradural transposition with removal of the posterior clinoid on one side can be completed with minimal morbidity.[29,30] Even with pituitary transposition, the exiting third nerve from the brainstem can block access to the AMZ (▶ Fig. 11.1, ▶ Fig. 11.2a).

The AMZ can be accessed safely through the interpeduncular cistern via the limited area on the cerebral peduncle between the oculomotor tract and nerve medially and the corticospinal tract (CST) laterally. This entry point takes advantage of CST fibers in the intermediate three-fifths of the peduncle and the location of the red nucleus and substantia nigra deep and medial to the entry zone.[31] The superior and inferior boundaries are the optic nerve and chiasm superiorly and the oculomotor nerve and superior cerebellar artery complex inferiorly (▶ Fig. 11.1, ▶ Fig. 11.2a). Laterally, the limitation to access via the endonasal approach is the cavernous carotid (▶ Fig. 11.3). This intracavernous carotid distance can be quite narrow in many individuals, and a medially coursing carotid can effectively block off access to the AMZ.[32]

Peritrigeminal Zone

The anterolateral surface of the pons, medial to the trigeminal nerve entry zone, lateral to the corticospinal tracks, and anterior to the motor and sensory nuclei of the trigeminal nerve, has been identified as the peritrigeminal safe entry zone (PTZ) within the pons[19,33,34,35] (▶ Fig. 11.2a, ▶ Fig. 11.4, ▶ Fig. 11.5). Utilizing an extended endoscopic transclival approach with removal of the anterior wall and floor of the sphenoid sinus allows for exposure of this safe pontine corridor. Sufficient lateral exposure is critical for this exposure, and the inferior petrosal sinuses represent the lateral borders of the exposure along the clivus (▶ Fig. 11.3). The medial border of the safe zone is the pyramidal tract. The inferior border of the PTZ are the roots of the CN VI medially and CNs VII and VIII laterally (▶ Fig. 11.2a, ▶ Fig. 11.5).

The downward trajectory of the abducens (CN 6) and facial nerve (CN 7) fibers through the pons necessitates taking an upward trajectory for any dissection, lateral and superior to the CN VI exit point (▶ Fig. 11.5, ▶ Fig. 11.6).

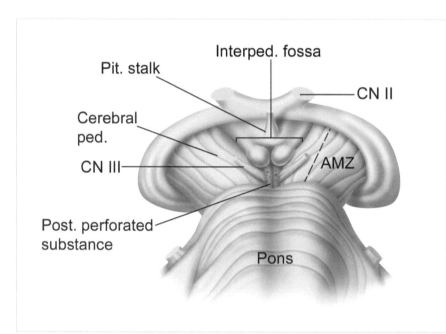

Fig. 11.1 A ventral view of the anterior mesencephalic safe-entry zone (AMZ).

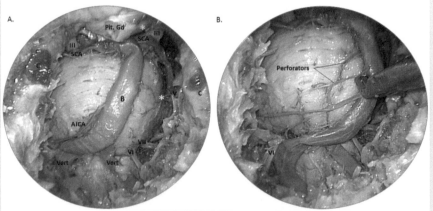

Fig. 11.2 (a) Endoscopic cadaveric view of the ventral brainstem after an endonasal transsphenoidal and transclival approach. *Green star:* AMZ, better accessed after unilateral pituitary transposition; *yellow star:* peritrigeminal zone (PTZ). III, oculomotor nerve; V, trigeminal nerve; VI, sixth nerve; VII, facial nerve; AICA, anteroinferior cerebellar artery; B, basilar trunk; C, carotid artery (intrapetrous); Pit. Gd, pituitary gland; SCA, superior cerebellar artery; Vert, vertebral artery. (b) Endoscopic view of the basilar perforators after displacing the basilar artery to the left.

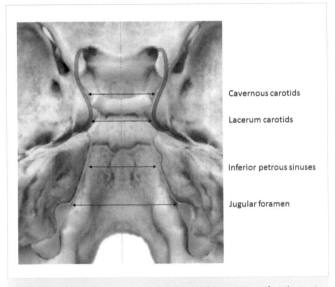

Fig. 11.3 Skull base projection of the lateral limitations of endoscopic exposure.

Cavernous carotids

Lacerum carotids

Inferior petrous sinuses

Jugular foramen

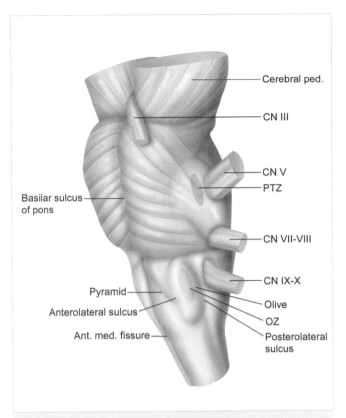

Cerebral ped.

CN III

CN V

PTZ

Basilar sulcus of pons

CN VII-VIII

CN IX-X

Pyramid

Olive

Anterolateral sulcus

OZ

Ant. med. fissure

Posterolateral sulcus

Fig. 11.4 Anterolateral view of the brainstem showing the location of the peritrigeminal zone (PTZ) and the olivary zone (OZ).

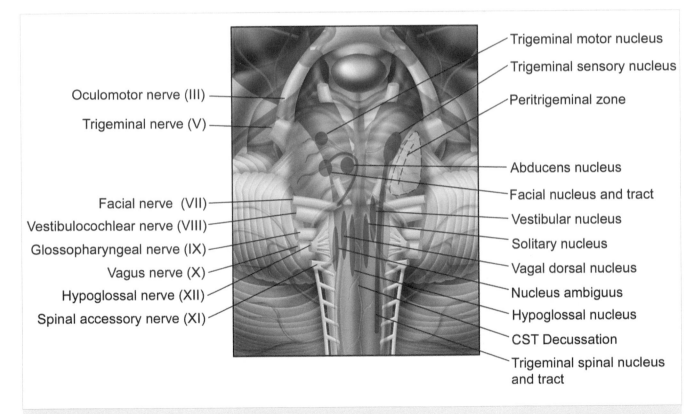

Oculomotor nerve (III)

Trigeminal nerve (V)

Facial nerve (VII)

Vestibulocochlear nerve (VIII)

Glossopharyngeal nerve (IX)

Vagus nerve (X)

Hypoglossal nerve (XII)

Spinal accessory nerve (XI)

Trigeminal motor nucleus

Trigeminal sensory nucleus

Peritrigeminal zone

Abducens nucleus

Facial nucleus and tract

Vestibular nucleus

Solitary nucleus

Vagal dorsal nucleus

Nucleus ambiguus

Hypoglossal nucleus

CST Decussation

Trigeminal spinal nucleus and tract

Fig. 11.5 Illustration demonstrating the corticospinal tract (CST) and deeper brainstem nuclei and tracts. The location of the peritrigeminal zone (PTZ) is shown.

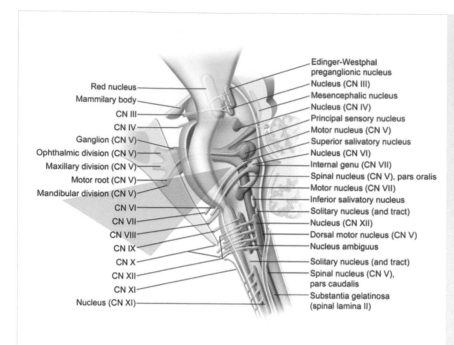

Red nucleus
Mammillary body
CN III
CN IV
Ganglion (CN V)
Ophthalmic division (CN V)
Maxillary division (CN V)
Motor root (CN V)
Mandibular division (CN V)
CN VI
CN VII
CN VIII
CN IX
CN X
CN XII
CN XI
Nucleus (CN XI)

Edinger-Westphal preganglionic nucleus
Nucleus (CN III)
Mesencephalic nucleus
Nucleus (CN IV)
Principal sensory nucleus
Motor nucleus (CN V)
Superior salivatory nucleus
Nucleus (CN VI)
Internal genu (CN VII)
Spinal nucleus (CN V), pars oralis
Motor nucleus (CN VII)
Inferior salivatory nucleus
Solitary nucleus (and tract)
Nucleus (CN XII)
Dorsal motor nucleus (CN V)
Nucleus ambiguus
Solitary nucleus (and tract)
Spinal nucleus (CN V), pars caudalis
Substantia gelatinosa (spinal lamina II)

Fig. 11.6 Brainstem sagittal section with the principal nuclei and tracts. The *blue triangle* represents the endoscopic upward dissecting trajectory inside the pons, avoiding the sixth and facial nerve fibers.

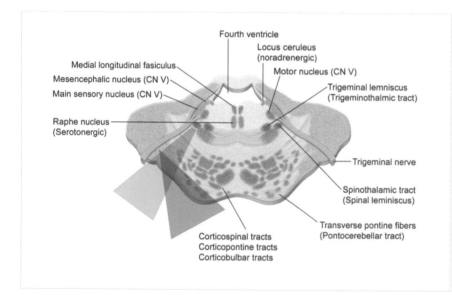

Medial longitudinal fasiculus
Mesencephalic nucleus (CN V)
Main sensory nucleus (CN V)
Raphe nucleus (Serotonergic)

Fourth ventricle
Locus ceruleus (noradrenergic)
Motor nucleus (CN V)
Trigeminal lemniscus (Trigeminothalmic tract)

Corticospinal tracts
Corticopontine tracts
Corticobulbar tracts

Trigeminal nerve

Spinothalamic tract (Spinal leminiscus)

Transverse pontine fibers (Pontocerebellar tract)

Fig. 11.7 Axial schematic representation of the microscopic and endoscopic exposure of the pons, at the level of the trigeminal nerve exit, with normal anatomy. The *blue triangle* represents the microsurgical view from a lateral approach; the *red triangle* represents the endoscopic view from a ventral midline approach.

While a transcranial subtemporal corridor affords a more direct approach to the PTZ, the endonasal endoscopic approach provides a wide midline to lateral view (▶ Fig. 11.7). This can be a difficult corridor to visualize and work through ventrally without the aid of angulated endoscopes, and makes the resection of deep-seated lesions very difficult. An additional consideration at the pontine level is the variance in the tortuosity of the basilar artery, and the lateral extent of basilar artery perforators that further limit access into the pons (▶ Fig. 11.2b).

Thus, the ventral endoscopic route is only safe for resection of small superficial lesions located anterior or lateral to the CSTs, or biopsy or debulking of larger exophytic lesions. While the superficial pontocerebellar fibers run in a *transverse* direction, incisions along the ventral aspect of the pons should follow a *longitudinal* course parallel to the CSTs coursing under them (▶ Fig. 11.2, ▶ Fig. 11.5).

In the future, MR tractography using diffusion-weighted imaging may prove helpful in identifying the location of the pyramidal tracts in relation to pontine lesions,[36,37] and ultimately guide approach.

Olivary Zone

The olivary zone proceeds through the olives on the anterolateral surface of the medulla. This zone is bordered medially by the anterolateral sulcus and the pyramids, and laterally by the posterolateral sulcus (▶ Fig. 11.4). Within the brainstem, the fibers of the hypoglossal nerve separate the olive from the pyramidal tracts medially and the medial lemniscus deeper (▶ Fig. 11.9).

Endoscopically, a wider exposure is attainable at this level as the inferior petrosal sinuses begin to splay laterally caudally along the brainstem. Exposure of the superior medulla is relatively straightforward with an endoscopic transclival approach, but exposure of the inferior medulla can be challenging. The hard palate can limit the entry angle of the endoscope and instruments caudally, and preoperative radiographic evaluation is crucial when planning a caudal medullary exposure.[38,39,40,41] The anterior arch of C1 and the odontoid tip (C2) can also be resected, if necessary, without causing significant cervical occipital instability in patients with no prior cervical kyphosis and healthy facet joints bilaterally.[42,43] The relatively small diameter of the medulla at this caudal extent allows for visualization of the hypoglossal nerve rootlets (CN XII) and olivary bodies (▶ Fig. 11.8). Thus, the olivary zone can be safely entered laterally via this approach, working in between the hypoglossal nerve rootlets (▶ Fig. 11.8, ▶ Fig. 11.9).

The relatively small size of the medulla and the superficiality of the CST tracts limits surgical maneuverability at this level. A midline approach through the caudal anterior median fissure is not recommended because of the decussating pyramidal fibers (CST + corticobulbar tract) in the medulla (▶ Fig. 11.8).

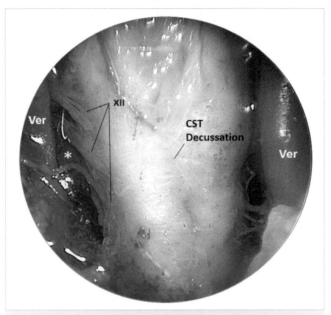

Fig. 11.8 Endoscopic view of the medulla. XII, hypoglossal nerve roots; Ver, vertebral artery. The asterisk symbol (*) indicates the olivary body.

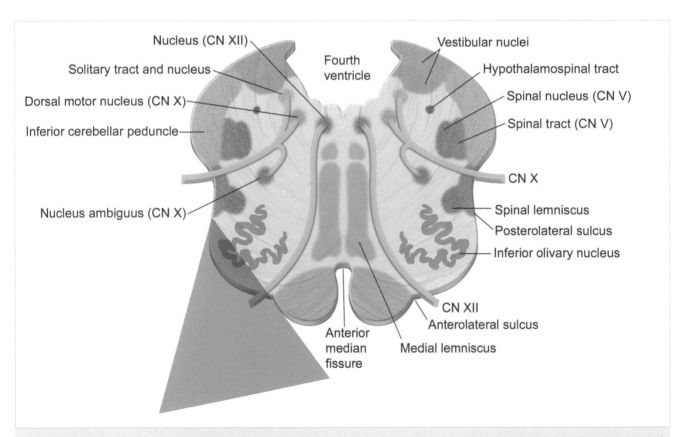

Fig. 11.9 Axial schematic representation of the medulla at the level of the hypoglossal nerve exit. The *red triangle* represents the endoscopic tangential view of the olivary body, with the hypoglossal roots in the way.

11.2.5 Closure Considerations

Resection of intraparenchymal pathology requires a wide dural opening, and depending on the pathology, can result in a high- or low-flow CSF leak. Adequate closure of the skull base after tumor resection is imperative to seal off the intracranial compartment from the sinonasal cavity and to prevent CSF rhinorrhea and intracranial infections. A multilayered closure, often involving fascia lata covered with a vascularized mucosal flap, such as the nasoseptal flap, works best to prevent leaks. CSF diversion using a lumbar drain or external ventricular drain

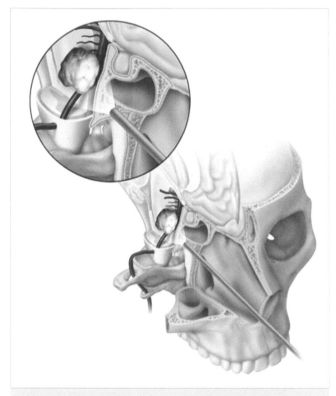

Fig. 11.10 An artist's depiction of the transclival approach using the transnasal corridor.

may increase the success of the closure by reducing the pressure of CSF pulsations on the new repair. A rigid buttress may also help counter CSF pulsations on the new repair and prevent herniation of the brain matter through the defect.[44] For a detailed review of the various options available for a multilayered closure, please refer to Chapter 29.

11.3 Case Examples

11.3.1 Transclival Approach for Ependymoma

A 16-year-old right-handed adolescent boy had undergone a subtotal resection of a posterior fossa mass at the age of 3 years. Gross total resection was not achieved because of brainstem invasion. Pathology revealed a WHO grade II ependymoma.[23] Subsequently, the patient underwent adjuvant therapy with stereotactic radiosurgery and chemotherapy, with serial MRI monitoring for residual disease.

The patient presented with headaches, dysphagia, and left hemiparesis. MRI demonstrated a 2.8 × 3.4 cm ventral intrinsic lesion at the pontomedullary junction with foci consistent with acute hemorrhage (▶ Fig. 11.11, **pre-op**).

The patient underwent an endonasal transclival approach for resection of this lesion (▶ Fig. 11.10). His fully pneumatized sphenoid sinus, laterally displaced basilar artery, and the direct ventral location of the exophytic disease all supported this choice of surgical corridor to achieve a palliative brainstem decompression of an incurable recurrence. The ventral exophytic lesion displaced the CSTs laterally, opening up a midline corridor into the brainstem for debulking this lesion (▶ Fig. 11.12, *red triangle*). A far lateral transcranial approach (▶ Fig. 11.12, *blue triangle*) would have placed the laterally displaced CSTs directly in way of the lesion.

Under endoscopic visualization with the aid of a 0-degree, 18-cm-long, 4-mm-diameter rigid endoscope (Karl Storz), a nasal septal flap was harvested based on the sphenopalatine artery and was tucked into the nasal pharynx. Bilateral superior and partial inferior turbinectomies, partial sphenoidectomy,

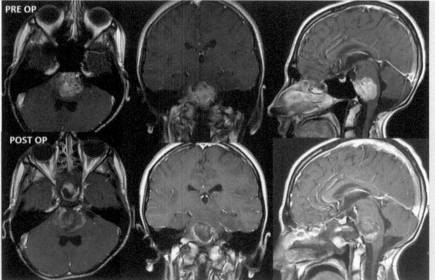

Fig. 11.11 Preoperative axial, coronal, and sagittal T1-weighted MRI images showing an enhancing intramedullary lesion in the pons and medulla. Postoperative imaging showing subtotal resection (STR) of lesion. The MEDPOR graft used for skull base reconstruction can be visualized (*blue arrow*).

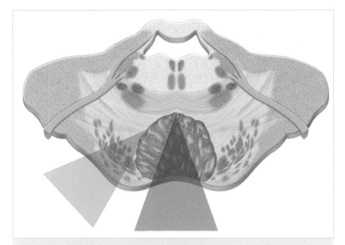

Fig. 11.12 Axial schematic representation of the microscopic and endoscopic exposure of the pons, at the level of the trigeminal nerve exit, with a ventral midline tumor. The corticospinal tracts (CSTs) are pushed laterally by the tumor, blocking off the microscopic corridor. The *blue triangle* represents the microsurgical view from a lateral approach; the *red triangle* represents the endoscopic view from a ventral midline approach. Exophytic lesions present a natural corridor to gain entry into the brainstem and debulk the lesions from within.

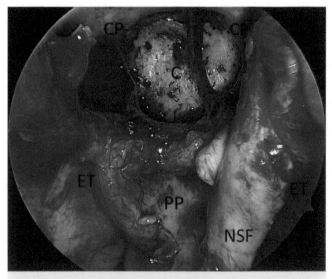

Fig. 11.13 Transnasal approach to the clivus. The nasoseptal flap (NSF) is harvested and stored in the oropharynx for use in skull base reconstruction. C, clivus; CP, carotid protuberance; ET, Eustachian tube; PP, posterior pharynx.

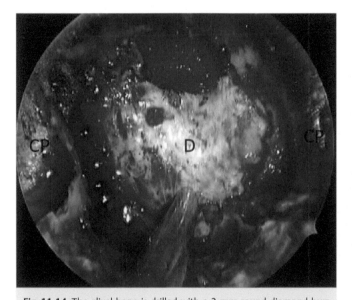

Fig. 11.14 The clival bone is drilled with a 3-mm round diamond burr and subsequently removed with a 2-mm Kerrison rongeur. The underlying dura (D) is exposed. CP, carotid protuberance.

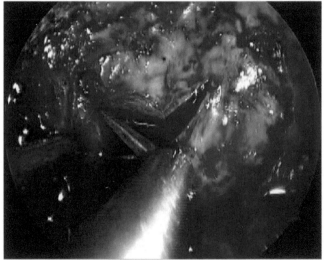

Fig. 11.15 Stellate opening of clival dura with angled scissors. The basilar artery course was traced using a Doppler on the right side of the image.

and partial ethmoidectomy were performed to widen the surgical corridor (▶ Fig. 11.13). The clival bone was drilled with a 3-mm round diamond burr and subsequently removed with a 2-mm Kerrison rongeur, exposing the dura (▶ Fig. 11.14).

A Doppler probe was used to map out the course of the basilar artery underneath the dura. Subsequently, a stellate opening was made in the clival dura over the projection of the tumor with angled scissors (▶ Fig. 11.15). The tumor was entered sharply using a number 11 blade (▶ Fig. 11.16), and it was debulked from within (▶ Fig. 11.17). Intraoperative neuromonitoring was used to guide extent of resection during the case.

For closure, an autologous fat graft was placed over the defect. A *gasket* seal was used for skull base reconstruction, using fascia lata and MEDPOR (Stryker, Kalamazoo, MI) (M) graft countersunk into the bony opening (▶ Fig. 11.18). The previously harvested pedicled nasoseptal flap was layered over this closure.

Postoperatively, the patient demonstrated significant neurological improvement in cranial neuropathies and hemiparesis soon after the procedure. The post-op MRI showed subtotal resection of the lesion (▶ Fig. 11.11, **post-op**). The tumor pathology was now consistent with a WHO grade III anaplastic ependymoma.

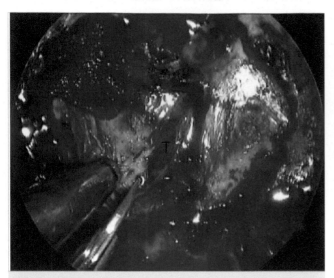

Fig. 11.16 Intramedullary opening using a number 11 blade, revealing grayish tumor (T).

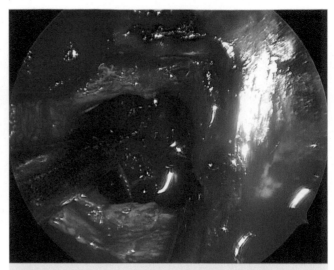

Fig. 11.17 Intramedullary resection of tumor. Intraoperative neuromonitoring was used to guide extent of resection during the case.

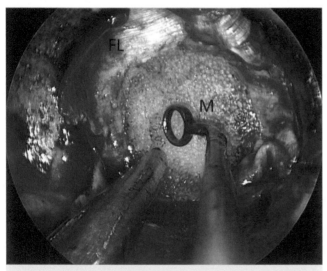

Fig. 11.18 Gasket seal used for skull base reconstruction, using fascia lata (FL) and MEDPOR (M) graft countersunk into the bony opening. The previously harvested pedicled nasoseptal flap was layered over this closure.

11.3.2 Transplanum Approach for Juvenile Pilocytic Astrocytoma

A 16-year-old adolescent girl presented with progressive headaches and visual loss (▶ Fig. 11.19). MRI showed a heterogeneously enhancing lesion arising from the suprasellar space and extending superiorly into the third ventricle (▶ Fig. 11.20, **pre-op**). The patient first underwent supraorbital tumor debulking, but limited resection could be performed. The diagnosis was juvenile pilocytic astrocytoma of the optic nerves and hypothalamus. She underwent fractionated radiation therapy and then presented with recurrence of her symptoms and further enlargement of her tumor. She was offered a transtuberculum, transplanum approach for debulking of this lesion. Subtotal resection was planned to preserve her vision and hypothalamic function.

An extended transsphenoidal transtuberculum approach was performed to widen the surgical corridor (▶ Fig. 11.21). The dura was sharply opened above and below the intercavernous sinus, and the sinus coagulated and cut (▶ Fig. 11.22). The tumor capsule was sharply opened with angled scissors (▶ Fig. 11.23), and the tumor was internally debulked using suction and the Myriad (NICO CORP, Indianapolis, IN), which has an oscillating side-cutting and aspirating tip (▶ Fig. 11.24). Care was taken to remain below the optic chiasm. Aggressive debulking was performed until CSF was reached, indicating the back of the third ventricle.

The tumor cavity was inspected and hemostasis achieved (▶ Fig. 11.25). The skull base was reconstructed using the Gasket technique with MEDPOR and fascia lata, followed by a nasoseptal flap.

The post-op MRI showed radical subtotal total resection of the juvenile pilocytic astrocytoma (JPA; ▶ Fig. 11.20, **post-op**). The patient made an excellent neurologic recovery, and her vision was preserved and her symptoms ameliorated.

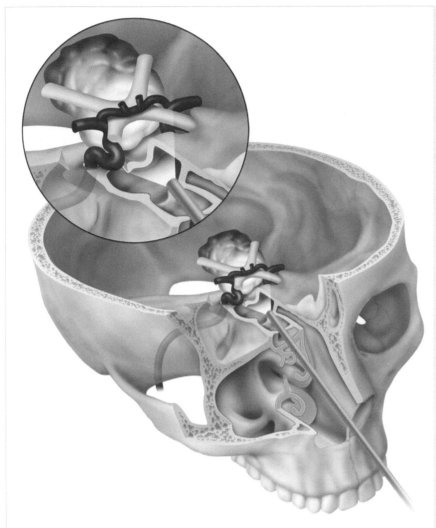

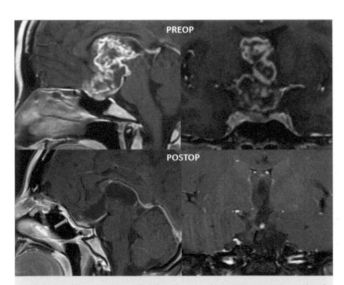

Fig. 11.20 Preoperative sagittal and coronal MRI images (T1 weighted with gadolinium) showing the juvenile pilocytic astrocytoma (JPA) postoperative images showing gross total resection of the JPA. The *blue arrow* shows the placement of the MEDPOR graft to reconstruct the skull base post resection.

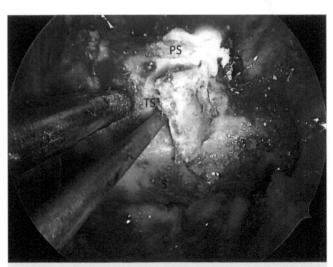

Fig. 11.21 The bone overlying the tuberculum sella (TS) and planum sella (PS) is drilled and removed. C, clivus; S, sella.

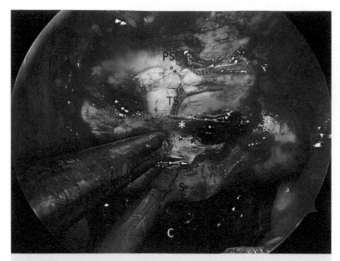

Fig. 11.22 The dura is sharply incised above and below the intercavernous sinus (*), and the sinus coagulated and incised.

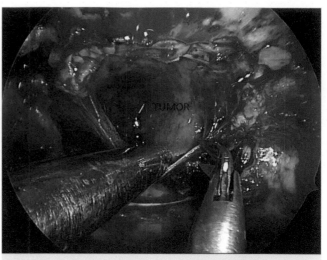

Fig. 11.23 The tumor capsule is opened leading us into the tumor.

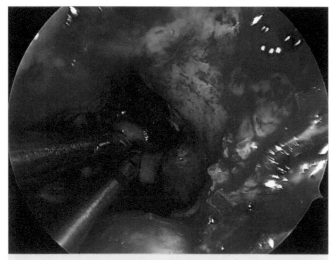

Fig. 11.24 The tumor is internally debulked using suction and the Myriad (NICO).

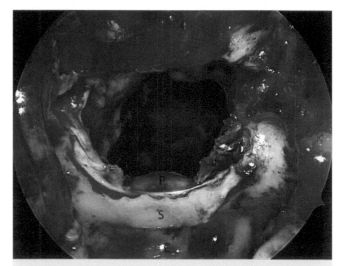

Fig. 11.25 The tumor cavity post resection. The pituitary gland (P) can be seen inside the sella (S). The skull base is reconstructed using the Gasket technique with MEDPOR and fascia lata, followed by a nasoseptal flap. The Gasket technique is illustrated later in this manual.

11.4 Conclusion

Endonasal surgery to address intraparenchymal pathology at the skull base and brainstem is feasible in the pediatric population. A thorough understanding of brainstem nuclei and tracts is required to operate successfully in this region. The use of classic anterolateral safe entry zones, such as peritrigeminal area in the pons and olivary bodies in the medulla, are not easily accessible when using the anterior endoscopic trajectory. This endoscopic window is safe only for approaching midline exophytic pontine lesions, but might also be extended to nonexophytic lesions strictly anterior to CSTs. Neuromonitoring and image guidance are valuable tools that can be utilized during the endoscopic resection of intraparenchymal oncologic pathology.

11.5 Authors' Contribution

Harminder Singh and Allen Ho contributed equally to the chapter.

References

[1] Thirumala PD, Kassasm AB, Habeych M, et al. Somatosensory evoked potential monitoring during endoscopic endonasal approach to skull base surgery: analysis of observed changes. Neurosurgery. 2011; 69(1) Suppl operative:64–76, discussion ons76

[2] Thirumala PD, Kodavatiganti HS, Habeych M, et al. Value of multimodality monitoring using brainstem auditory evoked potentials and somatosensory evoked potentials in endoscopic endonasal surgery. Neurol Res. 2013; 35(6): 622–630

[3] Little JR, Lesser RP, Lueders H, Furlan AJ. Brain stem auditory evoked potentials in posterior circulation surgery. Neurosurgery. 1983; 12(5):496–502

[4] Elangovan C, Singh SP, Gardner P, et al. Intraoperative neurophysiological monitoring during endoscopic endonasal surgery for pediatric skull base tumors. J Neurosurg Pediatr. 2016; 17(2):147–155

[5] Singh H, Vogel RW, Lober RM, et al. Intraoperative neurophysiological monitoring for endoscopic endonasal approaches to the skull base: a technical guide. Scientifica (Cairo). 2016; 2016:1751245

[6] Iaconetta G, de Notaris M, Cavallo LM, et al. The oculomotor nerve: microanatomical and endoscopic study. Neurosurgery. 2010; 66(3):593–601, discussion 601

[7] Abuzayed B, Tanriover N, Akar Z, Eraslan BS, Gazioglu N. Extended endoscopic endonasal approach to the suprasellar parachiasmatic cisterns: anatomic study. Childs Nerv Syst. 2010; 26(9):1161–1170

[8] Iaconetta G, de Notaris M, Benet A, et al. The trochlear nerve: microanatomic and endoscopic study. Neurosurg Rev. 2013; 36(2):227–237, discussion 237–238

[9] Benoit MM, Silvera VM, Nichollas R, Jones D, McGill T, Rahbar R. Image guidance systems for minimally invasive sinus and skull base surgery in children. Int J Pediatr Otorhinolaryngol. 2009; 73(10):1452–1457

[10] Khalili S, Palmer JN, Adappa ND. The expanded endonasal approach for the treatment of intracranial skull base disease in the pediatric population. Curr Opin Otolaryngol Head Neck Surg. 2015; 23(1):65–70

[11] Parikh SR, Cuellar H, Sadoughi B, Aroniadis O. Indications for image-guidance in pediatric sinonasal surgery. Int J Pediatr Otorhinolaryngol. 2009; 73(3):351–356

[12] Snyderman CH, Carrau RL, Prevedello DM. Technologic innovations in neuroendoscopic surgery. Otorhinolaryngol Clin North Am. 2009; 42(5):883–890

[13] Singh H, Rote S, Jada A, et al. Endoscopic endonasal odontoid resection with real-time intraoperative image-guided computed tomography: report of 4 cases. J Neurosurg. 2017:1–6

[14] Choudhri O, Mindea SA, Feroze A, Soudry E, Chang SD, Nayak JV. Experience with intraoperative navigation and imaging during endoscopic transnasal spinal approaches to the foramen magnum and odontoid. Neurosurg Focus. 2014; 36(3):E4

[15] Cavalcanti DD, Preul MC, Kalani MY, Spetzler RF. Microsurgical anatomy of safe entry zones to the brainstem. J Neurosurg. 2016; 124(5):1359–1376

[16] Abla AA, Lekovic GP, Turner JD, de Oliveira JG, Porter R, Spetzler RF. Advances in the treatment and outcome of brainstem cavernous malformation surgery: a single-center case series of 300 surgically treated patients. Neurosurgery. 2011; 68(2):403–414, discussion 414–415

[17] Abla AA, Benet A, Lawton MT. The far lateral transpontomedullary sulcus approach to pontine cavernous malformations: technical report and surgical results. Neurosurgery. 2014; 10 Suppl 3:472–480

[18] Hebb MO, Spetzler RF. Lateral transpeduncular approach to intrinsic lesions of the rostral pons. Neurosurgery. 2010; 66(3) Suppl operative:26–29, discussion 29

[19] Recalde RJ, Figueiredo EG, de Oliveira E. Microsurgical anatomy of the safe entry zones on the anterolateral brainstem related to surgical approaches to cavernous malformations. Neurosurgery. 2008; 62(3) Suppl 1:9–15, discussion 15–17

[20] Rhoton AL, Jr. The foramen magnum. Neurosurgery. 2000; 47(3) Suppl:S155–S193

[21] Dallan I, Battaglia P, de Notaris M, Caniglia M, Turri-Zanoni M. Endoscopic endonasal transclival approach to a pontine cavernous malformation: case report. Int J Pediatr Otorhinolaryngol. 2015; 79(9):1584–1588

[22] Kimball MM, Lewis SB, Werning JW, Mocco JD. Resection of a pontine cavernous malformation via an endoscopic endonasal approach: a case report. Neurosurgery. 2012; 71(1) Suppl operative:186–193, discussion 193–194

[23] Rajappa P, Margetis K, Sigounas D, Anand V, Schwartz TH, Greenfield JP. Endoscopic endonasal transclival approach to a ventral pontine pediatric ependymoma. J Neurosurg Pediatr. 2013; 12(5):465–468

[24] Sanborn MR, Kramarz MJ, Storm PB, Adappa ND, Palmer JN, Lee JY. Endoscopic, endonasal, transclival resection of a pontine cavernoma: case report. Neurosurgery. 2012; 71(1) Suppl operative:198–203

[25] Fujii T, Platt A, Zada G. Endoscopic endonasal approaches to the craniovertebral junction: a systematic review of the literature. J Neurol Surg B Skull Base. 2015; 76(6):480–488

[26] Kassam AB, Snyderman C, Gardner P, Carrau R, Spiro R. The expanded endonasal approach: a fully endoscopic transnasal approach and resection of the odontoid process: technical case report. Neurosurgery. 2005; 57(1) Suppl: E213–, discussion E213

[27] Essayed WI, Singh H, Lapadula G, Almodovar-Mercado GJ, Anand VK, Schwartz TH. Endoscopic endonasal approach to the ventral brainstem: anatomical feasibility and surgical limitations. J Neurosurg. 2017; 127(5):1139–1146

[28] Kassam AB, Prevedello DM, Thomas A, et al. Endoscopic endonasal pituitary transposition for a transdorsum sellae approach to the interpeduncular cistern. Neurosurgery. 2008; 62(3) Suppl 1:57–72, discussion 72–74

[29] Fernandez-Miranda JC, Gardner PA, Rastelli MM, Jr, et al. Endoscopic endonasal transcavernous posterior clinoidectomy with interdural pituitary transposition. J Neurosurg. 2014; 121(1):91–99

[30] Silva D, Attia M, Schwartz TH. Endoscopic endonasal posterior clinoidectomy. J Neurosurg. 2015; 122(2):478–479

[31] Bricolo A, Turazzi S. Surgery for gliomas and other mass lesions of the brainstem. Adv Tech Stand Neurosurg. 1995; 22:261–341

[32] Cheng Y, Zhang S, Chen Y, Zhao G. Safe corridor to access clivus for endoscopic trans-sphenoidal surgery: a radiological and anatomical study. PLoS One. 2015; 10(9):e0137962

[33] Cantore G, Missori P, Santoro A. Cavernous angiomas of the brain stem. Intra-axial anatomical pitfalls and surgical strategies. Surg Neurol. 1999; 52(1):84–93, discussion 93–94

[34] Ferroli P, Sinisi M, Franzini A, Giombini S, Solero CL, Broggi G. Brainstem cavernomas: long-term results of microsurgical resection in 52 patients. Neurosurgery. 2005; 56(6):1203–1212, discussion 1212–1214

[35] Porter RW, Detwiler PW, Spetzler RF, et al. Cavernous malformations of the brainstem: experience with 100 patients. J Neurosurg. 1999; 90(1):50–58

[36] Ulrich NH, Kockro RA, Bellut D, et al. Brainstem cavernoma surgery with the support of pre- and postoperative diffusion tensor imaging: initial experiences and clinical course of 23 patients. Neurosurg Rev. 2014; 37(3):481–491, discussion 492

[37] Yao Y, Ulrich NH, Guggenberger R, Alzarhani YA. Quantification of corticospinal tracts with diffusion tensor imaging in brainstem surgery: prognostic value in 14 consecutive cases at 3 T magnetic resonance. World Neurosurg. 2015; 83(6):1006–1014

[38] de Almeida JR, Zanation AM, Snyderman CH, et al. Defining the nasopalatine line: the limit for endonasal surgery of the spine. Laryngoscope. 2009; 119 (2):239–244

[39] La Corte E, Aldana PR, Ferroli P, et al. The rhinopalatine line as a reliable predictor of the inferior extent of endonasal odontoidectomies. Neurosurg Focus. 2015; 38(4):E16

[40] Singh H, Grobelny BT, Harrop J, Rosen M, Lober RM, Evans J. Endonasal access to the upper cervical spine, part one: radiographic morphometric analysis. J Neurol Surg B Skull Base. 2013; 74(3):176–184

[41] Singh H, Lober RM, Virdi GS, Lopez H, Rosen M, Evans J. Endonasal access to the upper cervical spine: part 2-cadaveric analysis. J Neurol Surg B Skull Base. 2015; 76(4):262–265

[42] Duntze J, Eap C, Kleiber J-C, et al. Advantages and limitations of endoscopic endonasal odontoidectomy. A series of nine cases. Orthop Traumatol Surg Res. 2014; 100(7):775–778

[43] Gladi M, Iacoangeli M, Specchia N, et al. Endoscopic transnasal odontoid resection to decompress the bulbo-medullary junction: a reliable anterior minimally invasive technique without posterior fusion. Eur Spine J. 2012; 21 Suppl 1:S55–S60

[44] Koutourousiou M, Filho FV, Costacou T, et al. Pontine encephalocele and abnormalities of the posterior fossa following transclival endoscopic endonasal surgery. J Neurosurg. 2014; 121(2):359–366

Part II

Pathology Specific to the Pediatric Skull Base

II

12 Meningoencephaloceles

Mehdi Zeinalizadeh, Seyed Mousa Sadrhosseini, Harley Brito da Silva, and Harminder Singh

Abstract

Congenital cranial base meningoencephaloceles are uncommon malformations characterized by a herniation of the brain and meninges through structural weaknesses in the bony structures of the skull base. The most frequent symptoms of anterior basal encephaloceles in neonates and infants are often overlooked, and cerebrospinal fluid rhinorrhea may be mistaken for runny nose and may finally be identified by recurrent episodes of meningitis. The majority of basal meningoencephaloceles are usually diagnosed in very young pediatric patients, due to respiratory distress caused by epipharyngeal obstruction. The surgical treatment of posterior basal encephaloceles in the pediatric population remains challenging. The advent of extended endoscopic cranial base surgery has allowed for a new endonasal approach for the treatment of cranial base encephaloceles, thereby minimizing patient morbidity. In this chapter, we review the endoscopic endonasal management of basal encephaloceles and present our experience regarding the effectiveness of endoscopic management in the pediatric population.

Keywords: congenital, meningoencephalocele, transsphenoidal encephalocele, endonasal, endoscopy, reconstruction, pediatric

12.1 Introduction

Trauma leading to fracture of the anterior skull base is a frequent cause of transethmoidal encephaloceles in the pediatric age group. Larger series in literature, however, report congenital encephaloceles as the most common variety.[1] A congenital encephalocele is defined as an extension of intracranial structures through a cranial defect resulting from an embryological malformation in a patient, with a medical history negative for secondary causes.[2] Encephaloceles can be meningoceles if they only contain meninges or meningoencephaloceles if they contain brain matter and meninges.[3]

Basal encephaloceles, especially the transsphenoidal type, are difficult to diagnose and to treat.[2] They have been traditionally treated by an open transcranial approach. The advent of extended endoscopic cranial base surgery has allowed for a new endonasal approach for the treatment of basal encephaloceles, thereby minimizing patient morbidity.

In this chapter, we review the endoscopic endonasal management of anterior basal encephaloceles and present our experience regarding the effectiveness of endoscopic management in the pediatric population.

12.2 Classification

Suwanwela and Suwanwela[4] proposed an origin-based classification for encephaloceles including congenital, spontaneous, or traumatic. Encephaloceles can also be classified according to their *localization* as anterior (frontoethmoidal or sincipital and basal) and posterior (infra- and supratorcular). Posterior or occipital types are the most common and compose 75% of the

encephaloceles. Frontoethmoidal and basal encephaloceles have also been defined as nasal encephaloceles. Frontoethmoidal types originate between the frontal and ethmoid bones, commonly at or anterior to the foramen cecum, and typically present as a facial mass over the nose and/or as an intranasal mass. Basal encephaloceles herniate posterior to the cribriform plate and present in the nasal cavity as opposed to external masses. Depending on the site of herniation, they are classified into five anatomic types[5]: sphenoethmoidal, transsphenoidal, spheno-orbital, transethmoidal, and sphenomaxillary (Table 12-1). Sphenoidal encephaloceles can be subdivided into *transsphenoidal* encephaloceles (▶ Fig. 12.1), which traverse the floor of the sinus and protrude into the nasal cavity or nasopharynx, and *intrasphenoidal* encephaloceles, which extend into the sphenoidal sinus. In the case of *intrasphenoidal* encephaloceles, most defects occur in the lateral wall of the sphenoidal sinus (▶ Fig. 12.2), the so-called temporosphenoidal encephaloceles.

12.3 Epidemiology, Embryology, and Pathogenesis

Encephaloceles occur in approximately 1 in 3,000 to 5,000 and the basal encephaloceles with an estimated incidence of 1 in every 35,000 live births. Nasal encephaloceles have a higher incidence in Southeast Asia than in Western countries and the Middle East.[6]

Basal encephaloceles, and the often-associated anomalies of midline structures of the brain and face, are considered to be sporadic abnormalities developed as a consequence of a neurulation disorder, or as a consequence of a mistake occurring in the complex process of ossification of the sphenoid bone.[2] Neural tissue overgrowth, viral infection, radiation, hyperthermia, hypervitaminosis, salicylates, trypan blue, hypoxia, and numerous other agents have been suggested as causes of persistent openings in the neural tube.[7]

12.4 Clinical Presentation

Unlike frontoethmoidal encephaloceles that mostly present at birth as skin-covered masses or visible protrusions on the face,

Table 12.1 Classification of basal encephaloceles

	Type of encephalocele	Definition
1	Spheno-ethmoidal	Herniation of cranial contents through the sphenoid and ethmoid bone into the posterior nasal cavity
2	Trans-sphenoidal	Herniation through the body of sphenoid bone into the sphenoid sinus or epipharynx
3	Spheno-orbital	Herniation through the superior orbital fissure or osseous defect into the orbit
4	Transethmoidal	Herniation through the lamina cribrosa into the anterior nasal cavity
5	Spheno-maxillary	Herniation through the inferior orbital fissure into the pterygopalatine fossa

over the nose, glabella, or forehead, basal encephaloceles are not externally visible, so the age of clinical diagnoses is determined by the large size of the encephalocele causing respiratory difficulties. The most frequent symptoms of anterior basal encephaloceles in neonates and infants (i.e., runny nose, nasal obstruction, mouth breathing, or snoring) are often overlooked. Cerebrospinal fluid (CSF) rhinorrhea may be mistaken for runny nose and may finally be identified by recurrent episodes of meningitis. Concomitant congenital malformations of the face, eyes, and brain are the most important clues for the diagnosis of basal encephalocele in the neonatal or infantile period.[2,6]

The majority of *transsphenoidal* meningoencephaloceles are usually diagnosed in very young pediatric patient due to manifestations such as respiratory distress caused by epipharyngeal

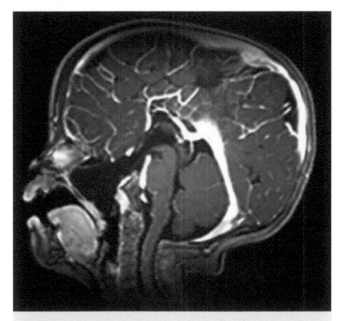

Fig. 12.1 Preoperative sagittal T1-weighted MRI with contrast injection revealing a midline soft-tissue mass without contrast enhancement consisting of mainly dysplastic brain tissue and cerebrospinal fluid extending from the suprasellar space and third ventricle through the body of the sphenoid bone into the nasopharynx, nasal cavity, and oropharynx.

obstruction, feeding difficulties, cranial midline defects with cleft lip or cleft palate, hypertelorism, optic malformations with anophthalmia, retinal abnormalities, optic nerve hypoplasia, unexplained bouts of recurrent meningitis, or endocrine abnormalities. They are commonly associated with pituitary dysfunction and visual problems attributable to the distension of the pituitary gland, hypothalamus, and optic pathways within the herniated sac. No mental retardation was seen in these patients.[2,3,7]

12.5 Diagnosis

MR imaging and CT scans are crucial preoperatively to assess associated brain abnormalities and to identify vital structures in the herniated sac. CT scans allow evaluation of bony anatomy and the associated craniofacial skeleton defects. The anterior skull base in infants is incompletely ossified or unossified. No consensus exists as to which imaging modality is considered to be most advantageous. Both CT and MRI are considered to be essential.[8] Biopsy is contraindicated for the diagnosis of nasal encephaloceles due to persisting intracranial communications.[3] Histologically, encephaloceles have shown to contain glial cells, cerebral tissue, nonfunctional neural tissue, choroid plexus, and ependymal cells.[6]

In the diagnosis of basal encephalocele, a complete hormone screening is necessary; diabetes insipidus is the most common finding of pituitary deficiency and is usually indicated by a variable thyroid hormone and cortisol response. Hormone profiles need to be monitored postoperatively and deficiencies may manifest many years after initial diagnosis.[9] Visual assessment is also recommended.

Differential diagnosis for a nasal mass should include nasal glioma, nasal polyp, or dermoid cysts. Though not restricted to the midline, a hemangioma is also included in the differential diagnosis of a pediatric nasal mass. Nasal gliomas are encephaloceles that lack a direct intracranial connection and occur as firm, noncompressible masses within the nasal cavity. In order to clinically distinguish these two entities, the Furstenberg test causes an encephalocele to enlarge due to its connection to the subarachnoid space but not a glioma.[10] Dermoid cysts present as nonpulsatile, noncompressible masses with a dimple

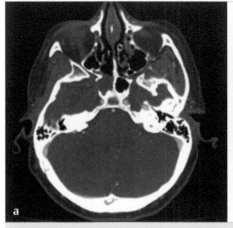
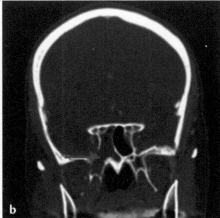
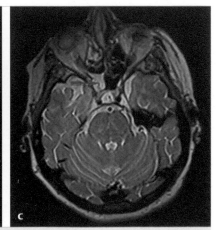

Fig. 12.2 (a–c) Preoperative axial and reconstructed coronal CT scan and axial T2-weighted MRI showing a defect (*red arrow*) at the right lateral wall of sphenoid bone through which the encephalocele has herniated.

containing a hair follicle.[4] Nasal polyps are rare in children and are usually associated with cystic fibrosis. The Furstenberg test is usually negative for most cases of nasal polyps and dermoid cysts.[6]

12.6 Treatment

Consensus management of basal encephaloceles, including the indication, timing, and the optimal mode of treatment, has yet to be established. The surgical treatment of posterior basal encephaloceles, particularly in the pediatric population, remains a challenge because of their close relationship with the opticochiasmatic structures, the hypothalamo–pituitary axis, and the proximity to the anterior and middle fossa vessels.[7] Some surgeons do not recommend the correction of encephaloceles, believing that this would result in worsening morbidity and mortality.[11] On the other hand, review of the literature reveals that a conservative approach to basal encephaloceles is associated with a progression of the signs and/or symptoms, and surgical treatment is associated with a better outcome in the long term.[2]

Surgery is the only treatment for these entities, but it requires excellent surgical skill. Strong indications for surgery include persistent CSF leak, recurrent meningitis, progression of neurological deficits, and respiratory obstruction.[11]

Reported surgical approaches for transsphenoidal encephaloceles include transpalatal, transcranial, endoscopic endonasal, or combined approaches.[11] Conventional anterior skull base surgery in children can potentially cause disruption of the growth centers in the craniofacial skeleton and result in facial asymmetry.[12] Endoscopic endonasal procedures achieve definitive repair of most anterior and middle cranial fossa CSF leaks.[13] In this sense, the lack of impact of pediatric sinus surgery on long-term facial development has been well documented.[14] Hence, endoscopic treatment allows minimizing surgical injury and consequently facilitates the management of these lesions at an earlier age.

In cases of transsphenoidal encephaloceles with large cleft palate defects, the transpalatal approaches are preferred by most authors. Performing palatal osteotomies and removing the hard palate may be technically challenging and create additional difficulties for the reconstruction of the skull base and closure of the mucosal layer. Furthermore, splitting of the palate can result in delayed palatal wound healing, palatal dehiscence, and prolonged enteral tube feeding due to velopharyngeal insufficiency.[2]

The transcranial subfrontal or pterional approach adds additional technical difficulties to a case of posterior basal encephalocele, particularly transsphenoidal type. The position of the sac in a sphenoethmoidal or transsphenoidal encephalocele is quite low and requires that a significant traction force be exerted on the frontal lobe. Therefore, these approaches are associated with high postoperative rates of morbidity, mortality, and hypothalamic dysfunction. Furthermore, infants are more susceptible to retraction injuries with subfrontal or frontotemporal approaches. In contrast to transcranial approaches, these limitations are not encountered with the endoscopic endonasal approach, because the sac is reached through natural cavities of the nostrils. Although the working space available in pediatric patients with an endoscopic approach is restricted, we have

used this approach even in children younger than 1 year.[7] Thin rigid endoscopes with an external diameter of 2.7 mm may need to be used in patients with small nares. In basal encephaloceles, except for transsphenoidal subtype, the endoscopic endonasal approach is relatively straightforward. Transsphenoidal encephalocele repair is more complicated, and we will discuss our preferred surgical technique in detail below.

12.6.1 Surgical Technique

The endoscopic endonasal approach with neuronavigation is usually used for most patients. Preparation of patients has been described in this book elsewhere. We routinely prepare the patient's right thigh and/or abdomen so that autologous fat or fascia lata can be harvested for graft reconstruction of the skull base defect, if needed. Depending on the type and location of the lesion, the extent of the approach and technical nuances may differ. Here, we describe the different endonasal approaches based on the type of the encephalocele.

Transethmoidal Encephaloceles

Direct paraseptal approach is performed for the lesion located in the cribriform plate. To gain access in some cases, it is necessary to perform an upper septoplasty and remove high septal bone. Every effort is made to preserve the middle turbinate. Once the lesion is visualized, the mucosal layer overlying the extruded dural sac is dissected from the surrounding structures to fully expose the bony defect at the skull base. Smaller encephaloceles can be shrunk with bipolar cautery, whereas larger encephaloceles presenting with neural tissue may need to be debulked with a suction-rotation microdebrider. In the majority of cases in this area, the encephalocele consists of nonfunctional neural tissue, which can be removed without neurological sequel. Once the encephalocele is minimized down to the level of the bony skull base defect, hemostasis is carefully obtained and the edges of the bony and dural defects are defined with an angled dissector or curette.

The method for closure of pure transethmoidal encephaloceles largely depends on the size of the defect being repaired. Defects of the cribriform plate smaller than 0.5 cm are usually repaired with a small onlay graft of fat, mucosa, or fascia. Defects sized 0.5 to 1 cm are usually repaired in a multilayer fashion with a piece of fat into the defect reinforced by an onlay fascia lata or free mucosal graft. The fat is pushed into the dural defect by using a blunt angled probe or curette followed by gentle pressure exerted using a cottonoid pledget. A second layer of fascia lata or free mucosal graft is subsequently used as an onlay graft. Larger defects with high-flow CSF leaks may require multilayered watertight closure accompanied by a pedicled flap.

Sphenomaxillary Encephaloceles

Endoscopic endonasal transpterygoid is the classic approach to sphenomaxillary and lateral recess sphenoid sinus encephaloceles. These types of encephaloceles usually occur in well-pneumatized sphenoid sinuses with large lateral recesses. After a maxillary antrostomy, to obtain full visualization of the pterygopalatine fossa (PPF) and associated neurovascular structures, the orbital process of the palatine bone and the posteromedial wall of the maxillary sinus must be removed. The contents of the PPF must be retracted laterally to allow exposure of the pterygoid process. With successful drilling of the pterygoid process, the lateral recesses of the sphenoid sinus should be widely exposed, with sufficient room to access and repair the skull base defect. The dural and bony defect should be reconstructed as described previously for transethmoidal encephaloceles.

Transsphenoidal and Sphenoethmoidal Encephaloceles

The surgical treatment of these types of encephaloceles, particularly in the pediatric population, is challenging. Therefore, we describe our surgical technique to treat these lesions in a stepwise fashion below.[7] An illustrative intraoperative video showcasing the technique is also attached:

- *Septal flap preparation*: A standard nasoseptal flap (NSF) is harvested on the right for reconstruction of the preexisting skull base defect (▶ Fig. 12.3a). With the help of a monopolar cautery and blunt dissection, the anterior attachment of the encephalocele to the posterior septum is disconnected.
- *Meningoencephalocele sac aspiration*: A 23-gauge spinal needle is introduced into the anteroinferior portion of the lesion, away from any critical neurovascular structures (▶ Fig. 12.3b), and CSF is gradually drained to decompress the meningoencephalocele sac. We usually do not use intraoperative lumbar drainage or external ventricular drainage for the procedure.
- *Dissection of the mucosal layer from meningoencephalocele sac*: The mucosa is dissected off the encephalocele sac in an anterior to posterior and superior to inferior direction (▶ Fig. 12.3c). Gradually, the sac is entirely separated from the

surrounding mucosal layer without any overt rupture; pinhole tears in the sac are unavoidable, however. Resection of anomalous herniated brain elements is *not* performed, except for taking a small biopsy from the most posteroinferior portion of the encephalocele wall.
- *Reduction of herniated encephalocele sac*: The herniated encephalocele sac is gradually pushed back into normal anatomic alignment to the floor of the cranial base dura (▶ Fig. 12.3d). When the dissection of the encephalocele sac is insufficient and not done circumferentially around the bony defect, it is difficult to reduce the sac completely.
- *Reconstruction of the bony cranial base defect*: The reduced encephalocele sac is covered by a fascia lata graft. A small flexible titanium mesh plate is fixed to the clivus inferiorly with screws, and is wedged underneath the bony edge anterosuperiorly, reconstructing the skull base (▶ Fig. 12.3e). Finally, the area is covered with a standard posterior pedicle nasoseptal flap.
- *Reconstruction of donor septal flap cartilage*: The septal flap donor site is reconstructed by using a free fascia lata graft[15] (▶ Fig. 12.3f).

Illustrative Case

A 24-month-old boy presenting with failure to thrive (FTT), cleft lip, nasal obstruction, polydipsia, and polyuria was referred for the treatment of nasal airway obstruction and cleft lip. The preoperative MRI and CT scan revealed agenesis of the corpus callosum, and a transsellar, transsphenoidal meningoencephalocele that protruded through a large skull base defect in the middle of the sphenoid bone (▶ Fig. 12.4 and ▶ Fig. 12.5a). The patient underwent surgical correction of the encephalocele through an

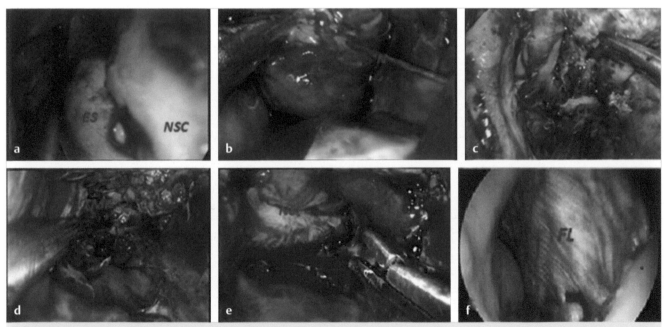

Fig. 12.3 Endoscopic view via the right nasal cavity demonstrating the technique for the repair of a transsphenoidal encephalocele. (a) Intraoperative view of denuded nasal septal cartilage (*NSC*) after harvesting the Hadad–Bassagaisteguy flap and exposing the anterior surface of the encephalocele sac (*ES*). (b) Aspiration of the sac by means of a spinal needle(*N*) number 23 to the anteroinferior portion of the lesion. (c) Pushback the sac to the normal anatomic position of the cranial base dura matter near the floor of sellar area and exposing the clivus (*CL*). (d) Reconstruction of the bony cranial base defect with a titanium (*TMP*) mesh plate fixed to the clivus. (e) The final position of the standard posterior pedicle nasoseptal flap (*NSF*). (f) Intraoperative view of donor septal site reconstructed with fascia lata graft (*FL*).

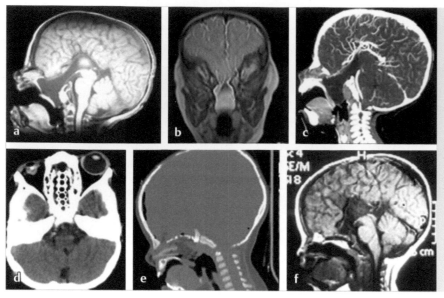

Fig. 12.4 (a,b) Preoperative sagittal T1- and coronal T2-weighted MR images demonstrating a transsphenoidal cephalocele. **(c)** Preoperative reconstructed sagittal CT scan with contrast injection revealing a large defect in body of the sphenoid bone with a transsphenoidal encephalocele. **(d,e)** Early postoperative axial and reconstructed sagittal CT scan showing the satisfied position of titanium mesh plate fixed into the clivus as well as a small amount of pneumocephalus in frontal area. **(f)** Postoperative MRI demonstrating reduction of encephalocele and a patent airway at 3 months.

endoscopic endonasal approach as described earlier for transsphenoidal encephaloceles (▶ Fig. 12.5b). The postoperative course was uneventful and the patient initiated oral diet on postoperative day 1. Postoperative CT scan (▶ Fig. 12.4d, e) was performed and the patient was discharged on postoperative day 7. Six months later, he underwent the repair of his cleft lip. MRI was performed at 6 month follow-up (▶ Fig. 12.4f). The patient completely regained the normal weight for his age, developed no CSF leak, and had no other complications at 2-year follow-up.

12.7 Complications

Surgical treatment of basal encephaloceles in the pediatric population has been associated with postoperative complications, including palatal dehiscence, recurrence of encephalocele, CSF leak, meningitis, epiphora, diabetes insipidus, recurrent meningitis, neurological deficits, development of seizures, panhypopituitarism, and even convulsions.[16] The main complication reported in the literature is postoperative meningitis.[2] A high risk of postoperative hypothalamic dysfunction and increased intracranial pressure has been reported after intracranial repair.[15]

Previous reports showed that the rates of mortality and morbidity/long-term severe disability, mainly through transcranial surgery, approached 50% and 70%, respectively.[17] These unsatisfactory results are considered to be partly due to insufficient dissection of the encephalocele at the posterior edge of the bony defect, and to resection of the encephalocele and its contents.[18] In contrast, repairing of anterior skull base defects with endoscopic endonasal techniques had significantly lower rates of complications such as meningitis, abscess/wound infection, and sepsis than open approaches.[19] We did not encounter any major complications in our series of patients.[7]

12.8 Conclusion

The surgical treatment of basal encephaloceles, especially transsphenoidal type with a descended voluminous sac into the naso-/oropharynx, remains a challenge. The endoscopic endonasal approach is not only feasible but also a minimally invasive, safe, and practical alternative. In this regard, the importance of a dedicated team consisting of an experienced otolaryngologist and neurosurgeon is critical for its success.

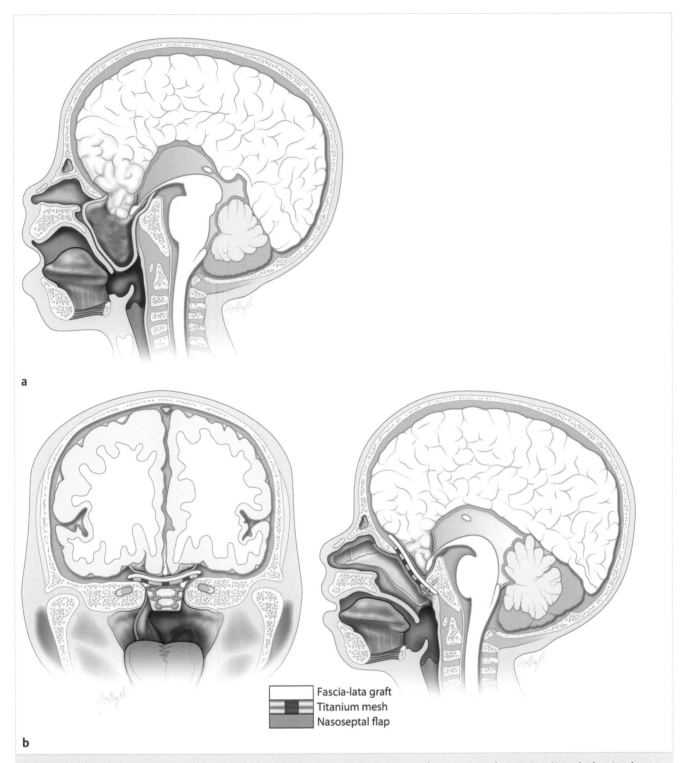

a

b

Fascia-lata graft
Titanium mesh
Nasoseptal flap

Fig. 12.5 **(a)** An artist's rendition of a transsphenoidal encephalocele in a pediatric patient, shown in sagittal projection. Note the herniated encephalocele sac crowding the naso- and oropharynx, which leads to respiratory distress. **(b)** Multilayered skull base closure after reduction of a transsphenoidal encephalocele in coronal and sagittal views.

References

[1] Keshri AK, Shah SR, Patadia SD, Sahu RN, Behari S. Transnasal endoscopic repair of pediatric meningoencephalocele. J Pediatr Neurosci. 2016; 11(1):42–45

[2] Spacca B, Amasio ME, Giordano F, et al. Surgical management of congenital median perisellar transsphenoidal encephaloceles with an extracranial approach: a series of 6 cases. Neurosurgery. 2009; 65(6):1140–1145, discussion 1145–1146

[3] Abdel-Aziz M, El-Bosraty H, Qotb M, et al. Nasal encephalocele: endoscopic excision with anesthetic consideration. Int J Pediatr Otorhinolaryngol. 2010; 74(8):869–873

[4] Suwanwela C, Suwanwela N. A morphological classification of sincipital encephalomeningoceles. J Neurosurg. 1972; 36(2):201–211

[5] Chen CS, David D, Hanieh A. Morning glory syndrome and basal encephalocele. Childs Nerv Syst. 2004; 20(2):87–90

[6] Tirumandas M, Sharma A, Gbenimacho I, et al. Nasal encephaloceles: a review of etiology, pathophysiology, clinical presentations, diagnosis, treatment, and complications. Childs Nerv Syst. 2013; 29(5):739–744

[7] Zeinalizadeh M, Habibi Z, Nejat F, Brito da Silva H, Singh H. Endonasal management of pediatric congenital transsphenoidal encephaloceles: nuances of a modified re-construction technique. J Neurosurg Pediatr. 2017; 19(3):312–318

[8] Huisman TA, Schneider JF, Kellenberger CJ, Martin-Fiori E, Willi UV, Holzmann D. Developmental nasal midline masses in children: neuroradiological evaluation. Eur Radiol. 2004; 14(2):243–249

[9] Morioka M, Marubayashi T, Masumitsu T, Miura M, Ushio Y. Basal encephaloceles with morning glory syndrome, and progressive hormonal and visual disturbances: case report and review of the literature. Brain Dev. 1995; 17(3):196–201

[10] Rahbar R, Resto VA, Robson CD, et al. Nasal glioma and encephalocele: diagnosis and management. Laryngoscope. 2003; 113(12):2069–2077

[11] Abe T, Lüdecke DK, Wada A, Matsumoto K. Transsphenoidal cephaloceles in adults. A report of two cases and review of the literature. Acta Neurochir (Wien). 2000; 142(4):397–400

[12] de Divitiis E, Cappabianca P, Gangemi M, Cavallo LM. The role of the endoscopic transsphenoidal approach in pediatric neurosurgery. Childs Nerv Syst. 2000; 16(10–11):692–696

[13] Castelnuovo P, Dallan I, Pistochini A, Battaglia P, Locatelli D, Bignami M. Endonasal endoscopic repair of Sternberg's canal cerebrospinal fluid leaks. Laryngoscope. 2007; 117(2):345–349

[14] Bothwell MR, Piccirillo JF, Lusk RP, Ridenour BD. Long-term outcome of facial growth after functional endoscopic sinus surgery. Otolaryngol Head Neck Surg. 2002; 126(6):628–634

[15] Yokota A, Matsukado Y, Fuwa I, Moroki K, Nagahiro S. Anterior basal encephalocele of the neonatal and infantile period. Neurosurgery. 1986; 19(3):468–478

[16] Baradaran N, Nejat F, Baradaran N, El Khashab M. Cephalocele: report of 55 cases over 8 years. Pediatr Neurosurg. 2009; 45(6):461–466

[17] David DJ. Cephaloceles: classification, pathology, and management–a review. J Craniofac Surg. 1993; 4(4):192–202

[18] Ogiwara H, Morota N. Surgical treatment of transsphenoidal encephaloceles: transpalatal versus combined transpalatal and transcranial approach. J Neurosurg Pediatr. 2013; 11(5):505–510

[19] Komotar RJ, Starke RM, Raper DM, Anand VK, Schwartz TH. Endoscopic endonasal versus open repair of anterior skull base CSF leak, meningocele, and encephalocele: a systematic review of outcomes. J Neurol Surg A Cent Eur Neurosurg. 2013; 74(4):239–250

[20] Zeinalizadeh M, Sadrehosseini SM, Barkhoudarian G, Carrau RL. Reconstruction of the denuded nasoseptal flap donor site with a free fascia lata graft: technical note. Eur Arch Otorhinolaryngol. 2016; 273(10):3179–3182

13 Sellar Arachnoid Cysts

Jason Chu, Joseph R. Keen, and Nelson M. Oyesiku

Abstract

Arachnoid cysts are benign cerebral fluid filled expansions of normal arachnoid mater. They are believed to be congenital lesions that develop in utero. Most often, they are found incidentally. Large intrasellar cysts can cause clinical symptoms by putting pressure on the optic nerves and pituitary gland. The intrasellar arachnoid cysts can be drained via the endoscopic transphenoidal approach, with or without cyst fenestration into the suprasellar subarachnoid space. In this chapter, the authors describe their preferred approach for treating intrasellar arachnoid cysts in pediatric patients.

Keywords: arachnoid cysts, intrasellular, suprasellular, sellar, pituitary gland, transsphenoidal, Rathke's cleft cyst, CFS leak

13.1 Introduction

Arachnoid cysts (ACs) are benign, cerebrospinal fluid (CSF) filled expansions of the normal arachnoid mater. The first known report of an intracranial AC was published by the English physician Richard Bright in 1831. He described these as "serous cysts forming in connection with the arachnoid and apparently between its layers."[1] Ultrastructural analysis conducted by Rengachary and Watanabe demonstrated four characteristic features of ACs: splitting of the arachnoid membrane at the cyst margin, hyperplastic arachnoid cells in the cyst wall, a thick collagen layer within the cyst wall, and the absence of traversing trabecular processes within the cyst.[2] ACs are believed to be congenital lesions that develop in utero, although there are rare reports of them having occurred after trauma, infection, or even de novo. Clinically, they typically have a benign natural history.

In the pediatric population, they are often found incidentally on imaging upon workup for other symptoms or head trauma. A recent study that analyzed over 12,000 pediatric MRI scans suggested that overall incidence of ACs in children is approximately 2.6%.[3] Their study also revealed a male and left-sided predominance. The middle fossa (47%) and posterior fossa (38%) were the two most common places ACs were observed in, with the remainder of the cysts seen in the quadrigeminal plate (6%), cerebral convexity (4%), anterior fossa (2%), sellar/suprasellar (2%) and interhemispheric (1%). Intrasellar arachnoid cyst (IAC) and suprasellar arachnoid cyst (SAC) deserve special attention due to their unique location and proximity to the pituitary gland, optic apparatus, hypothalamus, and third ventricle. These variants often produce clinical symptoms, including obstructive hydrocephalus, endocrine dysfunction, visual disturbances, and neurocognitive deficits. As a result, they require some form of neurosurgical intervention and the introduction of neuroendoscopy has shifted management, from CSF diversion devices and open microsurgical approaches to a minimally invasive approach. This chapter will focus on IACs and their endoscopic skull base management.

13.2 Epidemiology and Pathogenesis

The differential diagnosis for a cystic lesion in the sellar region should include Rathke's cleft cyst, craniopharyngioma, IAC, dermoid or epidermoid cysts, and empty sella syndrome. IACs are infrequently encountered and represent approximately 3% of all intracranial ACs.[2] Overall, there have been less than 100 cases reported in the English literature.[4] Moreover, the majority of those published have shown an adult predominance. Not only does this make these lesions exceedingly rare in the pediatric population, but it also suggests that the exact incidence and natural history of IACs in children remain unknown. Interestingly, this is in stark contrast to SAC, which have been well documented in children, and the reason for this discrepancy is unclear.

The development of any ACs may be due to a combination of mechanisms, and the prevailing theories include a one-way valve mechanism where CSF enters the cyst but cannot escape, an osmotic gradient enables fluid to collect in the cyst, and the normal arachnoid membranes may actively secrete fluid into the cyst. Within the sella, there is typically no arachnoid membrane below the diaphragma sellae and one theory for the formation of IACs involves the herniation of the basal arachnoid membranes through the diaphragma aperture.[5] The diaphragmatic aperture has been shown to have significant variation in size, with the aperture found to be larger than the pituitary stalk in approximately 40% of patients.[6] Hornig and Zervas postulated that the development of IACs must also involve a slit-valve mechanism from a diaphragmatic defect that allows unilateral transgression of CSF from the suprasellar area into the sella turcica.[7] The mechanism of a one-way valve was directly visualized by the authors during transsphenoidal fenestration of a sellar AC and they suggested that even a 1-mm slit perforation of the diaphragma could lead to the development of an IAC (▶ Fig. 13.1). Dubuisson et al observed that approximately 50% of their IACs in their series did not communicate with the suprasellar arachnoid space ("noncommunicating" cysts). They hypothesized that the site of CSF transgression may eventually close when intrasellar pressure counteracts the intracranial pressure due to apposition of the arachnoid membranes.[5] This closure has been speculated to be accelerated by infection, hemorrhage, or inflammatory events.

A histopathologic examination of an IAC was reported by Güdük et al, and they observed that the cyst wall was fibrous and contained a monolayer of flattened arachnoid cells on a reticulin rich basement membrane[4] (▶ Fig. 13.2). Immunohistochemistry was positive for epithelial membrane antigen (EMA) but negative for glial fibrillary acidic protein (GFAP), Ki-67, synaptophysin, and S-100. The combination of the histological and immunohistochemical findings aided in differentiating IACs from other epithelial cysts.

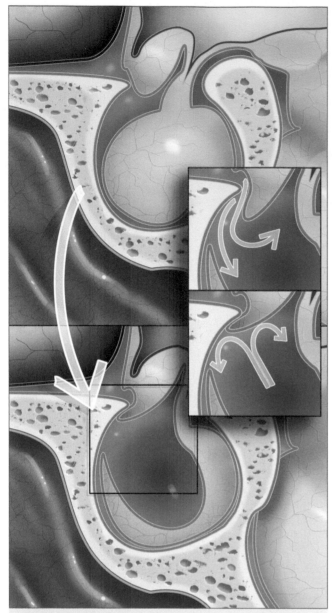

Fig. 13.1 Sellar arachnoid cysts may arise from the herniation of basal arachnoid membranes into the sella through a defect in the diaphragmatic aperture. The pulsatile cerebrospinal fluid (CSF) force drives suprasellar subarachnoid space into the sella. The pituitary stalk and gland participate in a slit valve–like mechanism for one way flow into the sella (inset). (Adapted from Dubuisson et al.[5])

13.3 Clinical Symptoms and Diagnostic Radiology Findings

The clinical symptoms of IAC are mainly due to their mass effect on the pituitary gland and the optic apparatus. Therefore, they may mimic those of a nonfunctional pituitary adenoma. Given the paucity of literature regarding IACs, Dubuisson et al conducted an extensive review and reported the clinical symptoms from 14 published papers on IACs between 1980 and 2007. A total of 51 patients (age range: 16–80 years; mean age: 47 years) were identified in their review and the main presenting

symptoms were visual disturbances (55%) and headache (41%).[5] While the visual symptoms may be explained by mass effect against the optic nerves and chiasm, the symptoms of headache are less specific, although some authors have attributed it to the dural distension caused by the cyst. Endocrine abnormalities were less common (22%) and symptomatic patients mainly had gonadotropic dysfunction (menstrual irregularity, decreased libido, impotence, and infertility), growth hormone insufficiency, or mild hyperprolactinemia. Bordo et al described severe hyponatremia (mean sodium level 115 ± 6 mmol/L) in three of eight patients with IACs as well as hypoadrenalism and hypothyroidism.[8]

ACs have a distinct appearance on both CT and MRI (▶ Fig. 13.3). On CT, they are well-circumscribed, nonenhancing masses that are typically hypodense. CT cisternography may also demonstrate communication with the subarachnoid space. MRI provides a definitive diagnosis, as they are well-demarcated fluid collections that should parallel CSF on all sequences. They are nonenhancing, isointense with CSF on T1- and T2-weighted imaging, exhibit T2 suppression on fluid attenuation inversion recovery (FLAIR) sequences, and lack diffusion restriction on diffusion-weighted imaging (DWI). In some instances, the IAC may appear slightly hyperintense to CSF on T1 sequences due to stagnation of fluid and elevated protein concentration.[9] IACs are isolated sellar lesions that may distort the pituitary gland, medial cavernous sinus walls, or the optic apparatus. Some studies suggest that the IAC may displace the pituitary gland posteroinferiorly, and this may be a differentiating factor from Rathke's cleft cyst, in which the pituitary gland may be distorted anteriorly.[5,9,10] Extension of an IAC into the suprasellar region has also been described.[5]

13.4 Management

The management of IACs is analogous to the management of a nonfunctioning pituitary adenoma. Asymptomatic lesions rarely require any form of intervention and can be followed with serial imaging.[11] Indications for surgical intervention include an enlarging cyst on serial imaging, visual compromise from mass effect on the optic nerves/chiasm, pituitary dysfunction, and severe headaches. The main goal of surgery is to decompress the cyst and relieve mass effect. Secondary goals include excision of all or part of the cyst membranes as well as fenestration of the cyst into the suprasellar cistern (cyst cisternostomy) in order to prevent recurrence. Given the location of IACs in the sella, the transsphenoidal approach to the cyst is favorable over a transcranial route and this can be accomplished via either the microscope or endoscope. Intraoperative findings should include egress of clear, CSF-like fluid after the cyst wall is opened. A normal pituitary gland, stalk, and diaphragma sellae may also be observed.[4] As part of the transsphenoidal approach, the sellar floor must be thoroughly packed and reconstructed at the end of the operation to prevent postoperative CSF leak. To our knowledge, there have not been any reports of cyst shunt placement for the treatment of IACs.

The outcomes after transsphenoidal approach to IAC have been favorable, and several reports suggest that recurrence is exceedingly rare,[4] although the exact rate remains unknown. The few reports that have documented recurrence suggest that it occurs in a delayed fashion and several years after the original

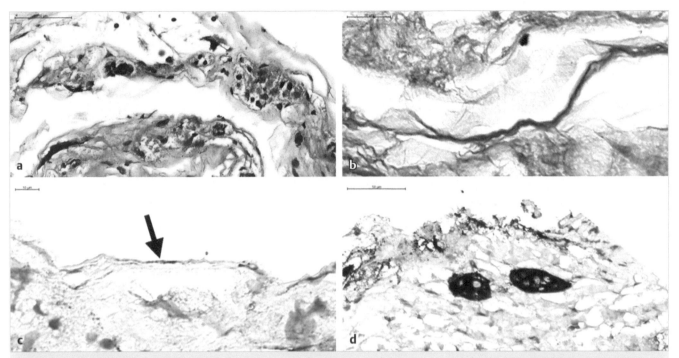

Fig. 13.2 Histopathology and immunohistochemistry of a sellar arachnoid cyst. **(a)** Flattened arachnoid cells lined on thin basement membrane (hematoxylin and eosin; ×59.7). **(b)** Basement membrane rich in reticulin fibers within the cyst wall (Gomori's reticulum stain, ×113.2). **(c)** Cyst wall lined with flattened arachnoidal cells stained with epithelial membrane antigen (EMA; *arrow*; biotinylated streptavidin complement, EMA, ×127.5). **(d)** Anterior pituitary cell cluster in close neighborhood of cyst wall (biotinylated streptavidin complement, synaptophysin, ×61.0). (Adapted from Güdük et al.[4])

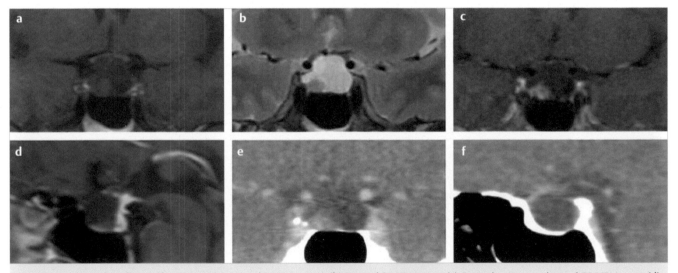

Fig. 13.3 Imaging of a sellar arachnoid cyst. **(a)** Coronal T1 MRI image. **(b)** Coronal T2 MRI image. **(c)** Coronal contrast-enhanced T1 MRI image. **(d)** Sagittal contrast-enhanced T1 MRI image. **(e,f)** Coronal and sagittal CT images. (Adapted from Güdük et al.[4])

operation.[4,12] Symptomatic IAC recurrence entails another operation through either a repeat transsphenoidal approach or transcranial approach. Murakami et al suggested that a craniotomy and transsylvian approach may be advantageous for reoperations, as it enabled wide cyst wall excision and communication between the cyst and the suprasellar cistern.[12] Visual deficits and partial pituitary dysfunction have both been reported to improve postoperatively.[5] Nonetheless, long-term follow-up after treatment of IACs has been recommended.

A delayed CSF leak following the transsphenoidal approach is a common postoperative complication, and the incidence has been reported to be as high as 21.4%.[13] CSF rhinorrhea typically presented 5 to 7 days after surgery; however, it was not uncommon outside this window. Any CSF leak is accompanied by an increased risk of meningitis and can be upward of 8% after the transsphenoidal approach for IACs.[4] Temporary CSF diversion with a lumbar drain is often employed as first-line treatment of CSF rhinorrhea; however, the current literature suggests that patients will often require a second operation to repair the site of the CSF fistula. Persistent CSF leaks may require a permanent CSF diversion device.[13] A rare, but feared, complication is one in which the optic apparatus prolapses into an empty sella with resultant blindness.[14] This has been reported, and the authors postulated that this could have been prevented if the sella was more efficiently packed at time of closure.

13.5 Role of Endoscopic Endonasal Surgery

The endoscope remains the instrument of choice for the transsphenoidal approach for the treatment of IACs and is a safe and viable option in the pediatric population as long as the sinuses are adequately pneumatized.[15] The details and advantages of this approach have been previously described in Chapter 7. As mentioned earlier, postoperative CSF leak after the transsphenoidal approach for IACs is common and higher than the standard rate of transsphenoidal surgery for other sellar lesions. A smaller durotomy may be required for cases of IACs and meticulous closure of the sella is imperative.

Given the high rate of postoperative CSF leak, Oyama et al recently described their technique for transsphenoidal cyst cisternostomy for IACs with a keyhole dural opening[16] (▶ Fig. 13.4 and ▶ Fig. 13.5). Their method was based on an extended transsphenoidal approach and involved a combination of the microscope and endoscope. In brief, a bony opening is made from the upper third of the sellar floor to the planum sphenoidale. A 1-cm-sized linear durotomy is made and with the assistance of a 30-degree endoscope, the prechiasmatic cistern is entered. The cyst wall, optic chiasm, and anterior communicating artery are identified. Cyst cisternostomy is completed along the anterior wall of the cyst and communicates the cyst with the prechiasmatic cistern. If the posterior wall is accessible, fenestration can connect it to the prepontine cistern. A duraplasty is then conducted with a fascia lata graft and 6–0 monofilament suture in a watertight fashion. The reconstructed area is then covered with a fat graft and fibrin glue. In their series, only one of seven patients developed a postoperative CSF leak that was successfully treated with 5 days of lumbar drainage. More importantly, all patients reported improvement in their preoperative visual defects and no new pituitary dysfunction or neurologic deficit was observed after surgery. Two patients were found to have

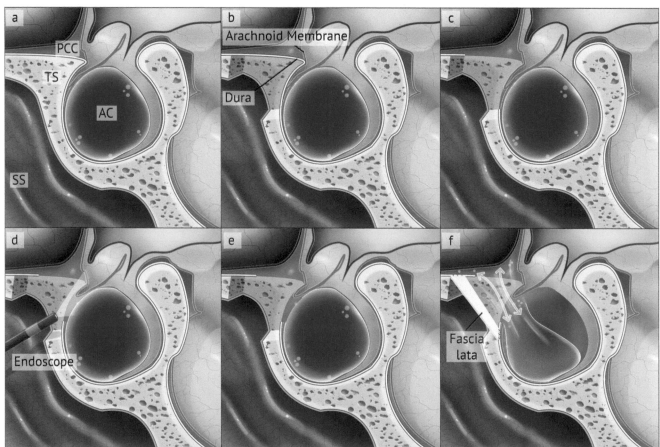

Fig. 13.4 An illustrated technique for transsphenoidal cyst cisternostomy with keyhole dural opening as described by Oyama et al.[16] **(a)** Schematic representation of a sellar arachnoid cyst (AC). A flattened pituitary gland (PG) is displaced posteriorly. PCC, prechiasmatic cistern; TS, tuberculum sellae; SS, sphenoid sinus. **(b)** The bony window is opened from the upper third of the enlarged sellar floor to the planum sphenoidale. **(c)** A 1-cm-long I-shaped keyhole dural opening is made by incising the dura from the upper edge of the sellar dura mater to the anterior skull base. Subsequently, the arachnoid membrane of the prechiasmatic cistern can be opened. **(d)** A 30-degree angled endoscope measuring 2.7 mm in diameter is inserted into the prechiasmatic cistern to confirm the position of the cyst wall, optic chiasm, and anterior communicating artery complex. **(e)** The anterior surface of the cyst wall can be opened, resulting in a communication between the cyst cavity and the prechiasmatic cistern. **(f)** Completion of our cyst-cisternostomy. A watertight duraplasty is performed using fascia lata, six to eight stitches with 6–0 monofilament sutures and fibrin glue. (Adapted from Oyama et al.[16])

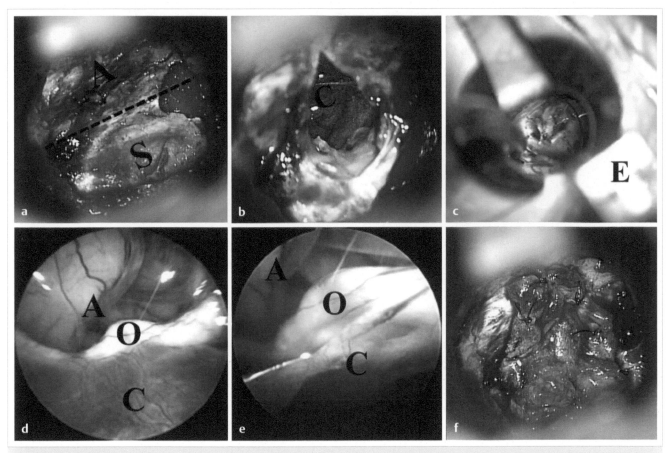

Fig. 13.5 Intraoperative images for a transsphenoidal cyst cisternostomy with keyhole dural opening as described by Oyama et al.[16] Microscopic (a–c, f) and endoscopic (d,e) are shown. (a) Dural surface after removal of the bone adjacent to the tuberculum sellae. A, dura of the anterior skull base; S, dura of the sella. The dotted line indicates the position of the removed tuberculum sellae. (b) An I-shaped keyhole dural opening is made. The arachnoid membrane of the prechiasmatic cistern is open and the cyst wall C is visible. (c) An angled endoscope E is inserted through the keyhole dural opening into the prechiasmatic cistern to confirm the relationship between the cyst wall and surrounding structures. (d,e) View of the 30-degree endoscope placed in the prechiasmatic cistern before (d) and after (e) cyst opening. A, anterior communicating artery complex; O, optic chiasm; C, cyst wall. (f) Duraplasty using fascia lata and eight stitches with 6–0 monofilament sutures. (Adapted from Oyama et al.[16])

recurrence at a mean follow-up period of 42.2 months; however, only one underwent reoperation. The authors concluded that this method is a safe and low-complication alternative to the standard transsphenoidal cyst cisternostomy, especially when it comes to postoperative CSF leaks.

13.5.1 Surgical Approach

Two general approaches have been adopted, one in which the communication between the AC and the subarachnoid space (SAS) is augmented, and the other, deliberately not. In both cases, however, the cyst cavity is obliterated and the floor of the sella is reconstructed with an extradural buttress or a nasoseptal flap. Both have been shown to have similar rates of postoperative CSF leakage and cyst recurrence.[5,17]

Our endonasal technique explicitly enlarges the communication between the AC and SAS to eliminate the ball-valve mechanism. We always advocate for a wide sphenoidotomy extending from one cavernous sinus to the other to allow for a wide dural opening, which is incised meticulously to preserve the underlying cyst capsule. Once identified, a plane between the cyst capsule and pituitary gland should be established to preserve the

gland, and extracapsular dissection will continue until points of herniation through the diaphragma are encountered. This will ensure the best chances for maximal cyst resection and preservation of pituitary function. Next, the cyst can be entered with the endoscope, inspected for the presence of tumor characteristics, and excised. Any remaining herniations through the diaphragma sella should be excised and fenestrated broadly into the SAS. Once hemostasis has been obtained and maximal cyst resection has been performed, the empty sella should be packed in layered fashion with adipose tissue, dural graft substitute, and a dural sealant. A pedicled, vascularized, nasoseptal flap can then be overlaid and sealed with another layer of dural sealant (▶ Fig. 13.6). We also advocate for CSF diversion via lumbar drainage for 3 to 5 days postoperatively.

The two main pitfalls include CSF rhinorrhea and cyst recurrence, which are usually the result of either an inadequately obliterated sellar cavity, failure, or inadequate nasoseptal flap, and/or persistence of the IAC-SAS communication. CSF leakage can typically be addressed with CSF lumbar drainage (10–15 mL/h) for 3 to 5 additional days. If leakage persists or the cyst recurs and is causing symptoms, the patient should undergo re-exploration to evaluate the integrity and adequacy of the nasoseptal flap and, in

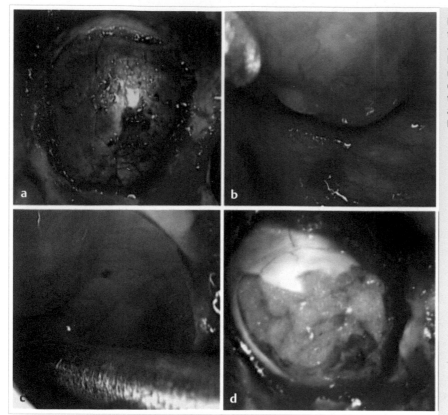

Fig. 13.6 Select images depicting the endoscopic technique for management of intrasellar arachnoid cysts. **(a)** View of the cystic intrasellar lesion through the dura using the endoscope. **(b,c)** View of the cyst's cavity using the endoscope. **(d)** Filling of the cavity with adipose tissue. A dural substitute with dural sealant is an alternative method for closure. (Adapted from McLaughlin et al.[17])

the case of cyst recurrence, re-resection of cyst wall and repeating the original closure techniques.

13.6 Conclusion

Sellar ACs are rare intracranial lesions, especially in the pediatric population. Nonetheless, they should be included in the differential diagnosis for any cystic lesion within the sella. Although they are believed to have a benign natural history, large IACs can produce clinical symptoms secondary to mass effect on the optic apparatus and pituitary gland. The preferred choice of surgical intervention is an endoscopic, endonasal transsphenoidal cyst cisternostomy. Postoperative CSF leak and meningitis are higher than standard transsphenoidal approaches, and surgeons should be vigilant about recognizing these complications early after surgery. Outcome after surgery is favorable with improvements in preoperative symptoms and low recurrence rate.

References

[1] Bright R. Serous cysts in the arachnoid. In: Rees O, Brown, Green, ed. Diseases of the Brain and Nervous System. Part I. London, UK: Longman Group Ltd; 1831

[2] Rengachary SS, Watanabe I. Ultrastructure and pathogenesis of intracranial arachnoid cysts. J Neuropathol Exp Neurol. 1981; 40(1):61–83

[3] Al-, Holou WN, Yew AY, Boomsaad ZE, Garton HJ, Muraszko KM, Maher CO. Prevalence and natural history of arachnoid cysts in children. J Neurosurg Pediatr. 2010; 5(6):578–585

[4] Güdük M, HamitAytar M, Sav A, Berkman Z. Intrasellar arachnoid cyst: a case report and review of the literature. Int J Surg Case Rep. 2016; 23:105–108

[5] Dubuisson AS, Stevenaert A, Martin DH, Flandroy PP. Intrasellar arachnoid cysts. Neurosurgery. 2007; 61(3):505–513, discussion 513

[6] Bergland RM, Ray BS, Torack RM. Anatomical variations in the pituitary gland and adjacent structures in 225 human autopsy cases. J Neurosurg. 1968; 28 (2):93–99

[7] Hornig GW, Zervas NT. Slit defect of the diaphragma sellae with valve effect: observation of a "slit valve.". Neurosurgery. 1992; 30(2):265–267

[8] Bordo G, Kelly K, McLaughlin N, et al. Sellar masses that present with severe hyponatremia. Endocr Pract. 2014; 20(11):1178–1186

[9] Meyer FB, Carpenter SM, Laws ER, Jr. Intrasellar arachnoid cysts. Surg Neurol. 1987; 28(2):105–110

[10] Nomura M, Tachibana O, Hasegawa M, et al. Contrast-enhanced MRI of intrasellar arachnoid cysts: relationship between the pituitary gland and cyst. Neuroradiology. 1996; 38(6):566–568

[11] Pradilla G, Jallo G. Arachnoid cysts: case series and review of the literature. Neurosurg Focus. 2007; 22(2):E7

[12] Murakami M, Okumura H, Kakita K. Recurrent intrasellar arachnoid cyst. Neurol Med Chir (Tokyo). 2003; 43(6):312–315

[13] Saeki N, Tokunaga H, Hoshi S, et al. Delayed postoperative CSF rhinorrhea of intrasellar arachnoid cyst. Acta Neurochir (Wien). 1999; 141(2):165–169

[14] Spaziante R, de, Divitiis E, Stella L, Cappabianca P, Donzelli R. Benign intrasellar cysts. Surg Neurol. 1981; 15(4):274–282

[15] Chivukula S, Koutourousiou M, Snyderman CH, Fernandez-Miranda JC, Gardner PA, Tyler-, Kabara EC. Endoscopic endonasal skull base surgery in the pediatric population. J Neurosurg Pediatr. 2013; 11(3):227–241

[16] Oyama K, Fukuhara N, Taguchi M, Takeshita A, Takeuchi Y, Yamada S. Transsphenoidal cyst cisternostomy with a keyhole dural opening for sellar arachnoid cysts: technical note. Neurosurg Rev. 2014; 37(2):261–267, discussion 267

[17] McLaughlin N, Vandergrift A, Ditzel, , Filho LF, et al. Endonasal management of sellar arachnoid cysts: simple cyst obliteration technique. J Neurosurg. 2012; 116(4):728–740

14 Odontoidectomy for Craniovertebral Junction Compression

Harminder Singh, Andrew Alalade, Jeffrey P. Greenfield, Vijay K. Anand, and Theodore H. Schwartz

Abstract

Endoscopic endonasal odontoidectomy, in appropriately selected patients, is safe and feasible in the pediatric population. Compared to transoral or transfacial approaches, endoscopic endonasal odontoidectomy results in less velopharyngeal insufficiency (VPI), leading to faster extubation and early oral intake post-surgery.

Intra-operative CT scan can help identify residual pathology, as well as the adequacy of surgical decompression at the cranio-cervical junction.

Right-handed surgeons operating predominately through the right nostril should pay attention to the contra lateral (left) side of the resection, where there is often a tendency towards residual pathology.

Keywords: craniovertebral junction, odontoidectomy, chiari malformation, endoscopic, transoral approach

14.1 Introduction

The craniovertebral junction (CVJ) is composed of both bony and neurovascular and ligamentous structures (▶ Fig. 14.1). The bony anatomy includes the clivus and dens ventrally, the condyles laterally, and the opisthion of the suboccipital bone and arch of C1 posteriorly.[1] The condyles articulate with C1 to create the atlantoaxial complex.[1] Abnormalities, many of them developmental, are common in this neuroanatomical region, particularly in the pediatric population. Down's syndrome, Chiari's malformation (CM), neoplasm, osteogenesis imperfecta, juvenile rheumatoid arthritis (JRA; Still's disease), achondroplasia, cleidocranial dysostosis, Klippel–Feil triad,[2] and Morquio's syndrome are often associated with CVJ abnormalities.[3]

Basilar invagination and cranial settling with resultant ventral brainstem compression are common indications for an odontoidectomy in pediatric patients. Basilar invagination

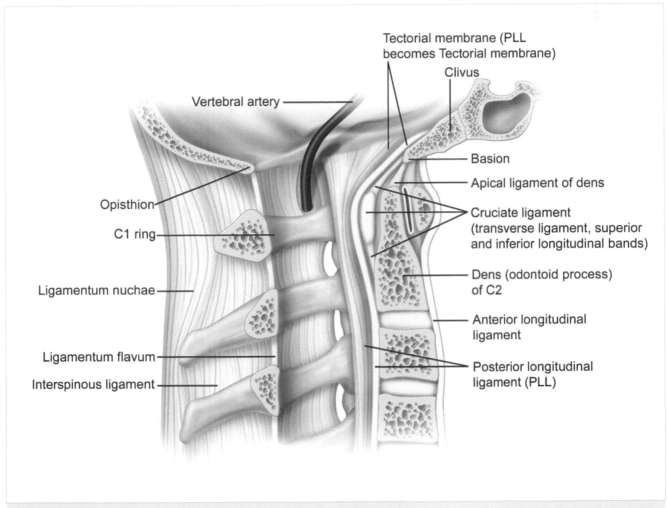

Fig. 14.1 A sagittal diagrammatic representation of ligaments at the craniovertebral junction.

occurs secondary to an upward migration of the odontoid process. Several factors define the severity and/or complexity of basilar invagination or brainstem compression: degree of upward migration of the odontoid process, degree of retroflexion of the odontoid process, volume of ligamentous pannus associated with the articulation over the dens, coincidence of atlantoaxial instability,[4] volume of the posterior fossa, surrounding soft tissue (normal or pathological), and associated pathological disorders.

CM is commonly associated with varying degrees of cerebellar herniation through the foramen magnum. CM has classically been defined as existing on a spectrum containing four types. Type I is the most common type, and is associated with the most favorable prognosis. It is by far the most commonly observed type in children, but is often first diagnosed only in adulthood. Characteristic features include tonsillar descent below the level of the foramen magnum, resulting in the possible disruption of normal cerebrospinal fluid (CSF) flow around and through the foramen magnum. Syringomyelia is present in 30% to 70% of these cases. Type II is more severe and is associated with myelomeningocele. Type III is usually associated with encephalomeningocele and is not compatible with life. Type IV is characterized by hypoplasia of cerebellar tissue.

Recently, the term "CM 1.5" has been used to identify a subgroup of patients with brainstem herniation (defined as obex below the level of the foramen magnum) in addition to tonsillar herniation. Data suggest patients with CM 1.5 frequently present with bulbar signs and symptoms, have distortion of the brainstem on sagittal MRI, and fail standard posterior decompression significantly more frequently than patients with CM without these features.[5] CM 1.5 patients are also at increased risk for requiring an occipitocervical fusion, following a standard decompressive procedure.[6] The combination of disruption of normal stabilizing forces as well as the common comorbid presence of connective tissue disorders is thought to underlie this morbidity of decompression.

Down's syndrome is also associated with ligamentous laxity (15%–20%) commonly resulting in atlantoaxial subluxation.[7] This finding can result in cervicomedullary compromise and myelopathic features. Surgical stabilization as well as odontoidectomy might be indicated in some cases.

JRA is the most common rheumatologic disease in children, and is one of the most common chronic disease conditions in childhood. It is defined as arthritis beginning before the age of 16 years, but the frequency is highest in children younger than 3 years.[8] The formation of a rheumatoid pannus at the odontoid–C1 articulation can cause symptomatic ventral compression of the brainstem in some children.

Tumors of the CVJ could be primary or secondary and either intradural or extradural. Congenital lesions like neurenteric cysts can also be encountered in this anatomical region. Other lesions include craniopharyngiomas, eosinophilic granulomas, neurofibromas, chordomas, chondrosarcomas, osteoblastomas, osteoid osteomas, and giant cell tumors. The clinical features range from headaches and neck pain to torticollis[4] and severe myelopathy. Other symptoms like drop attacks, migraines, and collapse could be due to vertebrobasilar insufficiency syndrome, in which case an angiographic study should be recommended as part of the preoperative evaluation.

14.2 Management Options: Medical, Surgical and Adjuvant

Medical, surgical, and adjuvant treatment options will vary by the specific pathology at the CVJ. Tumors in this region, although usually benign, are often chemo-/radioresistant, and surgical excision is often the treatment of choice. Several surgical approaches to the CVJ can be considered, including transfacial,[9,10] transoral, lateral extrapharyngeal, far lateral, transcondylar, and expanded endonasal endoscopic[11] (▶ Fig. 14.2).

The main indication for an odontoidectomy is radiologic and symptomatic ventral brainstem compression. Over the years, different radiographic criteria have been used to select patients who need odontoidectomies/ventral brainstem decompression. The basilar lines—Chamberlain's line,[2,12] McGregor's line,[2,13] Wackenheim's line,[14] McRae's line,[2,15] bimastoid line, etc.[16]—as well as other radiographic criteria[17] proposed by Ranawat et al,[18] Redlund-Johnell and Pettersson,[19] and Clark et al[20] have all been used for the assessment of basilar invagination.

Goel et al[21] classified basilar invagination, diagnosed using Chamberlain's line, into two groups based on their study of 190 surgically treated patients. Eighty-eight patients who had basilar invagination but no associated CM were assigned to group I; the remainder of the patients, who had both basilar invagination and CM, were assigned to group II. They highlighted that transoral decompression was the most suitable procedure for group I patients, while foramen magnum decompression was advised for group II patients.

Contrary to these data, Grabb et al[6] showed that in *pediatric* patients with Chiari I malformation as well as ventral brainstem compression from basilar invagination, a posterior decompressive procedure alone may not provide symptomatic relief and, in some cases, may lead to worsening of symptoms. They developed a novel method using sagittal MRI that measured objectively the encroachment by the odontoid and its investing tissues into the foramen magnum. They demonstrated that a value of 9 mm or greater was associated with a high risk for ventral brainstem compression, and some of these patients might warrant traction or transoral odontoidectomy before undergoing posterior fossa decompression.

Bollo et al[22] showed that patients with basilar invagination, CM 1.5, and craniocervical angulation (clivoaxial angle [CXA]) less than 125° are at increased risk of requiring an occipitocervical fusion procedure, either as an adjunct to initial surgical decompression or in a delayed fashion.

14.3 Endoscopic Endonasal Surgery

The transoral approach was the historical gold standard for ventral decompression at the CVJ by means of an odontoidectomy (▶ Fig. 14.3). Alfieri et al[23] developed the endoscopic endonasal approach (EEA) to the CVJ and odontoid process using cadaveric dissection in 2002.[23] Later, Kassam et al provided a description of EEA for resection of odontoid process and rheumatoid pannus in a patient with symptomatic cervicomedullary compression.[24] Since then, the EEA is now advocated by

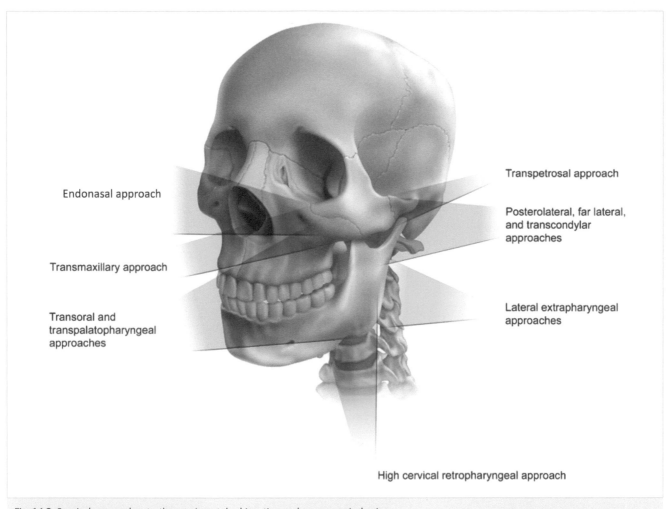

Fig. 14.2 Surgical approaches to the craniovertebral junction and upper cervical spine.

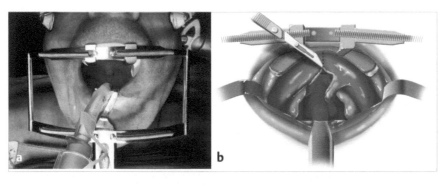

Fig. 14.3 The transoral approach using Dingman's or Crockard's oral retractors **(a)**. Note the placement of the endotracheal tube in relation to the retractor. The entrance to the oral cavity between the upper and lower incisors must be at least 2.5 to 3.0 cm in order to have adequate loupe or microscope visualization and introduce instruments. **(b)** If additional cephalad exposure is required, the soft palate may be incised in the midline starting on one side of the base of the uvula and then laterally retracted.

many surgeons as an alternative, as it avoids breaching the oropharynx and is an effective minimal-access technique for decompression of the cervicomedullary junction.[25,26,27]

When compared with the transoral approach,[28,29] endoscopic endonasal access presents four potential advantages: (1) excellent prevertebral exposure and lateral visualization in patients with small oral cavities, (2) a surgical corridor located above the hard palate that allows easy decompression of rostral pathological entities, (3) avoidance of the oral trauma and edema that follow oral retractor placement, and (4) avoidance of splitting the soft or hard palate and preservation of palatal function.[27,30]

The endonasal approach can provide excellent access to the clivus, C1, and C2 (odontoid) without the need for external inci-

sions, Le Fort osteotomy, mandibular split, or a circumglossal approach usually required for patients with a small oral cavity, trismus, or macroglossia. The incision used for the endonasal approach is more rostral in the nasopharynx (ideally at or above the level of the soft palate) than the posterior pharyngeal incision used for the traditional transoral approach. This spares the posterior pharynx musculature and mucosa, which may lead to a reduction in wound-healing complications and velopharyngeal incompetence.[11] There are several studies reporting that compared to the transoral approach, the endonasal approach to the CVJ leads to more rapid extubation and earlier time to feeding.[26,27,30]

Through radiographic and cadaveric morphometric analysis, Singh et al showed that the odontoid peg (comprising roughly two-thirds of C2 vertebral body in sagittal plane) can be endonasally accessed more than 90% of the time using a 0- or 30-degree endoscope, without splitting the hard or soft palate.[31,32] Similarly, other authors have also evaluated the inferior anatomic extent of odontoidectomy through an endonasal approach, which might be helpful in preoperative surgical planning.[33,34]

In pediatric patients, characteristic anatomical features like small nostrils, presence of adenoids, and absent or limited pneumatization of sinuses pose a different type of challenge to endoscopic surgeons, as discussed in Chapters 1 and 2. According to our experience, while the patient's age as well as size is not a significant limitation to the EEA,[35,36] a wider intercarotid distance (ICD) and shorter dens–nare distance predicts better outcomes and fewer complications.[37,38]

In our series of six pediatric patients who underwent endonasal odontoidectomies for CVJ compression, five of six patients had improvement in their modified Rankin's scale (mRS) scores on follow-up (▶ Table 14.1).[39]

14.3.1 Case Example

An 11-year-old with Ehlers–Danlos syndrome had cervical instability and brainstem compression from basilar invagination and a retroflexed odontoid. He also had a Chiari 1 malformation (▶ Fig. 14.4; ▶ Fig. 14.5a). His symptoms consisted of headaches and loss of feeling in his arms, hands, legs, and feet. He also had choking and gagging spells and poor balance.

He underwent a Chiari decompression and occipitocervical fusion, followed by endoscopic endonasal resection of the odontoid.

He was positioned supine and his head was pinned in three-point fixation in a radiolucent Mayfield head holder. Neuronavigation was set up using the intraoperative CT scanner. In the absence of an intraoperative CT scanner, registration coordinates may also be acquired using a preloaded MRI and/or CT scan of the patient. Neuromonitoring was set up, and motor and somatosensory evoked potentials were monitored throughout the surgery.

Table 14.1 Pediatric patients who underwent endonasal odontoidectomy for craniovertebral junction (CVJ) compression

No.	Age at surgery	Pre-op mRS	Post-op mRS	Follow-up duration (mo)
1	14	2	0	67
2	7	3	2	41
3	16	2	1	22
4	11	2	1	16
5	14	1	0	12
6	9	2	2	10

Abbreviation: mRS, modified Rankin's scale.

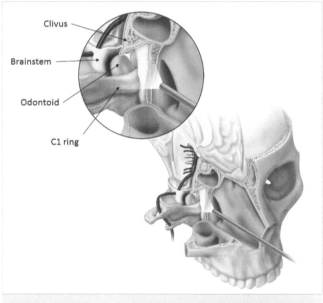

Fig. 14.4 Diagrammatic representation of the transodontoid approach using the endonasal corridor.

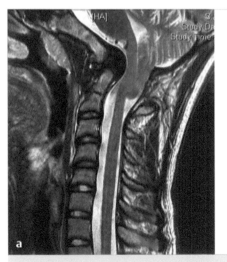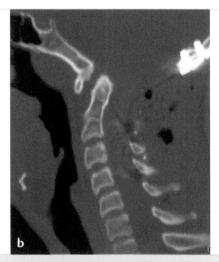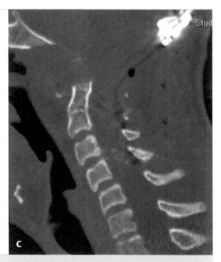

Fig. 14.5 Pre- and postoperative imaging (a). Preoperative T2-weighted sagittal MRI showing basilar invagination with compression of the medulla. **(b)** Sagittal noncontrast CT prior to the endonasal odontoid resection. Posterior decompression and occiput–C3 fusion is already done for this patient. **(c)** Sagittal noncontrast CT after endonasal odontoid resection. The cephalad portion of the odontoid, the caudal portion of the clivus, and the anterior portion of the C1 ring have been resected.

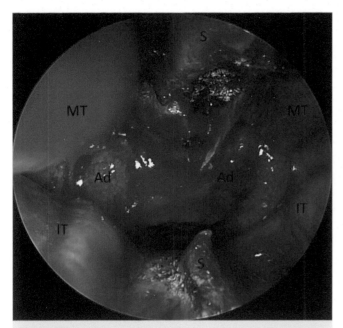

Fig. 14.6 A posterior septectomy is performed and the nasopharynx approached using a binostril approach. In pediatric patients, large adenoids (Ad) can occasionally obscure the choana. S, septum; MT, middle turbinate; IT, inferior turbinate.

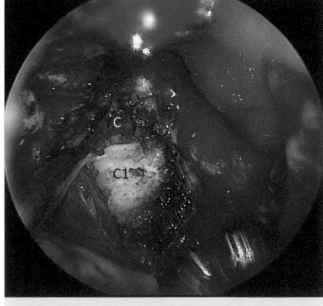

Fig. 14.7 The adenoids are resected and a vertical incision made in the posterior pharyngeal musculature using Bovie electrocautery. The anterior arch of the C1 ring can be seen underneath. The clival mucosa can also be cauterized to expose the clivus (C) above. In some cases of severe invagination, the inferior portion of the clivus might also need to be drilled and removed.

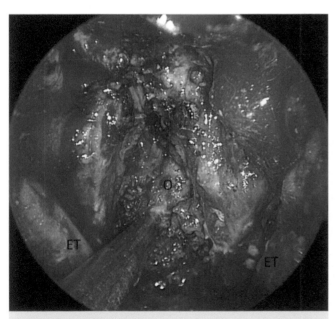

Fig. 14.8 The anterior arch of C1 is drilled off to expose the odontoid peg (O). The Eustachian tubes (ET) mark the lateral borders of the dissection.

A posterior septectomy is performed and the nasopharynx approached using a binostril approach. In pediatric patients, large adenoids (Ad) can occasionally obscure the choana (▶ Fig. 14.6).

The adenoids are resected for improved visualization and access to the posterior nasopharynx. A vertical incision is made in the posterior pharyngeal musculature using Bovie electro-cautery. The suction is used for dynamic retraction of the pharyngeal musculature and the anterior arch of the C1 ring is exposed. The incision can be extended cephalad to expose the inferior portion of the clivus as well. In some cases of severe invagination, the inferior portion of the clivus might also need to be drilled and removed (▶ Fig. 14.7).

The anterior arch of C1 is drilled off to expose the odontoid peg. The Eustachian tubes mark the lateral borders of the dissection (▶ Fig. 14.8).

The odontoid peg is hollowed out with a high-speed drill and then detached at the base. The remainder of the odontoid shell must be detached from the apical and alar ligaments superiorly and the cruciate ligament posteriorly for complete removal. Curettes and Kerrison rongeurs are helpful in dissecting the ligaments off the odontoid shell to remove it piecemeal (▶ Fig. 14.9).

Once the odontoid peg and cruciate ligament are removed, the glistening dura can be seen. Care must be taken to not cause a CSF leak while detaching the odontoid and cruciate ligament (along with the pannus) from the underlying dura (▶ Fig. 14.10). However, if a CSF leak is encountered, it can be repaired with autologous fat onlay and Tisseel fibrin glue, and held in place by suturing the overlying nasopharyngeal fascia utilizing chromic sutures.

The intraoperative CT scanner is now used to perform a second scan while acquiring new registration coordinates. This helps us access the adequacy of the bony decompression at the CVJ. If there is residual odontoid seen, further decompression is pursued using the newly acquired registration coordinates to localize the residual fragment.[40]

When the odontoidectomy is complete, the posterior pharyngeal musculature is approximated together using absorbable

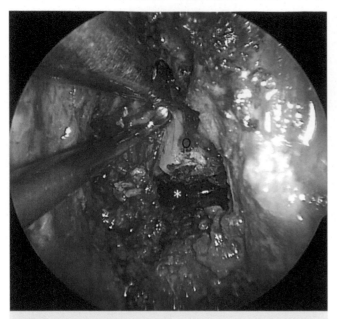

Fig. 14.9 The odontoid (O) peg is hollowed out with a high-speed drill and then detached at the base (*). The remainder of the odontoid shell must be detached from the apical and alar ligaments superiorly and the cruciate ligament posteriorly for complete removal.

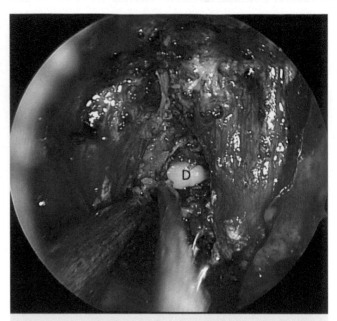

Fig. 14.10 Once the odontoid peg and cruciate ligament are removed, glistening dura (D) can be seen. Care must be taken to not cause a cerebrospinal fluid leak while detaching the odontoid and cruciate ligament from the underlying dura.

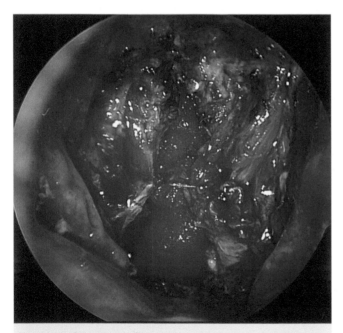

Fig. 14.11 The posterior pharyngeal musculature is approximated together using absorbable stitches. Some Floseal might be placed in the cavity to eliminate some of the dead space.

stitches. Some Floseal (Baxter, Deerfield, IL) might be placed in the cavity to eliminate some of the dead space (▶ Fig. 14.11).

All of our endoscopic odontoid resection patients who did not have occipitocervical fusion performed under the same anesthesia are extubated in the operating room. Patients who received combined fusion and odontoid decompression are electively extubated on the morning of postoperative day 1 to allow airway edema to subside after 8 to 10 hours of surgery, much of it in the prone position for the fusion portion of the case. Diet is resumed shortly thereafter.

Intraoperative CT has proven useful for delineating the adequacy of surgical decompression at the cervicomedullary junction by identifying residual bony fragments.[40,41,42] Whether these small residual fragments are clinically significant is unknown, but complete resection of the odontoid is more likely to relieve symptoms than a partial resection. Ongoing clinical assessments will try to elucidate these questions further.

Right-handed surgeons operating predominantly through the *right* nostril should pay special attention to the contralateral (left) side of the resection, where there is often a tendency toward residual pathology.[27,40] We hypothesize that this is because it is easier to retract the posterior pharyngeal musculature (using a suction) and drill the C1 ring and odontoid on the right than on the left where there is continuous overhang of the pharyngeal musculature.

Special attention should be paid to patients who are undergoing occipitocervical stabilization and fusion at the same time as the endonasal odontoidectomy. These patients should be fused in their neutral anatomic alignment presurgery. If they are fused in a flexed or posteriorly translated position, they can develop significant problems with swallowing postoperatively. The posterior pharyngeal edema postsurgery, in conjunction with the flexed and/or posteriorly translated position at the CVJ, can lead to airway compromise in severe cases (▶ Fig. 14.12).

14.4 Conclusion

Endoscopic endonasal odontoid resection is safe and feasible in the pediatric population. While the patient's age as well as size

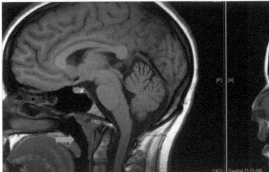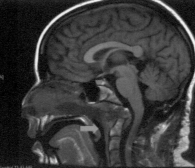

Fig. 14.12 Pre- and post-op T1 sagittal MRI sequences of a different pediatric patient who underwent endonasal odontoidectomy followed by occipitocervical fusion. Note the size of the airway (*blue arrow*) before (**a**) and after (**b**) surgery. The posterior pharyngeal edema, in conjunction with posterior translation at the craniovertebral junction, causes severe narrowing of the airway.

is not a significant limitation to the EEA, a wider ICD and shorter dens–nare distance predict better outcomes and fewer complications. Real-time intraoperative CT navigation provides accurate localization of pathology, thereby increasing the chance of a complete odontoidectomy and CVJ decompression.

14.5 Authors' Contribution

Haminder Singh and Andrew Alalade made equal contributions to the manuscript.

References

[1] Smoker WR. Craniovertebral junction: normal anatomy, craniometry, and congenital anomalies. Radiographics. 1994; 14(2):255–277

[2] Spillane JD, Pallis C, Jones AM. Developmental abnormalities in the region of the foramen magnum. Brain. 1957; 80(1):11–48

[3] Youssef CA, Smotherman CR, Kraemer DF, Aldana PR. Predicting the limits of the endoscopic endonasal approach in children: a radiological anatomical study. J Neurosurg Pediatr. 2016; 17(4):510–515

[4] Goel A. Goel's classification of atlantoaxial "facetal" dislocation. J Craniovertebr Junction Spine. 2014; 5(1):3–8

[5] Tubbs RS, Iskandar BJ, Bartolucci AA, Oakes WJ. A critical analysis of the Chiari 1.5 malformation. J Neurosurg. 2004; 101(2) Suppl:179–183

[6] Grabb PA, Mapstone TB, Oakes WJ. Ventral brain stem compression in pediatric and young adult patients with Chiari I malformations. Neurosurgery. 1999; 44(3):520–527, discussion 527–528

[7] Menezes AH, Ryken TC. Craniovertebral abnormalities in Down's syndrome. Pediatr Neurosurg. 1992; 18(1):24–33

[8] Sullivan DB, Cassidy JT, Petty RE. Pathogenic implications of age of onset in juvenile rheumatoid arthritis. Arthritis Rheum. 1975; 18(3):251–255

[9] Swearingen B, Joseph M, Cheney M, Ojemann RG. A modified transfacial approach to the clivus. Neurosurgery. 1995; 36(1):101–104, discussion 104–105

[10] Chandler JP, Silva FE. Extended transbasal approach to skull base tumors. Technical nuances and review of the literature. Oncology (Williston Park). 2005; 19(7):913–919, discussion 920, 923–925, 929

[11] Singh H, Harrop J, Schiffmacher P, Rosen M, Evans J. Ventral surgical approaches to craniovertebral junction chordomas. Neurosurgery. 2010; 66 (3) Suppl:96–103

[12] Chamberlain WE. Basilar impression (platybasia). A bizarre developmental anomaly of the occipital bone and upper cervical spine with striking and misleading neurologic manifestations. Yale J Biol Med. 1939; 11(5): 487–496

[13] McGreger M. The significance of certain measurements of the skull in the diagnosis of basilar impression. Br J Radiol. 1948; 21(244):171–181

[14] Thiebaut F, Wackenheim A, Vrousos C. New median sagittal pneumostratigraphical finding concerning the posterior fossa. J Radiol Electrol Med Nucl. 1961; 42:1–7

[15] McRae DL, Barnum AS. Occipitalization of the atlas. Am J Roentgenol Radium Ther Nucl Med. 1953; 70(1):23–46

[16] Almeida GG, Canelas HM, Lemmi H, Zaclis J. Value of Fischgold and Metzger's bimastoid line for radiological diagnosis of basilar impression. Arq Neuropsiquiatr. 1956; 14(4):285–298

[17] Wiesel SW, Feffer HL, Rothman RH. The development of a cervical spine algorithm and its prospective application to industrial patients. J Occup Med. 1985; 27(4):272–276

[18] Ranawat CS, O'Leary P, Pellicci P, Tsairis P, Marchisello P, Dorr L. Cervical spine fusion in rheumatoid arthritis. J Bone Joint Surg Am. 1979; 61(7): 1003–1010

[19] Redlund-Johnell I, Pettersson H. Radiographic measurements of the craniovertebral region. Designed for evaluation of abnormalities in rheumatoid arthritis. Acta Radiol Diagn (Stockh). 1984; 25(1):23–28

[20] Clark CR, Goetz DD, Menezes AH. Arthrodesis of the cervical spine in rheumatoid arthritis. J Bone Joint Surg Am. 1989; 71(3):381–392

[21] Goel A, Bhatjiwale M, Desai K. Basilar invagination: a study based on 190 surgically treated patients. J Neurosurg. 1998; 88(6):962–968

[22] Bollo RJ, Riva-Cambrin J, Brockmeyer MM, Brockmeyer DL. Complex Chiari malformations in children: an analysis of preoperative risk factors for occipitocervical fusion. J Neurosurg Pediatr. 2012; 10(2):134–141

[23] Alfieri A, Jho HD, Tschabitscher M. Endoscopic endonasal approach to the ventral cranio-cervical junction: anatomical study. Acta Neurochir (Wien). 2002; 144(3):219–225, discussion 225

[24] Kassam AB, Snyderman C, Gardner P, Carrau R, Spiro R. The expanded endonasal approach: a fully endoscopic transnasal approach and resection of the odontoid process: technical case report. Neurosurgery. 2005; 57(1) Suppl: E213-, discussion E213

[25] Laufer I, Greenfield JP, Anand VK, Härtl R, Schwartz TH. Endonasal endoscopic resection of the odontoid process in a nonachondroplastic dwarf with juvenile rheumatoid arthritis: feasibility of the approach and utility of the intraoperative Iso-C three-dimensional navigation. Case report. J Neurosurg Spine. 2008; 8(4):376–380

[26] Leng LZ, Anand VK, Hartl R, Schwartz TH. Endonasal endoscopic resection of an os odontoideum to decompress the cervicomedullary junction: a minimal access surgical technique. Spine. 2009; 34(4):E139–E143

[27] Goldschlager T, Härtl R, Greenfield JP, Anand VK, Schwartz TH. The endoscopic endonasal approach to the odontoid and its impact on early extubation and feeding. J Neurosurg. 2015; 122(3):511–518

[28] Hankinson TC, Grunstein E, Gardner P, Spinks TJ, Anderson RC. Transnasal odontoid resection followed by posterior decompression and occipitocervical fusion in children with Chiari malformation type I and ventral brainstem compression. J Neurosurg Pediatr. 2010; 5(6):549–553

[29] Nayak JV, Gardner PA, Vescan AD, Carrau RL, Kassam AB, Snyderman CH. Experience with the expanded endonasal approach for resection of the odontoid process in rheumatoid disease. Am J Rhinol. 2007; 21(5):601–606

[30] Komotar RJ, Raper DM, Starke RM, Anand VK, Schwartz TH. Endonasal versus transoral odontoid resection: a systematic meta-analysis of outcomes. Skull Base. 2011; 21:A051

[31] Singh H, Grobelny BT, Harrop J, Rosen M, Lober RM, Evans J. Endonasal access to the upper cervical spine, part one: radiographic morphometric analysis. J Neurol Surg B Skull Base. 2013; 74(3):176–184

[32] Singh H, Lober RM, Virdi GS, Lopez H, Rosen M, Evans J. Endonasal access to the upper cervical spine: part 2-cadaveric analysis. J Neurol Surg B Skull Base. 2015; 76(4):262–265

[33] de Almeida JR, Zanation AM, Snyderman CH, et al. Defining the nasopalatine line: the limit for endonasal surgery of the spine. Laryngoscope. 2009; 119 (2):239–244

[34] La Corte E, Aldana PR, Ferroli P, et al. The rhinopalatine line as a reliable predictor of the inferior extent of endonasal odontoidectomies. Neurosurg Focus. 2015; 38(4):E16

[35] Ali ZS, Lang SS, Kamat AR, et al. Suprasellar pediatric craniopharyngioma resection via endonasal endoscopic approach. Childs Nerv Syst. 2013; 29(11): 2065–2070

[36] Rigante M, Massimi L, Parrilla C, et al. Endoscopic transsphenoidal approach versus microscopic approach in children. Int J Pediatr Otorhinolaryngol. 2011; 75(9):1132–1136

[37] Banu MA, Guerrero-Maldonado A, McCrea HJ, et al. Impact of skull base development on endonasal endoscopic surgical corridors. J Neurosurg Pediatr. 2014; 13(2):155–169

[38] Banu MA, Rathman A, Patel KS, et al. Corridor-based endonasal endoscopic surgery for pediatric skull base pathology with detailed radioanatomic measurements. Neurosurgery. 2014; 10 Suppl 2:273–293, discussion 293

[39] Alalade AF, et al. A dual approach for the management of complex craniovertebral junction abnormalities: endoscopic endonasal odontoidectomy and posterior decompression with fusion. World Neurosurg. X. 2019; 24(2)

[40] Singh H, Rote S, Jada A, et al. Endoscopic endonasal odontoid resection with real-time intraoperative image-guided computed tomography: report of 4 cases. J Neurosurg. 2017; 16:1–6

[41] Gande A, Tormenti MJ, Koutourousiou M, et al. Intraoperative computed tomography guidance to confirm decompression following endoscopic endonasal approach for cervicomedullary compression. J Neurol Surg B Skull Base. 2013; 74(1):44–49

[42] Hum B, Feigenbaum F, Cleary K, Henderson FC. Intraoperative computed tomography for complex craniocervical operations and spinal tumor resections. Neurosurgery. 2000; 47(2):374–380, discussion 380–381

15 Rathke's Cleft Cysts

Matthew J. Shepard, Mohamed El Zoghby, and John Jane Jr.

Abstract

Rathke's cleft cysts (RCC) are benign cystic lesions of the pituitary that represent the commonest sellar lesion affecting the general population. Although RCCs are less commonly reported in the pediatric population, the reported incidence is rising. In the pediatric population, diagnosis is often made in the setting of severe, medically refractory headaches, a disturbance in the hypothalamic–pituitary axis (HPA), or visual disturbance. About one-third of pediatric patients who are diagnosed with an RCC fail conservative management and ultimately undergo surgical fenestration via an endoscopic transsphenoidal approach. While headache improvement is achieved in most cases, surgery is associated with new postoperative endocrinopathies in about one-fourth of patients. These rates are increased when aggressive cyst wall resection is attempted. Thus, cyst wall biopsy with concurrent fenestration is reasonable in instances with optic chiasmal compression with concurrent visual symptoms, instances of severe medical refractory headaches, progressive cyst growth toward the optic chiasm, or in cases where diagnostic uncertainty is present.

Keywords: Rathke's cleft cyst, endoscopic transsphenoidal surgery, pediatric sellar lesion

15.1 Introduction

Rathke's cleft cysts (RCC) represent the most common sellar lesion in adults and have been described to occur in up to one-third of individuals studied at autopsy.[1] Despite this, RCCs are often incidental findings and account for less than 10% of surgically treated sellar lesions.[1] Unlike their high prevalence in the adult population, these congenital lesions are uncommonly diagnosed in pediatric patients. While the prevalence of pediatric RCC is not precisely defined, less than 200 cases of symptomatic pediatric RCCs have been reported in the literature. In imaging studies of asymptomatic patients, cystic lesions of the pituitary were seen in 1.2% of patients younger than 15 years.[2] However, with increased access to advanced imaging, the diagnosis of smaller, incidental RCCs is rising, underscoring the need for the pediatric neurosurgeon or pituitary specialist to be familiar with their optimal diagnosis, natural history, and management. In this chapter, we will review the pathophysiology, diagnosis, and optimal management of these benign sellar lesions.

15.2 Pathophysiology

During development, Rathke's pouch develops from pharyngeal ectoderm that rises cranially to fuse with the descending infundibulum of neuroectodermal origin. Rathke's pouch forms the pars tuberalis within the suprasellar cistern, the pars distalis, and the pars intermedia. The pars distalis ultimately differentiates to become the anterior lobe of the pituitary, whereas the posterior lobe arises from the pars nervosa of the descending neuroectoderm.[1] In most instances, Rathke's pouch regresses. In some, however, a remnant persists and can become filled with cerebrospinal fluid (CSF) or proteinaceous fluid that leads to the development of an RCC. As such, RCCs are commonly sellar in location and are bound by the adenohypophysis anteriorly and the neurohypophysis posteriorly. RCC can expand into the suprasellar space or infrequently arise exclusively in the suprasellar cistern as remnants of the pars tuberalis. RCCs can enlarge and cause compression of the optic chiasm, leading to visual field deficits, or can disturb normal pituitary function, leading to a variety of hormonal syndromes.

15.3 Natural History

Much debate exists within the literature regarding the optimal management and natural history of RCCs. The majority of longitudinal studies of asymptomatic RCCs are relegated to the adult population. Culver et al reported a series of 75 patients who underwent conservative management for RCC.[3] Over a median follow-up of 24 months, 57% of the cysts had no growth and 11% of the cysts decreased in size. Aho et al similarly examined the natural history of incidental RCCs less than 1 cm in diameter.[4] In this series, 69% of patients had no growth of the cyst 9 years from the time of diagnosis. Thus, in the majority of patients with asymptomatic, incidental RCCs, watchful waiting with serial imaging studies is a reasonable strategy. Indeed, Amhaz et al reported 51 patients treated with RCC over a 9-year period.[5] Twenty-nine patients were managed conservatively, and serial imaging showed involution of RCCs in nine patients. Interestingly, of the seven patients who had presented with headaches, five had subjective improvement in symptoms at the time the cyst was found to have decreased in size. This response rate is similar to outcomes reported by Zada et al, who published an 88% response rate for headaches following cyst fenestration.[6] Not all RCCs have a benign course, however. In Aho et al's study, 31% of the patients at 9-year follow-up had developed an enlarging cyst, vision deficits, or pituitary hormonal dysregulation.[4] As such, surgical intervention may be warranted in some individuals.

In the pediatric population, headache, endocrinologic disturbance, and visual change are the most common manifestations of RCC. Disorders of the HPA in children frequently present with precocious puberty or growth delay, unlike the adult population, who exhibit pathology of the HPA via decreased libido, fatigue, menstrual irregularities, or altered mental status.[1,7] Aseptic meningitis or apoplexies have been reported in patients with RCC, but these presentations are relatively rare.[7] There have been several published retrospective literature reviews on RCCs in the pediatric population that are briefly summarized in ▶ Table 15.1. Of the 163 patients who have been previously described, 53% were females, the median age at the time of diagnosis was 10.9 years, and the median cyst size was 0.8 cm in maximum diameter. Pooled analysis of the reported cases shows that 47% of patients presented with headache, 50% presented with an underlying endocrinopathy, and 9% presented with visual disturbance. 16% of the lesions were

Table 15.1 Clinical characteristics of previously reported pediatric Rathke's cleft cyst

Study	Patients (n)	Median age (y)	Cyst size (cm)	Operative intervention	Follow-up (mo)
Hayashi et al 2016[8]	11	12.2	1.9	72%	85
Daubenbü et al 2015[13]	14	11.3	1.8	–	50
Oh et al 2014[7]	34	9.7	0.6	0%	–
Jahangiri et al 2011[2]	14	16	1.2	100%	38
Lim et al 2010	44	10.1	–	34%	16
Katavetin et al 2010[15]	13	14	1.2	31%	24
Evliyaoglu et al 2010[16]	1	7	0.7	100%	24
Locatelli et al 2010	4	10.5	–	–	–
Zada et al 2009	10	13	1.4	100%	34
Frazier et al 2008	1	14	3.0	100%	8
Takanashi et al 2005	4	2	0.6	0%	–
Kim et al 2004	1	11	1.6	100%	4
Im et al 2003	1	12	1.6	100%	26
Israel et al 2000	1	13	1.5	100%	5
Setian et al 1999	1	8	1.0	100%	–
Christophe et al 1993	7	4.3	1.4	29%	24
Voelker et al 1991	1	15	–	100%	1
Towbin et al 1987	1	10	–	–	–

incidental findings. In total, 37% of pediatric patients with a diagnosis of RCC in the literature underwent surgery, with the most common approach being via the transsphenoidal corridor.

15.4 Diagnosis and Management of RCC

RCCs are generally described as non–contrast-enhancing, midline cystic lesions of the sella situated between the anterior and posterior lobes of the pituitary. They are noncalcified and can have suprasellar extension in up to 30% to 50% of cases.[8,9] Diagnosis of an RCC on radiologic imaging alone can be challenging in some instances, given the variable appearance of cystic components on T1- and T2-weighted imaging (WI) on MRI. Although some heterogeneity does exist, RCCs generally are hyperintense on T2-WI MRI, whereas the T1-WI intensity is dependent upon whether or not the cystic contents are highly proteinaceous (hyperintense) or bland (hypointense). The major differential diagnosis on radiologic imaging for RCCs in the pediatric population is a cystic craniopharyngioma (CC), which is usually of the adamantinomatous subtype. The incidence of craniopharyngiomas in individuals younger than 18 years is greater than that of RCCs, and being able to differentiate between the two is imperative, as the optimal management for these two entities differs widely.[8] Classically, CCs, unlike RCCs, tend to have a contrast-enhancing nodular solid component, and the vast majority extend to the suprasellar space, with cystic components resembling cerebrospinal fluid on T1-WI and T2-WI. To further delineate differences between RCCs and CCs, Hayashi et al. performed a comparative study of RCCs and CCs based on MRI findings and concluded that RCCs tended to be smaller in size than CCs, regular in shape, and without calcification.[8] Byun et al further described that the presence of an intracystic nodule that was hyperintense on T1-WI and hypoin-

tense on T2-WI was characteristic of RCCs and represented deposits of cholesterol and protein on biochemical analysis.[9]

Histopathologic differentiation of RCCs versus CCs can likewise be difficult, and some have suggested that RCCs can progress toward CC formation via an intermediate entity known as RCC with squamous metaplasia.[8] RCCs resemble ectodermal tissue on histologic section and are characterized by the presence of a single layer of columnar or pseudostratified ciliated cuboidal epithelium.[1] CCs are divided into adamantinomatous and papillary subtypes. Both are characterized by proliferative stratified epithelium; however, the adamantinomatous subtype exhibits calcification and contains keratin debris with cholesterol clefts, while the papillary subtype is characterized by numerous papillae without dense keratin or calcification.[10] The papillary variant of RCC can be especially difficult to differentiate from RCCs, and genetic testing is important in their differentiation in certain cases. Papillary CCs contain the BRAF V600E mutation, while adamantinomatous variants of CC are characterized by intranuclear beta-catenin staining.[11] RCCs do not typically contain these genetic and molecular hallmarks, and thus their absence aids in the diagnosis of RCCs.

In the pediatric population, surgical intervention has been reported in approximately 60 cases, with the two largest individual series being documented by Jahangiri et al[2] and by Zada et al.[6] Jahangiri described 14 cases of pediatric RCCs treated by microsurgical transsphenoidal surgery for cyst fenestration.[2] Half of their reported cases described headaches, and one of the 14 patients endorsed visual disturbance. Postoperative outcomes were not documented for these patients, but the authors did note a 21% postoperative rate of diabetes insipidus (DI) and noted that none of the three patients with preoperative growth hormone (GH) or insulin-like growth factor (IGF-1) deficiencies had normalization of their GH or IGF-1 levels postoperatively. Zada et al described 10 cases of RCC treated by a transnasal transsphenoidal approach for cyst fenestration and aspiration.[6]

Table 15.2 Surgical outcomes of 60 patients undergoing surgery for Rathke's cleft cyst

Post-op pituitary improvement	25%
Post-op pituitary deterioration	27%
Post-op diabetes insipidus	27%
Gross total resection	82%
Mean follow-up	31 mo
Recurrence rate at follow-up	18%

Eighty-eight percent of the patients in their series with headaches had improvement of their symptoms postoperatively. Only one of their patients had visual disturbances preoperatively, and this patient had modest improvement following surgery. Two of the six patients with preoperative HPA dysfunction had improvement of their underlying endocrinopathy postoperatively, while three patients developed new hormonal deficiencies. Surgical outcomes for adults are better described in the literature, with improvements in headaches being documented in 70% to 90% of cases and visual field improvements being noted in 70% to 80% of cases.[1] Given the sparse data on surgery for pediatric RCCs, the 60 surgically described cases of RCC were pooled and collectively analyzed and are summarized in ▶ Table 15.2. In brief, 25% of patients had an improvement in a preoperative endocrinopathy; however, 27% had new anterior pituitary dysfunction postoperatively and an additional 27% had postoperative DI. Gross total resection was achieved in 82% of reported cases, and by the end of a 31-month follow-up, there was an 18% recurrence rate.

RCCs are not characterized by rapid division of multiplying cells, and as such, they are not sensitive to traditional chemotherapy or radiation. Medical therapy is mainly directed toward treating the underlying hormone excess or deficiency associated with an RCC, if any. In the pediatric population, this is most commonly aimed at treating GH deficiency (GHD) or precocious puberty. While some have advocated for surgery in these instances, surgical success in correcting underlying endocrinopathy as a result of RCC is limited, as noted earlier. Medical management for GHD involves GH supplementation, while gonadotropin-releasing hormone (GnRH) antagonists have been used to treat precocious puberty.[7] Oh et al showed that out of 26 pediatric patients with endocrinopathy associated with an underlying RCC, 27% were diagnosed with GHD, while 46% were diagnosed with central precocious puberty. At 1 year of treatment with either GH agonists or GnRH antagonists, outcomes were similar for age-matched controls with idiopathic GHD or central precocious puberty.[7]

Taking all of this into account, surgical resection for pediatric RCCs seems most reasonable in instances with optic chiasmal compression with concurrent visual symptoms, instances of severe medical refractory headaches, progressive cyst growth toward the optic chiasm, or in cases where diagnostic uncertainty is present. Medical therapy is directed at treating the underlying hormonal excess or deficiency in patients with RCCs, if present.

15.5 The Role of Endoscopic Endonasal Surgery

RCCs are slow-growing benign lesions that arise most commonly within the sella. As RCCs enlarge, the sella often expands, and as such, the endoscopic endonasal approach affords a clear pathway to the sella to facilitate cyst fenestration and drainage. There have been two varying points of view on the optimal surgical management of RCCs. Some authors advocate for aggressive cyst wall resection in order to decrease the rates of recurrence, while others advocate for a limited cyst fenestration, given the increased rates of postoperative hypopituitarism associated with radical cyst resection.[6,12] Aho et al, in one of the largest surgical series of RCCs, performed a radical cyst resection in the first 33 of 118 reported cases, which was accompanied by a 47% rate of postoperative DI.[4] The incidence of DI was reduced to 9% in the remaining 85 patients, who were treated with simple cyst fenestration. In their series, the recurrence rate was no different between the aggressive and limited cyst wall resection groups; advocating cyst fenestration and cyst aspiration is an effective and safer alternative to radical resection.

The endoscopic approach affords the surgeon the ability to access RCCs that are situated within both the sellar and suprasellar regions. Solari et al defined three types of RCCs. Type I RCCs reside within the sella exclusively, type II RCCs refer to cysts with both a sellar and a suprasellar component, while type III RCCs reside completely within the suprasellar cistern.[12] A standard endoscopic endonasal approach is utilized in type I and II RCCs, where the largest component of the cyst resides within the sella. In instances where the suprasellar cyst is the major feature of the RCC, as in type III RCCs and a subset of some type II RCCs, a transtuberculum/transplanum approach can be utilized.[12] In type III RCCs, the cyst is situated above the diaphragm sella and CSF leak is expected and prepared for with the harvest of a nasoseptal flap and possible lumbar drain placement preoperatively. For type I RCCs without CSF leak, some authors advocate for wide fenestration of the cyst and no sellar floor reconstruction to aid in cyst marsupialization to prevent recurrence. No large study has examined this in earnest, and many do advocate for sellar floor reconstruction.[1] The use of fat graft has been advocated by some authors who encounter CSF leak, but concern has been raised that this may be associated with an increased rate of RCC recurrence.[4]

The endoscopic, transnasal, transsphenoidal approach for RCC utilizes the standard binarial three-handed technique. The sellar face is exposed in the usual fashion, and a wide sphenoidotomy and posterior septectomy are both performed. A nasoseptal flap is deferred, except in instances where a type III RCC is expected based on preoperative imaging. After completion of the sphenoidotomy and dural opening, the RCC is often obscured by the anterior lobe of the pituitary, necessitating a vertical incision through the adenohypophysis. In most instances, this allows adequate exposure of the anterior cyst wall, which is biopsied and sent to pathology for permanent section. The cyst contents are evacuated using gentle suction and irrigation. The cyst cavity is then inspected using the endoscope to confirm adequate cyst decompression. Radical cyst wall resection is not advocated, given the high risk of hypopituitarism and DI. Reconstruction of the sella using fat graft or collagen matrix is performed only in instances where CSF leak is encountered. ▶ Fig. 15.1, ▶ Fig. 15.2, ▶ Fig. 15.3 detail the steps of resection of a standard sellar RCC.

As a guiding principle, the location of the RCC dictates the safest surgical corridor to the lesion, and simple cyst decom-

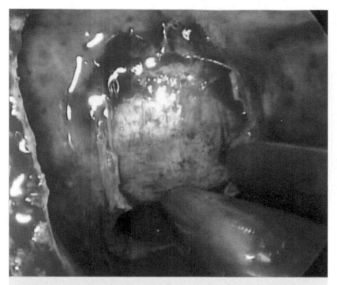

Fig. 15.1 The dura is opened sharply, maintaining the cyst capsule to facilitate adequate capsule sampling for pathologic review.

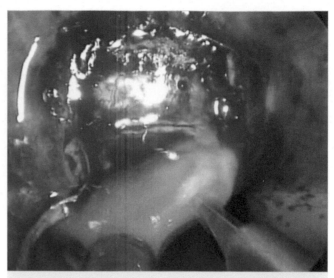

Fig. 15.2 After entering of the cyst wall, gelatinous cyst contents are encountered and evacuated using suction and irrigation.

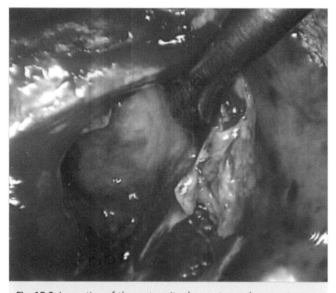

Fig. 15.3 Inspection of the cyst cavity does not reveal any cyst remnant; the posterior wall is not resected and the floor is not reconstructed to facilitate marsupialization of the cyst.

pression with or without sellar floor reconstruction is utilized most frequently in instances without CSF leak.

15.6 Conclusion

Pediatric RCCs are rare, benign, cystic lesions of the sella. The majority of these lesions are asymptomatic and are incidentally discovered, but a subset present to clinical attention with progressive growth, chiasmal compression, headaches, or disturbances of the HPA. In most cases, RCCs can be managed conservatively, but in instances of medically refractory headaches, diagnostic uncertainty, or visual changes, cyst drainage without radical cyst wall resection is a viable option.

References

[1] Han SJ, Rolston JD, Jahangiri A, Aghi MK. Rathke's cleft cysts: review of natural history and surgical outcomes. J Neurooncol. 2014; 117(2):197–203

[2] Jahangiri A, Molinaro AM, Tarapore PE, et al. Rathke cleft cysts in pediatric patients: presentation, surgical management, and postoperative outcomes. Neurosurg Focus. 2011; 31(1):E3

[3] Culver SA, Grober Y, Ornan DA, et al. A case for conservative management: characterizing the natural history of radiographically diagnosed Rathke cleft cysts. J Clin Endocrinol Metab. 2015; 100(10):3943–3948

[4] Aho CJ, Liu C, Zelman V, Couldwell WT, Weiss MH. Surgical outcomes in 118 patients with Rathke cleft cysts. J Neurosurg. 2005; 102(2):189–193

[5] Amhaz HH, Chamoun RB, Waguespack SG, Shah K, McCutcheon IE. Spontaneous involution of Rathke cleft cysts: is it rare or just underreported? J Neurosurg. 2010; 112(6):1327–1332

[6] Zada G, Ditty B, McNatt SA, McComb JG, Krieger MD. Surgical treatment of Rathke cleft cysts in children. Neurosurgery. 2009; 64(6):1132–1137, author reply 1037–1038

[7] Oh YJ, Park HK, Yang S, Song JH, Hwang IT. Clinical and radiological findings of incidental Rathke's cleft cysts in children and adolescents. Ann Pediatr Endocrinol Metab. 2014; 19(1):20–26

[8] Hayashi Y, Kita D, Fukui I, et al. Pediatric symptomatic Rathke cleft cyst compared with cystic craniopharyngioma. Childs Nerv Syst. 2016; 32(9):1625–1632

[9] Byun WM, Kim OL, Kim D. MR imaging findings of Rathke's cleft cysts: significance of intracystic nodules. AJNR Am J Neuroradiol. 2000; 21(3):485–488

[10] Alomari AK, Kelley BJ, Damisah E, et al. Craniopharyngioma arising in a Rathke's cleft cyst: case report. J Neurosurg Pediatr. 2015; 15(3):250–254

[11] Schweizer L, Capper D, Hölsken A, et al. BRAF V600E analysis for the differentiation of papillary craniopharyngiomas and Rathke's cleft cysts. Neuropathol Appl Neurobiol. 2015; 41(6):733–742

[12] Solari D, Cavallo LM, Somma T, et al. Endoscopic endonasal approach in the management of Rathke's cleft cysts. PLoS One. 2015; 10(10):e0139609

[13] Daubenbüchel AM, Hoffmann A, Gebhardt U, Warmuth-Metz M, Sterkenburg AS, Müller HL: Hydrocephalus and hypothalamic involvement in pediatric patients with craniopharyngioma or cysts of Rathke s pouch: impact on long-term prognosis. Eur J Endocrinol. 2015; 172 (5):561–569

[14] Lim HH, Yang SW: Risk factor for pituitary dysfunction in children and adolescents with Rathke s cleft cysts. Korean J Pediatr. 2010; 53(7):759–765

[15] Katavetin P, Cheunsuchon P, Grant E, Boepple PA, Hedley-Whyte ET, Misra M, et al: Rathke s cleft cysts in children and adolescents: association with female puberty. J Pediatr Endocrinol Metab. 2010; 23(11):1175-1180

[16] Evliyaoglu O, Evliyaoglu C, Ayva S: Rathke cleft cyst in seven-year-old girl presenting with central diabetes insipidus and review of literature. J Pediatr Endocrinol Metab. 2010; 23(5):525-529

16 Craniopharyngioma

Harminder Singh, Walid I. Essayed, and Theodore H. Schwartz

Abstract

Craniopharyngiomas represent up to 4% of pediatric intracranial tumors. Their operative and postoperative management continue to be challenging, particularly in the pediatric population. In this chapter, we discuss the natural history and different management options deployed for the treatment of these tumors, with a specific focus on endoscopic endonasal surgical techniques, and an illustrative case summarizing the different surgical steps. The primary goal of the endoscopic approach is to achieve maximum resection while avoiding hypothalamic and optic apparatus injuries. The pituitary function should be preserved as much as possible, but should not impede gross total resection when achievable.

Keywords: Craniopharyngioma, epithelial tumor, opticochiasmatic compression, hypothalamic, cystic

16.1 Prevalence

Craniopharyngiomas represent between 1% and 4% of diagnosed pediatric tumors and are the most-diagnosed tumors involving the sellar and suprasellar region.[1] These tumors tend to progress slowly and are often diagnosed between 5 and 14 years of age.[1,2] Craniopharyngiomas are rare tumors, with less than 100 pediatric cases a year in the United States,[3] making it difficult to evaluate the different treatment strategies applied across institutions.

16.2 Natural History

Craniopharyngiomas are benign epithelial tumors rising from ectopic remnants of Rathke's pouch. Therefore, they are almost exclusively localized to sellar and suprasellar regions. However, some tumors are purely intrasellar (5%), while others are purely suprasellar (20%).[1,4] Though benign, these tumors tend to damage surrounding structures by their growth. Opticochiasmatic compression, hypothalamic involvement, and intraventricular progression are the main reasons for presenting symptoms. Pituitary dysfunction is less prominent in pediatric patients, but can often lead to the diagnosis, particularly with linear growth impairment with growth hormone (GH) deficiency, and puberty delay due to follicle-stimulating hormone (FSH)/luteinizing hormone (LH) deficiencies.[4,5] Pediatric craniopharyngiomas usually have solid and cystic components, whereas in adults, they tend to be more solid. The cystic dilation of the tumor can be responsible for a rapid increase in the tumor size, inducing life-threatening symptoms (hydrocephalus), and necessitating rapid surgical treatment.[6]

16.3 Management Options: Medical, Surgical, and Adjuvant

Surgical treatment represents the gold standard of care for craniopharyngiomas. The surgical objective is to achieve gross total resection with minimum morbidity.[6,7,8] Classic resection of a craniopharyngioma is done through open transcranial microscopic surgery. Purely intraventricular tumors are usually resected through a transcallosal transventricular approach, while for the other lesions, multiple surgical corridors have been described in the literature. These range from anterior (subfrontal), anterolateral (pterional), to lateral (subtemporal transtentorial, posterior petrosal) approaches, and their different modifications.[6,8] Each approach has its advantages and limitations; however, they all require some degree of brain retraction, resulting in an increased risk of contusions and seizures. Moreover, craniopharyngiomas are midline tumors, and lateral approaches can create blind spots, since the surgeon is often working around critical neurovascular structures.

Aggressive resection resulting in bilateral hypothalamic injury can lead to severe functional impairment. Hyperthermia, thirst sensation deficit, hyperphagia leading to morbid obesity, as well as severely debilitating neurocognitive issues are of major concern, particularly in pediatric patients.[9] Injury to the mammillary bodies, particularly in retrochiasmatic tumors, can also lead to cognitive and memory disturbances. The lack of infrachiasmatic visualization is shared by all cranial microscopic approaches, putting the optic apparatus at risk for iatrogenic injury or vascular disruption of the optic chiasm. Intraoperative identification of the stalk, superior hypophyseal arteries, and normal pituitary tissue can be challenging, which, together with the frequent infiltration of the stalk, severely impedes postoperative pituitary function.

These unsatisfactory postoperative morbidities, along with the evolution of adjuvant treatment options (radiotherapy, radiosurgery, intracystic treatment, etc.), have led to divergent opinions over the balance between obtaining a complete resection and avoiding postoperative morbidity. No consensus is currently available over management strategies; some authors advocate less invasive procedures in conjunction with adjuvant therapy, in hope to preserve pituitary and hypothalamic function, while others insist on the importance of total resection as a definitive cure for a pathology where reoccurrences are even more delicate to manage. In general, if gross total resection can be achieved without damaging the hypothalamus, it should be attempted, particularly in tumors with infradiaphragmatic origin and no fluid-attenuated inversion recovery (FLAIR) signal in the hypothalamus.

Hypothalamic injuries are difficult to manage. Hypothalamic invasion is frequent and can be found in more than 90% of pediatric patients.[5] It is best assessed on MRI on T2 and FLAIR sequences, and if present, can help the surgeon preoperatively plan for a subtotal resection strategy associated with postoperative adjuvant treatment.[10] On the other hand, pituitary function, even though important, can be intentionally sacrificed to achieve gross total resection. This decision should be guided by thorough preoperative evaluation. Preoperative pituitary deficiencies and transinfundibular growth of the craniopharyngioma, classically signifying invasion of the pituitary stalk, are indicative of a poor postoperative functional preservation outcome. Furthermore, postoperative pituitary insufficiency is relatively frequent even in the subset of patients with subtotal resections. Since pituitary insufficiency can be medically managed, pituitary and stalk preservation should not get in the way of achieving gross total resection.

The adjuvant treatments currently available for postoperative management are mainly based on radiation and intracystic chemotherapy. Multiple radiation therapy algorithms are available with equivalent results in decreasing the recurrence rate in partially resected tumors.[1] Radiation is also useful if only biopsy was attempted in supposedly unresectable tumors. However, this local control is understandably associated with regional radiation toxicity. Already precarious endocrine equilibrium can be destabilized; visual complications are not uncommon, and long-term neurocognitive impairment is a major concern in pediatric cases, particularly with irradiation of the hypothalamus. Radiation-induced neoplasms and moyamoya can also occur in the pediatric population.[1] Stereotactic radiosurgery seems to be associated with less morbidity, but long-term results are still under investigation.[11] Accordingly, even though radiotherapy is a useful option, it should be delayed if possible in pediatric patients. Even though secondary surgery is usually more difficult, recurrences judged safe to resect should not be irradiated.

Pediatric craniopharyngiomas are frequently cystic. The cyst can represent the major component of a primitive or recurrent tumor and might display an accelerated growth pattern. Historically, intracystic chemotherapy was first developed in patients with reservoir-drained lesions. Many drugs, such as radioactive isotopes, bleomycin, and interferon, display varying degrees of efficiency but are unfortunately limited to the cystic portion of the tumor.[12] Currently, intracystic interferon-α instillation via an Ommaya reservoir is one of the most effective therapies.[13] Even though treatment modalities are still heterogeneous, multiple reports support the conclusion that intracystic interferon-α provides durable cyst shrinkage beyond the obvious benefit of repeated fluid aspirations.[13]

16.4 Endoscopic Endonasal Surgery

The anatomically sensitive location of craniopharyngiomas dictates this surgical approach. The position of the tumor in relation to the sellar diaphragm, optic chiasm, third ventricle, and infundibulum is important for the preoperative planning of surgery. Given the midline origin of most craniopharyngiomas, the endoscopic endonasal approach is often the best-suited approach for a majority of craniopharyngiomas. Recent data support the potential of endoscopic endonasal surgery in decreasing previously mentioned morbidities.[14] Contraindications for the endoscopic approach are tumors extending lateral to the cavernous sinus or carotid bifurcation, where gross total resection is the goal of surgery. Purely intraventricular tumors are a relative contraindication, since the floor of the third ventricle may be intact and violated through the endonasal endoscopic approach. The floor is formed by hypothalamic structures. In most cases, the floor is often extremely attenuated, making the endonasal approach safe. However, the degree of attenuation of the third ventricular floor can be difficult to determine on preoperative MRI scans.

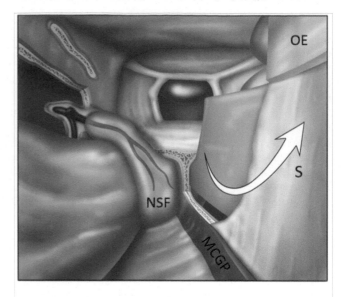

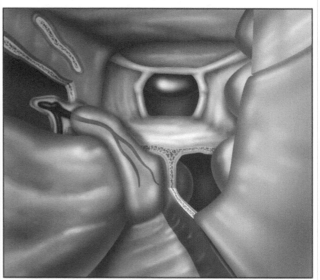

Fig. 16.1 The contralateral mucosal "swing" flap is used to cover the denuded septum. The olfactory epithelium (OE) and maxillary crest growth plate (MCGP) should be preserved in pediatric patients.

Pediatric considerations should be evaluated preoperatively. The sinus cavities are less developed in children, offering little room during surgery. Adenoidal resection may also be necessary when they limit access to the posterior nasopharynx. Care should be taken to preserve the olfactory epithelium (OE) as well as the maxillary crest growth plate (MCGP) when preparing the nasoseptal flap (NSF) and performing the posterior septostomy. The contralateral septal mucosal flap can then be cut and swung around to cover the denuded septum (from harvesting the NSF) on the ipsilateral side (▶ Fig. 16.1).

The infundibulum-based classification is the most pertinent when discussing endoscopic approaches.[8,10] The amount of skull base bony exposure should be tailored to the size and location of the tumor.[9] Transversely, opening the sella "from carotid to carotid" is important to offer maximum room for bimanual dissection. In the sagittal plane, the bony opening can be variable. For a purely intrasellar lesion, a limited classic opening of the anterior wall of the sella may be sufficient. On the other hand, preinfundibular lesions usually grow between the optic chiasm and the pituitary stalk, occupying the suprasellar and infrachiasmatic cisterns, and variably extending into the prechiasmatic cistern. For exposing these lesions, an extension of the drilling through the sphenoidal tuberculum as well as planum is usually necessary.[8,9] For transinfundibular tumors, further anterior exposure might be necessary to follow the tumor inside the third ventricle.[8,9] Retroinfundibular lesions can be resected by working on either side of the stalk. If the tumor extends into the prepontine cistern behind the dorsum sellae, the bone opening can be extended inferiorly along the clivus with removal of the posterior clinoid process.[8,9,10]

Once the bony opening is completed, the dura is opened, and tumor resection is started. The tumor can usually be quickly identified, allowing for internal debulking of the tumor as the first surgical step. The decompression allows the early identification of neurovascular structures and thus safer tumor dissection. Bimanual technique is employed for gentle and sharp progressive dissection from surrounding structures. Careful dissection of the anterior arterial communicating complex is important when attacking the prechiasmatic extension of the tumor. Preservation of the optic apparatus vasculature is also mandatory when dissecting this anterior extension of the tumor from the optic chiasm.[9] The dissection is then carried away from the anterior part, circumferentially to the lateral sides of the tumor, allowing progressive downward retraction to expose its superior aspect. This step is crucial for optimal close evaluation of the extent of hypothalamic invasion. Clear demarcation between the tumor and hypothalamic reactive gliosis can be difficult, but as we emphasized earlier in this chapter, maximal preservation of the hypothalamus is a key factor for maintaining patient functional outcome. Early identification of the pituitary stalk and superior hypophyseal arteries is important when attempting to preserve pituitary function. A branch of this artery can also extend up to the chiasm, which should be preserved. The decision to sacrifice the stalk should be left until the final stage of the resection. The use of angled endoscopes can help evaluate the extent of invasion of the surrounding structures along the resection cavity, and also for final inspection once the tumor is removed.

The progressive improvement in closure techniques have drastically reduced the postoperative rates of cerebrospinal fluid (CSF) leaks in endoscopic endonasal procedures. The systematic use of vascularized nasoseptal flaps in conjunction with postoperative lumbar drainage also helps in decreasing this risk. Various closure tactics have been reported, from the "gasket-seal" technique using MEDPOR and fascia lata[15] to the "bilayer-button" technique using two pieces of fascia lata stitched together in the center.[16] Some centers also advocate the use of intrathecal fluorescein to stain the CSF to better identify and repair intraoperative leaks.[17] Even so, in most craniopharyngioma series, the postoperative CSF leak rates are still around 10 to 15%.[9] The most successful closure has been the gasket seal combined with an NSF and a lumbar drain with leak rates on the order of 0 to 3%.[15,18,19] Close monitoring for postoperative diabetes insipidus is important, particularly since patients can experience both pituitary dysfunction and hypothalamic thirst deregulation.

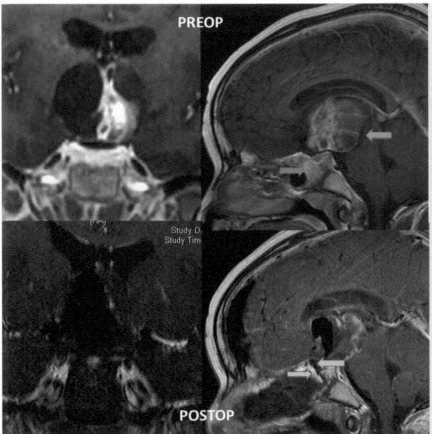

Fig. 16.2 Preoperative coronal and sagittal T1-weighted MRI images show an enhancing cystic *suprasellar* lesion with extension into the third ventricle and adherence to the hypothalamus (*blue arrow*). Conchal pattern of pneumatization of the sphenoid is seen (*orange arrow*). Postoperative imaging show subtotal resection (STR) of lesion. The MEDPOR graft used for skull base reconstruction can be visualized (*yellow arrow*), as well as the nasoseptal flap (*green arrow*). Note that some portions of the tumor are adherent to the hypothalamus and are left behind.

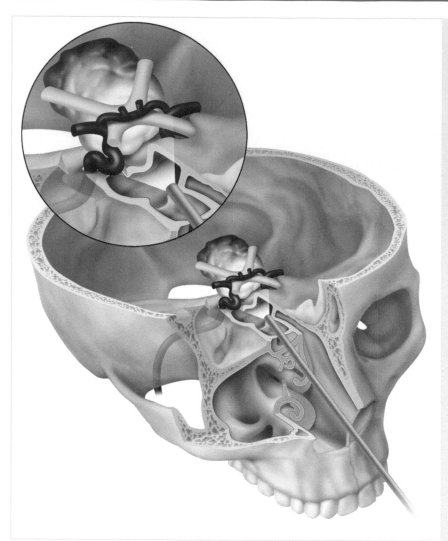

Fig. 16.3 The transtuberculum approach, through the transsphenoidal corridor, is used to approach most craniopharyngiomas.

16.4.1 Case Example

A 7-year-old boy was diagnosed with a large cystic craniopharyngioma. He underwent endoscopic intraventricular biopsy, cyst fenestration, and placement of a ventriculoperitoneal shunt at an outside institution. However, the patient continued to have increasing memory problems, and the cysts continued to grow in size (▶ Fig. 16.2). Therefore, the decision to proceed with endoscopic endonasal resection of this lesion was made.

The transtuberculum approach, through the transsphenoidal corridor, was used to approach the craniopharyngioma (▶ Fig. 16.3).

There was incomplete pneumatization (conchal type) of the sphenoid sinus. This soft, cancellous bone was drilled to reach the sella (▶ Fig. 16.4).

The bone over the sella and tuberculum was removed to expose the underlying dura, and the underlying intercavernous sinus was visualized. Laterally, the dura was exposed from one cavernous sinus to another for a panoramic exposure of the skull base (▶ Fig. 16.5).

The dura was opened above and below the intercavernous sinus, over the sella and the tuberculum sella. The optic chiasm and pituitary gland were visualized. The pituitary stalk was also seen (▶ Fig. 16.6).

Working on both sides of the pituitary stalk and under the optic chiasm, the tumor was mobilized from the third ventricle, (▶ Fig. 16.7) and removed in a piecemeal fashion (▶ Fig. 16.8).

The majority of the tumor and its capsule was resected in this fashion. Small fragments of the tumor capsule that were adherent to the hypothalamus were left behind to avoid injury to the hypothalamus (▶ Fig. 16.9).

A "gasket seal" was used for skull base reconstruction, using fascia lata and MEDPOR graft wedged into the bony opening (▶ Fig. 16.10). The previously harvested pedicled nasoseptal flap was layered over this closure, for a multilayer closure of the *skull base.*

16.5 Conclusion

Pediatric craniopharyngiomas can pose several management dilemmas. Does one aim for gross total resection or maximal functional preservation? What is the role of radiotherapy in children? How about adjuvant treatment modalities?

Since pediatric craniopharyngiomas are such a rare entity, there is no consensus regarding treatment algorithms (▶ Fig. 16.11). Ultimately, the treatment should be tailored to the child's presenting symptoms, his or her unique pathology, and the expectations of the parents. Hypothalamic injury can

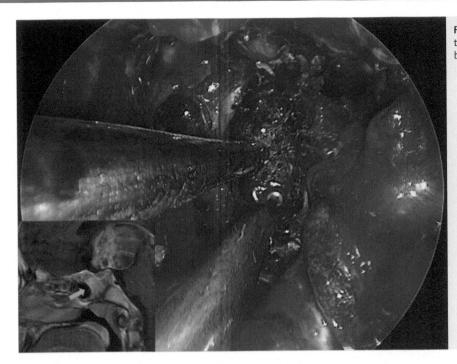

Fig. 16.4 Incomplete pneumatization (Conchal type) of the sphenoid is seen. This cancellous bone can be easily drilled to reach the sella.

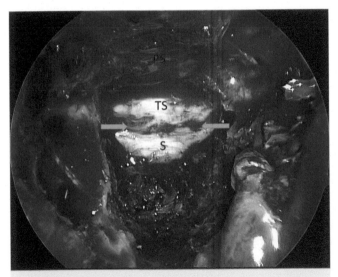

Fig. 16.5 The dura over the sella (S), tuberculum sella (TS), and planum sphenoidale (PS) is exposed. The intercavernous sinus is visualized (*blue arrows*).

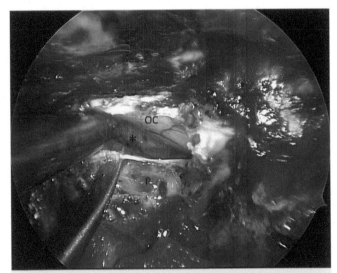

Fig. 16.6 The dura is opened above and below the intercavernous sinus, over the sella and the tuberculum sella. The optic chiasm (OC) and pituitary gland (P) are visualized. The pituitary stalk (*) is also seen. The green staining of the cerebrospinal fluid is from the fluorescein dye, which was injected via a lumbar puncture prior to the start of the case.

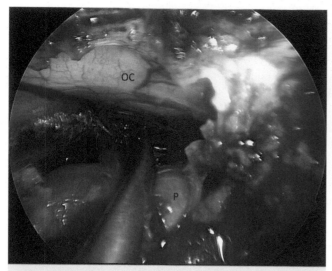

Fig. 16.7 The tumor is mobilized from the third ventricle, posterior to the pituitary stalk (*).

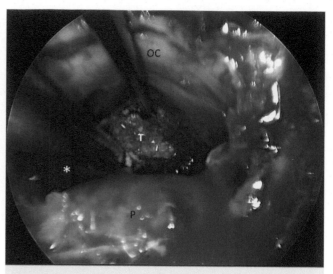

Fig. 16.8 The tumor (T) is resected in a piecemeal fashion. The pituitary stalk (*) is indented over the suction.

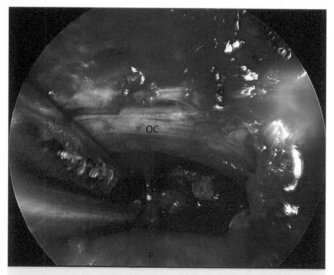

Fig. 16.9 The last few fragments of tumor are removed. The thinned out pituitary stalk (*) is seen. Small fragments of the capsule are stuck to the hypothalamus and are left behind.

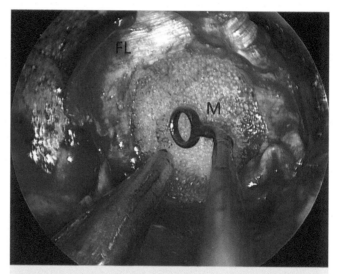

Fig. 16.10 A "gasket seal" is used for skull base reconstruction, using fascia lata (FL) and MEDPOR (M) graft wedged into the bony opening. The previously harvested pedicled nasoseptal flap is layered over this closure.

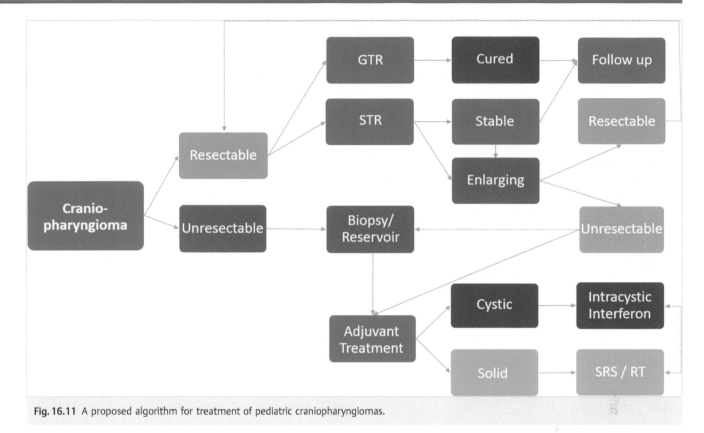

Fig. 16.11 A proposed algorithm for treatment of pediatric craniopharyngiomas.

lead to severe functional impairment in young children and should be avoided, even if it means leaving some residual tumor behind. Pituitary stalk and function may be sacrificed if it allows for a gross total resection, since recurrences are so difficult to manage in the pediatric population. Finally, the role of the BRAF mutation and the possible use of chemotherapy either in the neoadjuvant or recurrent setting is an area of future research that could change our management algorithm.[20]

16.6 Authors' Contribution

Harminder Singh and Walid I. Essayed contributed equally to the manuscript.

References

[1] Clark AJ, Cage TA, Aranda D, et al. A systematic review of the results of surgery and radiotherapy on tumor control for pediatric craniopharyngioma. Childs Nerv Syst. 2013; 29(2):231–238

[2] Bunin GR, Surawicz TS, Witman PA, Preston-Martin S, Davis F, Bruner JM. The descriptive epidemiology of craniopharyngioma. J Neurosurg. 1998; 89(4): 547–551

[3] Bunin GR, Surawicz TS, Witman PA, Preston-Martin S, Davis F, Bruner JM. The descriptive epidemiology of craniopharyngioma. Neurosurg Focus. 1997; 3 (6):e1

[4] Müller HL. Craniopharyngioma. Endocr Rev. 2014; 35(3):513–543

[5] Cohen M, Bartels U, Branson H, Kulkarni AV, Hamilton J. Trends in treatment and outcomes of pediatric craniopharyngioma, 1975–2011. Neuro-oncol. 2013; 15(6):767–774

[6] Komotar RJ, Roguski M, Bruce JN. Surgical management of craniopharyngiomas. J Neurooncol. 2009; 92(3):283–296

[7] Cavallo LM, Solari D, Esposito F, Villa A, Minniti G, Cappabianca P. The role of the endoscopic endonasal route in the management of craniopharyngiomas. World Neurosurg. 2014; 82(6) Suppl:S32–S40

[8] Fernandez-Miranda JC, Gardner PA, Snyderman CH, et al. Craniopharyngioma: a pathologic, clinical, and surgical review. Head Neck. 2012; 34(7):1036–1044

[9] Conger AR, Lucas J, Zada G, Schwartz TH, Cohen-Gadol AA. Endoscopic extended transsphenoidal resection of craniopharyngiomas: nuances of neurosurgical technique. Neurosurg Focus. 2014; 37(4):E10

[10] Raza SM, Schwartz TH. How to achieve the best possible outcomes in the management of retroinfundibular craniopharyngiomas? World Neurosurg. 2014; 82(5):614–616

[11] Niranjan A, Kano H, Mathieu D, Kondziolka D, Flickinger JC, Lunsford LD. Radiosurgery for craniopharyngioma. Int J Radiat Oncol Biol Phys. 2010; 78 (1):64–71

[12] Bartels U, Laperriere N, Bouffet E, Drake J. Intracystic therapies for cystic craniopharyngioma in childhood. Front Endocrinol (Lausanne). 2012; 3:39

[13] Dastoli PA, Nicácio JM, Silva NS, et al. Cystic craniopharyngioma: intratumoral chemotherapy with alpha interferon. Arq Neuropsiquiatr. 2011; 69(1):50–55

[14] Komotar RJ, Starke RM, Raper DM, Anand VK, Schwartz TH. Endoscopic endonasal compared with microscopic transsphenoidal and open transcranial resection of craniopharyngiomas. World Neurosurg. 2012; 77(2):329–341

[15] Garcia-Navarro V, Anand VK, Schwartz TH. Gasket seal closure for extended endonasal endoscopic skull base surgery: efficacy in a large case series. World Neurosurg. 2013; 80(5):563–568

[16] Luginbuhl AJ, Campbell PG, Evans J, Rosen M. Endoscopic repair of high-flow cranial base defects using a bilayer button. Laryngoscope. 2010; 120(5):876–880

[17] Raza SM, Banu MA, Donaldson A, Patel KS, Anand VK, Schwartz TH. Sensitivity and specificity of intrathecal fluorescein and white light excitation for detecting intraoperative cerebrospinal fluid leak in endoscopic skull base surgery: a prospective study. J Neurosurg. 2016; 124(3):621–626

[18] Leng LZ, Greenfield JP, Souweidane MM, Anand VK, Schwartz TH. Endoscopic, endonasal resection of craniopharyngiomas: analysis of outcome including extent of resection, cerebrospinal fluid leak, return to preoperative productivity, and body mass index. Neurosurgery. 2012; 70(1):110–123, discussion 123–124

[19] Patel KS, Raza SM, McCoul ED, et al. Long-term quality of life after endonasal endoscopic resection of adult craniopharyngiomas. J Neurosurg. 2015; 123 (3):571–580

[20] Brastianos PK, Shankar GM, Gill CM, et al. Dramatic response of BRAF V600E mutant papillary craniopharyngioma to targeted therapy. J Natl Cancer Inst. 2015; 108(2):djv310

17 Pituitary Adenomas: Functional

Davide Locatelli, Nurperi Gazioglu, and Paolo Castelnuovo

Abstract

Pediatric pituitary adenomas are rare lesions, for which endoscopic surgical treatment represents a feasible and effective choice. We report our personal experience in treating these lesions, describing the surgical technique in endoscopic-extended approaches, outcome, complications, and future perspectives.

Keywords: pituitary adenomas, endoscopic extended approaches, remission, outcome, skull base

17.1 Introduction

Pituitary adenomas represent uncommon lesions in the pediatric age group, accounting for approximately 3% of intracranial supratentorial tumors, with a mean annual incidence of 0.1 per million children.[1,2,3,4,5] The age range used to define "pediatric" is an important issue, as some authors report the upper age limit varying from 16 to 20 years. Therefore, the incidence of lesions of the sellar region ascribed to the pediatric population is affected by the upper age limit used to define "pediatric."[3,4] Pituitary adenoma is relatively rare in childhood, and the incidence increases from adolescence through 19 years of age.[6,7] Despite the rarity of these tumors, they can dramatically impact normal growth and cognitive maturation in young patients by causing changes in hormonal function and determining a significant effect on quality of life during a critical period of development.[4,8] This is especially true in younger children who are in periods of rapid sexual and skeletal development. Early evaluation and intervention, either medical or surgical, is necessary to avert permanent consequences of pituitary-related endocrinopathy.[9]

17.1.1 General Classification and Incidence

Historically, these tumors have been classified according to their size as being micro, macro, or giant adenomas. However, this classification has been enforced by a more comprehensive system based on immunohistochemistry and electron microscopy.[1] Pituitary adenomas can be classified further as functional or nonfunctional, depending on their hormonal activity in vivo. Pituitary adenomas in the pediatric population are usually hormonally active microadenomas, manifesting with an endocrinopathy rather than with a mass effect. They cause different endocrine symptoms than in adults, with primary amenorrhea, pubertal and/or growth delay, except in growth hormone (GH) secreting adenomas. Prolactinomas are the most frequent histologic subtype in children, followed by corticotrophin-secreting tumors and somatotropinomas.[5] Thyroid-stimulating hormone (TSH) secreting adenomas are only rarely reported as unique cases.[1,10] Functioning gonadotroph adenomas are extremely rare. Recent review has only found two case reports of adolescent girls. Nonsecreting adenomas are very rare in children, accounting for only 3% to 6% of all pituitary

tumors. This distribution is opposite to that observed in adults, where nonfunctioning adenomas predominate.[11]

An increased prevalence of pituitary adenomas in female patients has been reported, which most likely reflects the relative predominance of the two main types of adenomas: prolactin (PRL) and adrenocorticotropic hormone (ACTH) secreting adenomas.[4,12]

Childhood-onset pituitary adenomas can be associated with a variety of genetic syndromes, the most common being multiple endocrine neoplasia type 1 (MEN-1).

17.1.2 Clinical Presentation General Features

Clinical onset of pediatric pituitary tumors is generally related to endocrine dysfunction rather than mass effect. Tumors that grow rapidly, even if they are hormonally inactive, are capable of producing symptoms of an intracranial mass, such as visual field disturbances.[2] Rarely, pituitary adenomas present with pituitary apoplexy, an acute syndrome caused by infarction and hemorrhage. Small, slow-growing, hormonally inactive lesions are sometimes identified as incidental findings on radiologic or postmortem examinations, whereas small, slow-growing lesions with hormonal overproduction can manifest clinically as typical syndromes.

Pituitary Apoplexy in the Pediatric Population

Literature regarding pituitary apoplexy in the pediatric or adolescent population is restricted to case reports or individual cases; however, gaps remain in our knowledge of the differences between adults and children in the presentation, severity of symptoms, and outcomes of this disease.[13] Pituitary apoplexy is a clinical syndrome recognized by the onset of abrupt signs and symptoms that are associated with changes at the histologic level, consisting of infarction, hemorrhage, or a combination of both in pituitary tumors.[1,4,5,14,15,16] Some authors, like Mehrazin, reported a higher chance of pituitary apoplexy in pediatric invasive pituitary tumors.[17]

Diagnosis of this entity is based on clinical and imaging features. Cornerstones of management include hormonal replacement with steroids, followed by rapid surgical decompression.

Giant Pituitary Adenomas

Giant pituitary adenomas (GPAs) are rare entities in the group of pituitary adenomas. A majority are functional tumors and are distinct from their adult counterparts, with prolactinomas being the most common subtype followed by GH-secreting adenomas.

Some authors have described a high invasiveness of pituitary adenomas in younger patients. GPAs present more frequently with mass effect, offering a surgical challenge, considering their close proximity to optic pathways, intracavernous carotid artery, and oculomotor nerves, therefore making a radical resection more difficult. In a study of 12 children with GPAs, it was noted that symptoms due to local mass effect were predominant, presenting with visual deterioration (73%) and headache (64%).[18] Transsphenoidal surgical removal of the adenoma is a first choice, improving vision in 44% of pediatric patients.

GPAs present a higher complication rate compared with nongiant adenomas. In the study population presented in the literature, there is a high incidence of morbidity (25%), mortality (8%), poor outcome (50%), and preoperative (18%) and postoperative (8%) pituitary apoplexy.[18] The higher rate of pituitary apoplexy in this group of tumors confirms the aggressive nature of these lesions.

17.2 Indications for Surgical Treatment

There are no consensus statements nor guidelines available for the treatment of pediatric patients with pituitary adenomas. Although medical treatment can be effective, surgery is accepted as the first-line treatment in patients with gigantism or Cushing's disease (CD). It is also indicated when lesions cause mass effect and cranial neuropathy, mostly affecting visual function, or if the side effects of medical therapy are intolerable and endocrinologic disorders become unmanageable. The goal of surgery is radical excision of the tumor while preserving the normal pituitary gland. Tumor recurrence depends mostly on whether the patients undergo total or subtotal resection. In a retrospective review of 20 patients younger than 20 years old with pituitary adenomas, the authors describe the necessity of further surgical treatment in 5 of the 8 cases of subtotal resection; on the other hand, only 2 of the 12 patients who underwent total resection documented recurrent disease (17%).[4] Other authors like Mindermann and Wilson have described a recurrence rate of 10% in cases of subtotal resection.[3]

17.3 Anatomical Peculiarities in Pediatric Population

Endoscopic transsphenoidal surgery is generally accepted as the surgical method of choice for the resection of pituitary adenomas, especially if they are large and invasive. Standard and expanded endonasal approaches (EEAs) have demonstrated their efficacy in managing sellar and parasellar skull base lesions in younger patients. Some anatomic features have to be considered when endoscopically treating sellar lesions and pituitary adenomas in the pediatric population. They are potentially limited by several bony sinonasal landmarks and critical neurovascular structures such as piriform aperture, sphenoid sinus pneumatization, and intercarotid distances.

Piriform aperture width is significantly different between patients younger than 2 years (17.2 ± 0.5 mm) and adults (22.2 ± 1.3 mm); $p < 0.00003$.[14] It is significantly narrower in patients up to 6 to 7 years of age compared with adults ($p < 0.002$); there is no significant difference among patients 9 to 10 years of age and older.

Sphenoid bone pneumatization begins after 2 years of age at the anteroinferior wall of sphenoidal bone; by 6 to 7 years of age, the anterior sphenoid wall, the anterior sellar wall (77%), and 32% of the sellar floor are pneumatized. Therefore, incomplete pneumatization of the sphenoid sinus is common in

pediatric patients; this factor does not restrict resection of sellar region tumors for most of the authors via EETA (endoscopic endonasal transsphenoidal approach). The sphenoid sinus is well pneumatized in patients 10 years of age and older, and sphenoidal septations in pediatric patients older than 10 years are comparable to those in adults. Intercarotid distance is significantly narrower in patients up to 6 to 7 years old (10.2 ± 1.0 mm) compared with adults (12.6 ± 0.9), with $p < 0.003$ at the level of the cavernous sinus. There is no significant difference among patients 9 to 10 years of age and older ($p > 0.36$). At the level of superior clivus, there is no statistical difference between adults and any of the pediatric cohorts ($p > 0.18$).[14]

These three major anatomical parameters do not represent a limitation to the use of EEAs in pediatric patients. Piriform aperture constitutes a limit only in the youngest patients (younger than 2 years); incomplete sphenoid pneumatization needs more drilling during the access; assessing the intercarotid distance during the intervention is supported by modern devices like micro-Doppler and neuronavigational systems.

Considering the developmental stage of the skull in children and the inconsistency of specific anatomic landmarks compared with the fully developed cranium of adults, endonasal surgical procedures in children are technically challenging and present higher surgical risk than in adults. This demonstrates the importance of smaller, dedicated instruments, together with a specific preoperative neuroimaging assessment. These anatomical peculiarities constitute an even greater limitation for the transsphenoidal microsurgical technique. The use of microdrills is impossible when working within a speculum indispensable for the microsurgical technique. In addition, several severe complications, such as skull base fractures and blindness, have been reported due to the use of a speculum.

Although the cranio-orbitozygomatic skeleton reaches 85% of adult size by 5 years of age, the size of the nasoseptal flap (NSF) area is a potential limitation in reconstructing skull base lesions.[19] Recent literature has suggested that the NSF is only a viable option in patients older than 6 to 7 years.[20] A recent retrospective review of 16 pediatric patients evaluated the viability of NSF reconstruction in endoscopic endonasal approaches (EEA) for intracranial suprasellar neoplasms. Radiographic analysis demonstrated that septal lengths even in children younger than 10 years were adequate to cover the defects created by the suprasellar resections.[20] With adequate radiographic measurements, the authors demonstrated that the flap reconstruction length is adequate for EEA reconstruction in suprasellar lesions.

17.4 Surgical Management

The EETA to the sellar region for the removal of pituitary adenomas and other neoplasms of this area has proven its efficacy in the adult population over the last 20 years. It is safe and effective thanks to its favorable peculiarities, that is, its minimal invasiveness and decreased peri- and postoperative complications, including lower rates of cerebrospinal fluid (CSF) leak, septal perforation, and lower neurovascular damage, if associated with modern intraoperative instruments as Doppler and neuronavigation.

The use of endonasal transsphenoidal endoscopic surgery is increasingly reported as the technique of choice for the treatment of sellar and suprasellar lesions in the pediatric population as well. The association with minimal surgical trauma is a recognized feature in these patients. Children report lower pain perception after endoscopic pituitary surgery compared with traditional transsphenoidal surgery.[21,22] They also reported a lower rate of access to ICU and lower rate of perioperative blood transfusions.

17.4.1 Endoscopic Approaches and Surgical Technique

Depending on the site of extension of the lesion, endoscopic approaches include direct paraseptal transsphenoidal approach to sellar region, usually bilateral, transethmoidal sphenoidal approach, transethmoidal-pterygoidal-sphenoidal approach (TEPSA).

The direct bilateral paraseptal transsphenoidal approach to the sellar region is the preferential approach to the sellar cavity, providing a direct access to the sphenoid sinus; it has been described as standard for space-occupying lesions in sellar and suprasellar spaces, according to specific anatomy.

A transethmoidal-sphenoidal approach is adopted for sellar lesions with extension to the medial parasellar region, the lateral recess of the sphenoid sinus, and the posterolateral ethmoid, as well as accessing the posterior ethmoid, orbital apex, lateral wall of the sphenoid sinus, and medial component of the cavernous sinus. This approach starts with an ethmoidectomy with partial resection of the middle and superior turbinates, which, in combination with resection of posterior ethmoidal cells, allows for the exposure of the anterior wall of the sphenoid sinus, orbital apex, and the base of the pterygoid. The anterior wall of the sphenoid sinus is removed, and the sphenopalatine artery (SPA) is electrocauterized.[23]

TEPSA is dedicated for surgical excision of lesions extended to the lateral part of the cavernous sinus, the base of the middle cranial fossa, and the infratemporal fossa. Depending on the site of maximum lateral extension, TEPSA can be performed monolaterally with a paraseptal transsphenoidal approach contralaterally.

Surgical Steps in Paraseptal Transsphenoidal Approach

In the nasal stage, if NSF reconstruction is planned, the flap is harvested before sphenoidotomy, preserving the flap pedicle and blood supply by SPA in its septal branches (rescue flap). First described in 2006, the NSF has become the standard for adult and, more recently, pediatric skull base reconstruction.[24] Pedicled on the posterior septal branches of the SPA, this mucoperiosteal and mucoperichondrial flap is reliable for most skull base sites of reconstruction. The pedicle courses across the inferior sphenoid sinus face, and flap harvesting should occur before sphenoidotomy, as removal of the sphenoid face before this maneuver could interrupt the pedicle.[25] The maximal size of an NSF depends on nasal growth, an important consideration with the pediatric population.

A study of craniofacial CT scans suggests that although the width of the NSF is likely sufficient at any age, the length may be insufficient for a transsellar/transplanum defect until age 6 to 7 years, a transcribriform defect until age 9 to 10 years, and insufficient for a clival defect at all pediatric ages.[16]

During the procedure, many important anatomical landmarks should be taken into account in order to be preserved. Identification of the choanal margin, the superior turbinate, and the sphenoid ostium, the latter of which is visible in the region medial to the tail of superior or supreme turbinate, represents the first step to safely accessing the sphenoid sinus. The secure site to access the sphenoid sinus is located at the junction of two lines: the first vertical and parallel to the interchoanal septum and the second horizontal (parallel to the tail of the superior turbinate).[23] Access to sphenoidal sinus is gained by drilling medially to this secure anatomical site. On the contrary, in widening and opening inferiorly, attention must be paid to septal branches of SPA, which need to be electrocoagulated in case of damage.

If trimming/drilling of the superior turbinate is needed to enlarge access, attention must be paid to preserve the superolateral attachment and the tail of superior turbinate (axilla), preventing iatrogenic injury to the olfactory neuroepithelium, causing hyposmia.

After bilateral sphenoidotomy and drilling of the sphenoidal rostrum and intrasphenoidal septum, the next step is represented by identification of intrasphenoidal key landmarks. Enlarging the sphenoid sinus facilitates locating the intracavitary position of the internal carotid artery (ICA) and optic nerves bilaterally. Complete bilateral sphenoidotomy allows complete removal of the entire anterior wall of the sphenoid sinus, joining the two ostia, removing the intersphenoidal septum, and exposing the sellar floor. Once the entire sphenoid sinus cavity is exposed, the sellar floor must be opened.[23] Removal of the sellar floor involves prior anatomical localization of specific landmarks to avoid major iatrogenic injuries. Varying according to the type of sphenoid anatomy, the surgeon must identify the bony prominence covering both paraclival ICAs, depression of the wall of the clivus, the bony prominence of the cavernous tract of the ICAs, chiasmatic protrusions, and interoptic carotid recesses. Anatomical landmarks are checked during the intervention using Doppler sound and neuronavigation systems. When the central bony part of the sellar floor has been removed, the periosteal dural layer is incised to gain access to the lesion.

The intrasellar surgical technique consists of classical curettage for tumor excision in sellar cavity. The use of different graded scopes is essential to check a 360-degree tumor extension in the sellar, parasellar, and suprasellar spaces.

In the sellar stage, care must be taken to enlarge the approach laterally. Control with a micro-Doppler is important in order not to injure vital neurovascular structures.

Depending on the consistency of the lesion, hydrodissection can be sufficient to complete tumor excision in very soft tumors. In fibrous lesions or hard consistency tumors, microsurgical sharp dissection is needed, and fibrous or calcific components could require Sonopet® or cavitron® ultrasonic aspirator (CUSA) use.

Lesion removal is completed by planned endoscopic "diving" exploration of the sellar and parasellar spaces; this technique is useful to complete and evaluate the radical removal of sellar lesions, providing a faster and safer removal of sellar and suprasellar lesions. We described this technique in view of our experience in neuroendoscopic transcranial approaches to the ventricular system in the early 1990s.[26] Diving technique optimizes vision using the dynamic fluid film lens principle, becoming useful to go beyond mere visualization of the surgical field, to complete the removal of the lesion, improving hemostasis, CSF leakage, and lesion removal detection. The diving technique is particularly useful to detect small infiltrations to the cavernous sinus and in checking the integrity of the pituitary stalk when instruments are introduced into the sella.

Hemostasis is conducted during the whole procedure with warm water irrigation, the use of cottonoids, and the attempt to preserve normal mucosa. In the presence of abundant bleeding, sealants and hemostatic matrices such as thrombin-derived products can improve bleeding control and can be placed in the surgical site.

EEA to skull base lesions requires correct reconstruction of skull base defect in case of CSF leakage, and if there is intraoperative evidence of cisternal opening into the sphenoid, in case of extended surgical approach. The technique requires multilayer reconstruction strategy using different kinds of materials. The choice of material depends on the type of surgical approach and the patient's anatomy. The authors prefer autologous materials such as temporal fascia, septal or turbinate mucoperiosteum, quadrangular cartilage, and turbinate bone. If, during access, the middle turbinate has to be removed (as in TEPSA), it can be used as a free graft. Reconstruction techniques require placement of the intrasellar layer of connective fascia, a second layer of bone or cartilage (underlay), and a third extracranial layer of mucoperiosteum on the sellar floor (overlay); these layers can be reduced to two (underlay and overlay), and the fascia may also be used alone.

The authors believe that in standard direct paraseptal approach, reconstruction is not mandatory.

Final placement of hemostatic material and Merocel packing are useful to complete closure, together with bilateral paraseptal Silastic sheets to help re-epithelialization and avoid synechiae.

17.4.2 Intraoperative and Postoperative Complications

Possible complications are related to sinonasal function, neurovascular injury, CSF leak, central nervous system (CNS) infection (meningitis, abscess), and damage to CNS tissue (endocrinopathy, motor, or sensory dysfunction). Neurovascular complications include intraoperative acute bleeding (hemorrhage from ICA and its branches, SPA bleeding), stroke, and cranial nerve damage, especially the sixth cranial nerve, causing diplopia.

An important consideration in pediatric patients is the potential impact of skull base surgery on craniofacial growth. Endoscopic skull base surgery is safe in well-trained skull base teams with little impact on craniofacial growth.

CSF leakage is one of the most adverse complications described for EETA. Published CSF leak rates in adults range from 1.3% to 15% and in the pediatric age from 8% to 10.5%.[27] Higher rates in adults may be associated with extended procedures, with greater subarachnoid dissection required to access the lesions. Many techniques have been described to prevent CSF leakage after endoscopic transsphenoidal approaches, but we prefer multilayer reconstruction with autologous material and pedicled NSF as described in the previous section.[20] Its efficacy in preventing postoperative CSF leaks in adult population has already been proven and described in the literature. Less is known about reconstruction in the pediatric population.

Mucocele represents another possible complication in this kind of surgery. The basic etiologic problem is the compromised ventilation of sinuses. Children may be particularly at risk for mucocele formation because of the pediatric anatomical features with incomplete sinus development. A recent study in traumatic cases has described the importance of proper positioning of the graft in endoscopic repair of frontal recess fractures.[28] Pediatric cases of mucocele are also described decades after the initial trauma. Endoscopic sinonasal procedures such as functional endonasal endoscopic surgery have been proven to raise the risk of nasofrontal duct stenosis and mucocele formation. This type of approach, in particular transethmoidal approach, might play a role in mucocele pathogenesis. Avoiding trauma of the healthy mucosa, especially in the middle meatus region, as well as meticulous postoperative cleaning and debridement of the ethmoid cavity might decrease the risk for middle meatus adhesion and mucocele formation.[28] When the middle turbinate is used for the repair, care must be taken to strip off both the mucosa surrounding the defect and the skull base facing turbinate mucosa, to avoid any mucosal inclusion, as it may generate a future mucocele.[29]

Other endonasal complications include local crusting (treated with softening medications), scarring, and synechiae, prevented with placement of Silastic sheets at the end of surgical procedure. Short-term sinonasal dysfunction requiring debridement and saline irrigation is expected, but long-term issues are possible and include synechiae, nasal obstruction, chronic sinusitis, septal perforation, and altered olfaction.

Transient diabetes insipidus (DI) is a described complication after EETA, ranging from 0.4% to 48.8% for transient DI. Permanent DI rates range from 2.3% to 8.1%. DI is neurogenic from injury to the magnocellular neurons in the hypothalamus where arginine-vasopressin is produced and transported to the posterior pituitary gland. Factors including lesion size, adherence to surrounding structures, and histopathology, and surgical approach can result in DI. Care should be taken during surgery to preserve neurovascular structures in close proximity to the lesion.

Hypopituitarism occurred in 1.4% to 19.8% of cases reported in the literature. It can be associated with dysfunction of the anterior pituitary gland, requiring hormonal replacement therapy.[15,19,30]

17.5 Histological Subtypes

17.5.1 Prolactin-Secreting Adenomas

Prolactinomas are the most frequent pituitary tumors in childhood, and their frequency varies with age and sex, occurring mostly in adolescents for pediatric age group and in women between the ages of 20 and 50 years.

Criteria for Prolactin-Secreting Adenomas

PRL-secreting adenomas are usually diagnosed at the time of puberty or in the postpubertal period.[5,14,30] Clinical manifestations vary, depending on the age and sex of the child. Girls of prepubertal age generally present with a combination of headache, visual disturbances, growth failure, and primary amenorrhea.

The differential diagnosis of hyperprolactinemia should consider any process interfering with dopamine synthesis, its transport to the pituitary gland, or its action at lactotrophic dopamine receptors. A single measurement of PRL levels is unreliable, because PRL secretion is markedly influenced by physical and emotional stress. To obtain a diagnostic value of PRL concentrations, at least three to six samples are necessary, taking into consideration the mean value. PRL levels are parallel to the tumor volume, and differential diagnosis of hyperprolactinemia caused by pituitary microadenoma hypersecretion or with so-called stalk effect of a nonfunctioning macroadenoma or craniopharyngioma is important for the management of the lesion. Contrarily, a macroprolactinoma with a very high PRL secretion can be misdiagnosed due to the so-called hook effect, consisting of a measurement error in the chemiluminometric method. In case of a macroadenoma with PRL below 200 ng/mL, measurement of serum PRL after 1:100 dilution is recommended in order to clarify whether there is a hook effect.

Dopamine agonists are very effective in the treatment of the majority of prolactinomas. Surgery is only recommended for drug-resistant or intolerant caes.

17.5.2 Adrenocorticotropic Hormone–Secreting Adenomas

In children between 11 and 15 years of age, ACTH-secreting adenomas are the most frequent cause of adrenal hyperfunction and the second most frequent pituitary adenoma after prolactinomas. A macroadenoma is rarely the cause of CD in children.

Criteria for Cushing's Disease

The clinical manifestations of CD are mostly the consequence of cortisol overproduction. The clinical presentation is highly variable, with signs and symptoms that can range from subtle to obvious. Diagnosis is generally delayed because frequently a growth rate decrease may be the only symptom for a long time. Growth failure in patients with CD may be due to a decrease of free insulin-like growth factor 1 levels and/or a direct negative effect of cortisol on the growth plate.

Other physical manifestations of CD include facial plethora, purple striae in the abdomen, legs and arms, muscular weakness, hypertension, and osteoporosis. Children with CD may also have impaired carbohydrate tolerance (although diabetes mellitus is uncommon). Excessive adrenal androgens may cause acne and excessive hair growth, or premature sexual development in the first decade of life. Besides, hypercortisolism may cause pubertal delay in adolescent patients. Peculiarly, young patients with CD may present with neuropsychiatric symptoms that differ from those of adult patients. Frequently, they tend to be obsessive and are high performers at school.

The differential diagnosis of CD includes adrenal tumors, ectopic ACTH production (rare in the pediatric population), and ectopic corticotropin-releasing hormone (CRH)-producing tumors. In a child/adolescent with suspected CD, the diagnosis is based on the measurement of basal and stimulated levels of cortisol and ACTH. Measurement of 24-hour urinary free cortisol is elevated, and a low dose of dexamethasone at midnight does not induce suppression of morning serum cortisol concentrations[31]. Suppression of the spontaneous circadian variations of serum cortisol is another feature of CD. Suppression of

cortisol by more than 50% after administration of high-dose dexamethasone given at midnight will confirm that hypercortisolism is ACTH dependent. On enhanced MRI, ACTH-secreting pituitary adenomas are significantly smaller than all other types of adenomas, and therefore even high-quality pituitary MR images may fail to visualize the tumor.

In some cases, diagnosis of CD is based on the initial clinical and laboratory data. In uncertain cases of CD, inferior petrosal sinus sampling can have a high specificity, but it carries a high rate of false-positive results.[32,33] Cavernous sinus sampling is another method of venous sampling, and because it is less influenced by variations of the venous anatomy, it is more reliable for lateralization of the lesion within the pituitary gland.[34] This procedure can also be difficult in children, both from a technical standpoint and because of the risk of morbidity from the intervention and anesthesia.[33] If a patient exhibits a lateralizing ACTH gradient of 2:1 or greater, removal of the appropriate half of the anterior pituitary gland will be curative in 80% of cases.[35] According to Kunwar and Wilson,[9] in the presence of negative findings on surgical exploration, the use of inferior petrosal sinus sampling as a guide to the localization of a pituitary adenoma can be successful and curative. Patients who failed for remission after transsphenoidal surgery have to receive adjunctive medical treatment. In case of persistent disease, bilateral adrenalectomy and/or radiotherapy are the last options.

17.5.3 Growth Hormone–Secreting Adenomas

In childhood, GH-secreting adenomas account for 5% to 15% of all pituitary adenomas. In less than 2% of the cases, excessive GH secretion is caused by a hypothalamic or ectopic GH-releasing hormone-producing tumor (i.e., a bronchial or pancreatic carcinoid).

Criteria for GH-Secreting Adenomas

In adults, chronic GH hypersecretion causes acromegaly, which is characterized by hyperostosis. In children and adolescents, it leads to gigantism due to associated secondary hypogonadism, which delays epiphyseal closure, thus allowing long-bone growth. The two disorders may be considered part of a spectrum of GH oversecretion, with principal manifestations determined by the developmental stage in which this originates.[27] Diagnosis of acromegaly and gigantism is usually clinical and can be promptly confirmed measuring circulating insulin-like growth factor 1 concentrations, correlated to the integrated 24-hour GH secretion levels.[8]

17.5.4 Thyroid Stimulating Hormone–Secreting Adenomas

This tumor type is rare in adulthood and even rarer in childhood and adolescence, with only a few case reports in the literature.[5] It is frequently a macroadenoma presenting with mass effect symptoms such as headache and visual disturbance, together with symptoms and signs of hyperthyroidism. TSH-secreting adenomas must be differentiated from thyroid hormone resistance. In most cases, the classic criteria of lack of TSH response to

TRH stimulation, elevation of serum alpha-subunit levels, and a high alpha-subunit/TSH ratio, along with a pituitary mass on MR images, are diagnostic of TSH-secreting adenoma.

17.5.5 Gonadotropin-Staining Adenomas

The incidence of follicle-stimulating hormone (FSH) and luteinizing hormone (LH)-secreting tumors with a clinical picture of hormone hypersecretion is very rare in the pediatric population.[3]

17.6 Differential Diagnosis

Locating the lesions in the sellar and suprasellar spaces is important in order to differentiate pituitary adenomas from other benign lesions like Rathke's cleft cysts (RCC), which usually remain asymptomatic. When clinically relevant, they cause headache (32.1–80%), endocrine disturbances (30–69.4%), and visual impairment (14.3–55.8%).

A study evaluating MR images in a group of 341 patients younger than 15 years revealed only 4 pituitary cystic lesions.[34] Regarding differentiation from pituitary adenomas, location is an important factor, in that RCCs typically lie centrally in the pars intermedia between the anterior and posterior lobes, whereas pituitary adenomas are often eccentric and typically located within the adenohypophysis. Furthermore, as far as MRI is concerned, apparent diffusion coefficient (ADC) values of RCC are significantly higher than those of the cystic components of craniopharyngiomas and hemorrhagic components of pituitary adenomas, providing a useful information in the differential diagnosis.

Incidentalomas may create management difficulties. Incidental identification of a small cyst in the pituitary gland of a child must be considered an incidental finding in the absence of signs or symptoms referable to pituitary dysfunction.[25]

17.7 Authors' Experience

Considering a total series of 1,500 transsphenoidal procedures for sellar tumor excision from 1997 to 2016, we analyzed our cases and found 23 cases of pediatric pituitary adenomas (unpublished series). We include in this series patients operated in three different university hospitals by three senior skull base neurosurgeons and otolaryngologists. Medical records were evaluated retrospectively, recording the clinical presentation, surgical strategies, histology, and follow-up.

The total population of 23 cases consists of 14 females and 9 males (female:male of 14:9), with a minimal age of 4 years and maximal age of 18 years (median age 15.13 years).

All 23 cases were operated by transsphenoidal surgery; 7 of them microscopically, before 2007 and the other 14 cases by EETA. Only one case was first operated by microscopic surgery then by EETA for recurrence.

Of the total population, 56.5% (13/23) were microadenomas, 13% (8/23) were macroadenomas, and 8.6% (2/23) were not radiologically visible. Of all macroadenomas, 50% presented with cavernous sinus invasion (4/8).

Of all cases, 13 cases presented with Cushing's syndrome (56%; 13/23: 2 macroadenomas, 9 microadenomas, and 2 not

visible), 5 patients presented with hyperprolactinemia (21.7%; 5/23: 3 macroadenomas, 2 microadenomas), and 2 adolescents presented with gigantism (8.7%; 2/23: macroadenomas with cavernous sinus invasion).

Nonfunctioning adenomas represented 3 of 23 cases (13.4%; 2 macroadenomas, 1 microadenomas). Total resection was achieved in 17 cases (17/23; 73.9%). Complications included 2 cases of CSF fistula requiring a second EETA for closure and 1 transient DI. There was no mortality nor neurological morbidity in this series.

17.7.1 Illustrative Case

We report the case of a 4-year-old male presenting with fast weight gain, irritability, and abdominal pain (▶ Fig. 17.1a, b); his physical examination showed a height of 95 cm (height standard deviation [SD]: 1.24), weight of 22.5 kg with central obesity (BMI: 25 kg/m^2; BMI > 95%), plethora, moon face, buffalo hump, and purple striae. Neurological examination was normal.

Hormonal tests showed the following: cortisol greater than 59.8 mcg/dL, ACTH 53.6 pg/mL, dehydroepiandrosterone sulfate

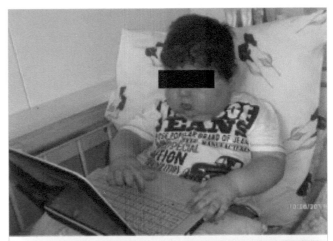

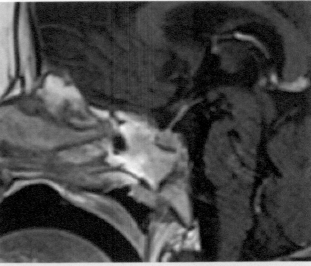

Fig. 17.1 (a) The child presented with weight gain; physical examination showed a height of 95 cm and weight of 22.5 kg with a central obesity. **(b)** Enhanced sellar MRI showed a suspect microadenoma.

(DHEA-SO$_4$) 496.1 mcg/dL, 24-hour urinary free cortisol (UFC) greater than 1,000 mcg, TSH 0.5 mIU/mL, fT4 1 ng/dL, fT3 1.8 pg/mL, Testosterone 92 ng/dL.

Suppression tests showed the following: 1-mg dexamethasone suppression (DST)—cortisol greater than 59.8 mcg/dL, ACTH 53.24 pg/mL; at 2 days 2-mg DST—cortisol 40 mcg/dL, 24-hour UFC greater than 1,000 mcg; 8-mg DST—cortisol greater than 59.8 mcg/dL and ACTH 7.02 pg/mL.

Radiological investigations showed normal adrenal gland. Enhanced sellar MRI showed a suspect microadenoma.

The patient underwent an endoscopic transsphenoidal exploration of pituitary gland with biopsies on suspected areas. Laboratory tests on cavernous sinus sampling are shown in ▶ Table 17.1.

Pathology showed normal adeno- and neurohypophysis on the right side and Crooke's cell positivity on the left side.

There were no postoperative complications; the patient is in remission (follow-up time of 4.5 years). The postoperative height at 6.7 years was 117 cm, with a BMI of 15.3 kg/m^2 (BMI SD: –0.07). Pituitary function is within normal ranges; postoperative MRI showed no residuals or relapses (▶ Fig. 17.2a–c).

Table 17.1 Cavernous sinus sampling (CSS)

ACTH levels with CSS	Right CS	Left CS	Peripheral sample
Initial	70.97	67.66	44.74
1 min after CRH	54.61	77.79	46.06
2 min after CRH	50.84	65.53	41.94
5 min after CRH	61.36	61.41	44.27
10 min after CRH	95.38	54.18	38.16

Abbreviations: ACTH, adrenocorticotropic hormone; CRH, corticotropin-releasing hormone; CS, cavernous sinus.

17.8 Discussion and Conclusion

Pediatric pituitary adenomas represent a rare pathology, and the literature about surgical approaches and series on this issue remains poor. Reasons for that include the fact that tumors in the sellar region are more frequently craniopharyngiomas, pituitary adenomas being relatively infrequent; anatomic features in pediatric population may sometimes restrict surgical indication for endoscopy; and the age range applied to define "pediatric" has been reported inconsistently, with the upper age limit varying from 16 to 20 years, so that the incidence of lesions of the sellar region ascribed to pediatric populations is affected by the upper age limit used to define "pediatric."[7]

Considering the particular age range in which these lesions may develop, some distinctive features have to be analyzed. Different clinical presentation, that is, different endocrine symptoms than adults, growing facial skeleton, and some particular anatomical characteristics have to be considered and discussed before surgery to optimize the access.

Endoscopic endonasal transsphenoidal surgery has proven its safety and efficacy in the treatment of pituitary lesions in the pediatric group, considering its relatively minimal invasiveness; it is useful in preserving anatomical and functional integrity of the hypothalamic–pituitary axis and is essential to child growth and maintaining good sinonasal functionality.

Dedicated instruments for pediatric age are necessary to the surgeons in order to perform procedures targeted on the growing skull base, but at the same time demand a lifelong training for every skull base surgeon.

In conclusion, skull base pathologies in the pediatric population, including pituitary adenomas, are rare and require particular management in order to offer the best surgical treatment and to avoid significant morbidity. Some anatomical typical

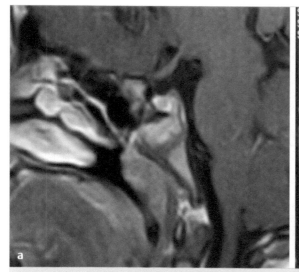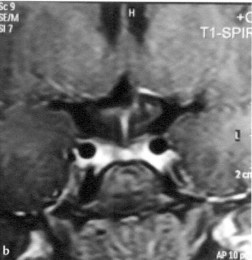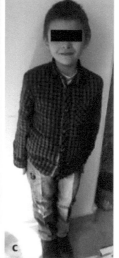

Fig. 17.2 Surgical procedure consisted in endoscopic transsphenoidal exploration of pituitary gland with biopsies on suspected areas. **(a,b)** Postoperative MRI showed no residuals or relapses. **(c)** There were no postoperative complications; the patient is in remission. Pituitary function is within normal range.

peculiarities have to be considered when planning a surgical intervention in the sellar and suprasellar spaces in pediatric patients. The improved techniques of endoscopic endonasal skull base surgery and intraoperative guidance have provided promising perspectives in the treatment of this kind of pathologies.

Multidisciplinary well-trained skull base teams represent today the best management option to achieve ideal candidate selection and optimize patient surgical treatment.

17.9 Acknowledgments

We thank Olcay Evliyaoğlu, MD, for providing the endocrinological data of our illustrative case; Oya Ercan, MD, for providing endocrine support to the pediatric patients operated in Cerrahpasa Medical Faculty Department of Neurosurgery; and Necmettin Tanriover, MD, one of the two senior neurosurgeons operating on pediatric pituitary adenomas. We also thank Desiree Lattanzi, MD, and Lidia Bifone, MD, both residents in neurosurgery working in Neurosurgery Unit, Ospedale di Circolo e Fondazione Macchi-ASST Sette Laghi, Varese, Italy, for their kind support in researching, providing data, and collaborating in manuscript editing.

References

[1] Artese R, D'Osvaldo DH, Molocznik I, et al. Pituitary tumors in adolescent patients. Neurol Res. 1998; 20(5):415–417

[2] Haddad SF, VanGilder JC, Menezes AH. Pediatric pituitary tumors. Neurosurgery. 1991; 29(4):509–514

[3] Mindermann T, Wilson CB. Pediatric pituitary adenomas. Neurosurgery. 1995; 36(2):259–268, discussion 269

[4] Webb C, Prayson RA. Pediatric pituitary adenomas. Arch Pathol Lab Med. 2008; 132(1):77–80

[5] Jagannathan J, Dumont AS, Jane JA, Jr, Laws ER, Jr. Pediatric sellar tumors: diagnostic procedures and management. Neurosurg Focus. 2005; 18 6A:E6

[6] Jagannathan J, Dumont AS, Jane JA, Jr. Diagnosis and management of pediatric sellar lesions. Front Horm Res. 2006; 34:83–104

[7] Zhan R, Xin T, Li X, Li W, Li X. Endonasal endoscopic transsphenoidal approach to lesions of the sellar region in pediatric patients. J Craniofac Surg. 2015; 26(6):1818–1822

[8] Cannavò S, Venturino M, Curtò L, et al. Clinical presentation and outcome of pituitary adenomas in teenagers. Clin Endocrinol (Oxf). 2003; 58(4):519–527

[9] Kunwar S, Wilson CB. Pediatric pituitary adenomas. J Clin Endocrinol Metab. 1999; 84(12):4385–4389

[10] Ezzat S, Asa SL, Couldwell WT, et al. The prevalence of pituitary adenomas: a systematic review. Cancer. 2004; 101(3):613–619

[11] Tindall GT, Barrow DL. Disorders of the Pituitary. St. Louis, MO: CV Mosby; 1986

[12] Blackwell RE, Younger JB. Long-term medical therapy and follow-up of pediatric-adolescent patients with prolactin-secreting macroadenomas. Fertil Steril. 1986; 45(5):713–716

[13] Jankowski PP, Crawford JR, Khanna P, Malicki DM, Ciacci JD, Levy ML. Pituitary tumor apoplexy in adolescents. World Neurosurg. 2015; 83(4):644–651

[14] Tatreau JR, Patel MR, Shah RN, et al. Anatomical considerations for endoscopic endonasal skull base surgery in pediatric patients. Laryngoscope. 2010; 120 (9):1730–1737

[15] Berker M, Hazer DB, Yücel T, et al. Complications of endoscopic surgery of the pituitary adenomas: analysis of 570 patients and review of the literature. Pituitary. 2012; 15(3):288–300

[16] Shah MV, Haines SJ. Pediatric skull, skull base, and meningeal tumors. Neurosurg Clin N Am. 1992; 3(4):893–924

[17] Mehrazin M. Pituitary tumors in children: clinical analysis of 21 cases. Childs Nerv Syst. 2007; 23(4):391–398

[18] Sinha S, Sarkari A, Mahapatra AK, Sharma BS. Pediatric giant pituitary adenomas: are they different from adults? A clinical analysis of a series of 12 patients. Childs Nerv Syst. 2014; 30(8):1405–1411

[19] Ghosh A, Hatten K, Learned KO, et al. Pediatric nasoseptal flap reconstruction for suprasellar approaches. Laryngoscope. 2015; 125(11):2451–2456

[20] Shah RN, Surowitz JB, Patel MR, et al. Endoscopic pedicled nasoseptal flap reconstruction for pediatric skull base defects. Laryngoscope. 2009; 119(6):1067–1075

[21] Massimi L, Rigante M, D'Angelo L, et al. Quality of postoperative course in children: endoscopic endonasal surgery versus sublabial microsurgery. Acta Neurochir (Wien). 2011; 153(4):843–849

[22] Frazier JL, Chaichana K, Jallo GI, Quiñones-Hinojosa A. Combined endoscopic and microscopic management of pediatric pituitary region tumors through one nostril: technical note with case illustrations. Childs Nerv Syst. 2008; 24 (12):1469–1478

[23] Castelnuovo P, Locatelli D. The Endoscopic Surgical Technique. Two Nostrils-Four Hands. Tuttlingen, Germany: Endo-Press; 2008

[24] Hadad G, Bassagasteguy L, Carrau RL, et al. A novel reconstructive technique after endoscopic expanded endonasal approaches: vascular pedicle nasoseptal flap. Laryngoscope. 2006; 116(10):1882–1886

[25] Rastatter JC, Snyderman CH, Gardner PA, Alden TD, Tyler-Kabara E. Endoscopic endonasal surgery for sinonasal and skull base lesions in the pediatric population. Otolaryngol Clin North Am. 2015; 48(1):79–99

[26] Locatelli D, Canevari FR, Acchiardi I, Castelnuovo P. The endoscopic diving technique in pituitary and cranial base surgery: technical note. Neurosurgery. 2010; 66(2):E400–E401, discussion E401

[27] Kassam A, Thomas AJ, Snyderman C, et al. Fully endoscopic expanded endonasal approach treating skull base lesions in pediatric patients. J Neurosurg. 2007; 106(2) suppl:75–86

[28] Verillaud B, Genty E, Leboulanger N, Zerah M, Garabédian EN, Roger G. Mucocele after transnasal endoscopic repair of traumatic anterior skull base fistula in children. Int J Pediatr Otorhinolaryngol. 2011; 75(9):1137–1142

[29] Frank G, Pasquini E. Endoscopic endonasal cavernous sinus surgery, with special reference to pituitary adenomas. Front Horm Res. 2006; 34:64–82

[30] Mamelak AN, Carmichael J, Bonert VH, Cooper O, Melmed S. Single-surgeon fully endoscopic endonasal transsphenoidal surgery: outcomes in three-hundred consecutive cases. Pituitary. 2013; 16(3):393–401

[31] Magiakou MA, Mastorakos G, Oldfield EH, et al. Cushing's syndrome in children and adolescents. Presentation, diagnosis, and therapy. N Engl J Med. 1994; 331(10):629–636

[32] Liu C, Lo JC, Dowd CF, et al. Cavernous and inferior petrosal sinus sampling in the evaluation of ACTH-dependent Cushing's syndrome. Clin Endocrinol (Oxf). 2004; 61(4):478–486

[33] Oldfield EH, Doppman JL, Nieman LK, et al. Petrosal sinus sampling with and without corticotropin-releasing hormone for the differential diagnosis of Cushing's syndrome. N Engl J Med. 1991; 325(13):897–905

[34] Takanashi J, Tada H, Barkovich AJ, Saeki N, Kohno Y. Pituitary cysts in childhood evaluated by MR imaging. AJNR Am J Neuroradiol. 2005; 26(8):2144–2147

[35] Gazioglu N, Ulu MO, Ozlen F, et al. Management of Cushing's disease using cavernous sinus sampling: effectiveness in tumor lateralization. Clin Neurol Neurosurg. 2008; 110(4):333–338

18 Pituitary Adenoma: Nonfunctional

Wenya Linda Bi, Edward R. Smith, Ian F. Dunn, and Edward R. Laws Jr.

Abstract

Nonfunctional adenomas are uncommon amongst pediatric pituitary tumors, with experience inferred largely from their more common adult counterparts. Nonfunctional adenomas are associated with lack of biochemical or clinical evidence of hormone hypersecretion, allowing them to grow until mass effect from compression of abutting neurovascular structures heralds their existence. A thorough history and physical examination, including perturbation of developmental milestones, may lend insight into the trajectory of these tumors. When intervention is indicated, surgery is the treatment of choice for nonfunctional adenomas. Very young children may have anatomic limitations that challenge a transsphenoidal approach. The ultimate decision for a transcranial or transnasal transsphenoidal route is dictated by the growth pattern of the tumor, its consistency, involvement of the optic apparatus and circle of Willis, and the surgeon's experience and preference. Following surgery, close monitoring of hormone status and electrolyte balance is critical, especially as children may not be able to compensate for rapid fluid shifts as readily as adults. Long-term follow-up and multidisciplinary care remains essential to the optimal outcome of children with nonfunctional pituitary adenomas.

Keywords: pituitary adenoma, nonfunctional adenoma, endoscopic endonasal surgery

18.1 Introduction

Sellar lesions in the pediatric population encompass a diverse gamut of pathologies, including craniopharyngioma, Rathke's cleft cyst, germ cell tumor, chordoma, adenoma, and others. As compared to adults, pediatric pituitary adenomas are relatively uncommon and are most frequently horomone-producing, or "functional," with the diagnosis of nonfunctional adenomas being rare (▶ Table 18.1).[1,2,3,4,5] When encountered, sporadic pituitary adenomas are associated with a higher rate of associated genetic mutations in children as compared to adults.[6]

Table 18.1 Relative incidence of pituitary adenoma subtypes in pediatric surgical series[a]

Pituitary adenoma subtype	Incidence (%)
Nonfunctional adenoma	6
Hypersecreting adenoma	94
Prolactin secreting	61
ACTH secreting	33
GH secreting[b]	15

Abbreviations: ACTH, adrenocorticotropin hormone; GH, growth hormone; PRL, prolactin.
[a]While hypersecreting adenomas typically express only one hormone, a small number may produce more than one hormone.
[b]GH-secreting adenomas in children either secrete GH alone or are frequently observed in the setting of plurihormonal expression.

These include germline and somatic mutations in *MEN1, AIP, CDKN1B,* and *PRKAR1A,* which may occur as part of a familial syndrome or in isolated cases.[7,8,9,10]

Given the low incidence of nonfunctional adenomas in children, the natural history of these particular tumors is inferred from their more common adult counterparts, with sparse experience documenting their clinical course and response to treatment in a solely pediatric population. Nonfunctional pituitary adenomas are associated with lack of clinical or biochemical evidence of hormone hypersecretion and encompass null cell adenoma, oncocytoma, silent corticotroph adenoma subtypes 1 and 2, silent subtype 3, nonfunctional gonadotroph adenoma, and silent somatotroph adenoma.[11,12] The absence of endocrinologic symptoms common to hypersecreting tumors cloaks the growth of nonfunctional adenomas until mass effect results from compression of adjacent neurovascular structures. Headache, visual disturbance, and subtle symptoms referable to hypopituitarism or compression of the infundibulum with diabetes insipidus may be elicited from the history. Following a thorough history and physical examination with growth charts, preoperative evaluation should include endocrinologic testing, formal neuro-ophthalmologic assessment (including visual field testing, specifically looking for bitemporal hemianopsia and any differences between left and right optic nerve function), and imaging (commonly a thin-cut MRI of the brain and skull base, with and without contrast). Biochemical data, abnormalities in developmental milestones, and progress through puberty may lend clinical insight for young patients from whom detailed symptoms may not be elicitable.

18.2 Management Options

Upon diagnosis of a sellar mass, observation, surgical resection, adjuvant radiation, and medical management may be considered. Indications for intervention include mass effect causing neurologic compromise, systemic sequelae from hormone hypersecretion, derangement of normal pituitary function from compression, and the need for a diagnosis. Surgery is the primary treatment of choice for nonfunctional adenomas. The goals of surgery mirror the indications for treatment, with aims focused on tissue diagnosis and maximal safe resection without compromising function (▶ Table 18.2). Reoperation for a residual or recurrent tumor is made more complex by the obscuring of surgical planes by scarring, adhesions increasing the risk of iatrogenic injury, and greater likelihood of cerebrospinal fluid

Table 18.2 Goals of pituitary surgery

Relief of mass effect

Procurement of a histopathologic diagnosis

Cytoreduction and minimization of tumor recurrence (particularly if nonsecreting)

Normalization of excess hormone secretion (if hypersecreting)

Preservation or restoration of normal pituitary function (if possible)

(CSF) leakage. Therefore, every effort to optimize the surgical approach for resection of tumor should be made at the initial surgery. Some large invasive or recurrent pituitary tumors may not be fully resectable, and may be addressed by a staged approach or adjuvant therapies. In such a situation, decompression of tumor from the optic apparatus and other vital structures should be prioritized during surgical resection.

A residual or recurrent tumor following initial surgery may be observed over time, especially if the pace of tumor growth is indolent. Repeat resection may be favored over radiotherapy with slow progressive growth, especially given the adverse long-term consequences of radiation in young children. Postoperative radiotherapy is typically administered only in the case of rapid tumor regrowth or persistent tumor-derived hormonal hypersecretion,[13] and may be equally effective as delayed salvage therapy, justifying its use in these clinical scenarios.[14]

Pharmacotherapy options for nonfunctioning adenomas remain sparse. The presence of dopamine and somatostatin receptors in nonfunctioning pituitary adenomas has prompted trials with inhibitors such as bromocriptine, cabergoline, and quinagolide, all with limited efficacy in reducing the tumor burden.[15]

Throughout the course of any treatment, especially following surgical resection, fluid balance and hormonal status should be closely monitored. Since pediatric adenomas manifest as macroadenomas more frequently than as microadenomas,[1] perturbation of the infundibular stalk is a distinct risk of surgery. Children may not be able to compensate for rapid fluid shifts as readily as adults and require closer vigilance in postoperative electrolyte and fluid balance monitoring. In particular, infants and toddlers may not have the cognitive skills to communicate symptoms as well as older children, prompting a more proactive use of laboratory testing to assess fluid balance in this population.

18.3 The Role of Endoscopic Endonasal Surgery

Surgical approaches to the pituitary region are generally classified into transcranial and endonasal categories. The choice of a transcranial or transnasal approach is dictated by several critical factors: the anticipated extent of resection; the origin and pattern of growth of the tumor as well as its consistency; involvement of the optic apparatus, circle of Willis, and other neurovascular structures; prior surgical interventions or radiation; and the surgeon's experience and preference (▶ Table 18.3).[16] Of important note, very young children may

Table 18.3 Considerations in choice of a transnasal versus transcranial approach for resection of pituitary adenoma

Factors influencing the choice of surgical approach for a sellar mass
Origin, growth pattern, and consistency of the tumor
Neurovascular involvement, particularly of the optic apparatus and circle of Willis
Anticipated extent of resection
Prior surgery or radiation
Surgeon's preference

have anatomic limitations that add to the difficulty of the endoscopic approach, including small nares, a non-pneumatized sphenoid, and a small working corridor between the carotid arteries. That said, the transnasal transsphenoidal route is increasingly accepted as the standard of care for most pituitary pathologies and will be the focus of discussion here.

18.3.1 Anatomic Considerations in Children

The natural axis of pituitary tumor growth favors surgical resection via an endonasal trajectory. The pituitary is bounded by the sella turcica, diaphragma sellae, and cavernous sinuses. Circumferential growth of adenomas results in thinning of the sellar walls, compression or invasion of the cavernous sinuses and their contents, encroachment on the optic apparatus, and potential obstruction of CSF flow into the third ventricle. Such pathologic changes to the normal anatomy should be accounted for in designing the surgical approach.

In children, specific surgical approach considerations include a smaller midface and nasal corridor, and often the absence of a fully pneumatized sphenoid sinus. Sphenoid bone pneumatization starts at 10 months of age, accelerates between ages 3 to 6 years, and continues until the third decade of life.[17] A non-pneumatized sphenoid sinus requires significantly more bony removal during an endonasal transsphenoidal approach to the pituitary. Availability of sufficient nasoseptal tissue for a potential vascularized flap may also be a concern. In some cases, sublabial approaches may afford a more accessible working corridor when nares are particularly small.

Operative Approach

We employ a two-surgeon, three-handed endoscopic endonasal surgical technique, as previously described.[18] In brief, the operating table is turned approximately 170° from the anesthesia team, with the surgeon to the patient's right, the scrub nurse to the patient's left, and anesthesia colleagues and apparatus at the feet (▶ Fig. 18.1). The patient is positioned supine in a reclining lawn chair position, with the torso elevated 30° to minimize venous congestion. The dorsum of the nose is positioned to be parallel to the lateral walls of the room, as well to the floor to maintain spatial orientation; the face is tilted slightly to the right to minimize reach over the torso during surgery. For tumors with significant intracranial extension beyond the sellar region, slight extension of the head facilitates access to the planum sphenoidale and cribriform plate; alternatively, moderate flexion improves visualization of the clival region. The nose is prepared with intranasal oxymetazoline (0.05% solution; Afrin) spray preoperatively and is packed with cotton pledgets saturated with oxymetazoline, alternating with pledgets of 1% lidocaine with 1:200,000 epinephrine following induction of anesthesia. An abdominal site (usually subumbilical) is prepared to allow for potential fat-graft harvest should a CSF leak be encountered. Frameless stereotaxy is a useful adjunct to surgery, and placement of the viewing screen in the line of sight of the primary surgeon is important. If a magnetic field is used as the tracking mechanism (vs. the more common line-of-sight infrared systems), then a nonmetallic headframe may be needed to prevent interference.

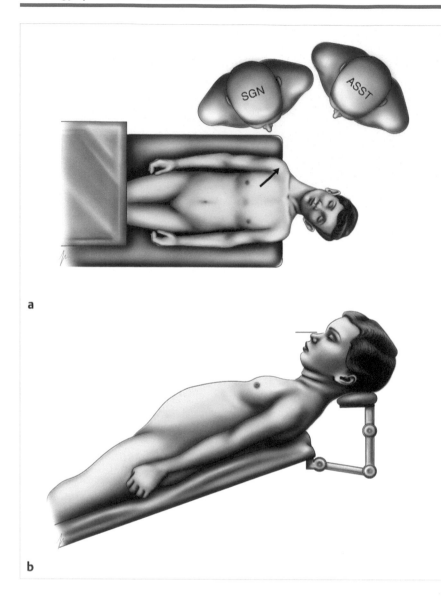

Fig. 18.1 Endoscopic transsphenoidal surgery operative room setup. **(a)** The patient is positioned to maximize exposure to the sellar region while maintaining surgeon comfort and spatial orientation. The table is turned 170°, with the surgeon (SGN) on the patient's right side and the assistant (ASST) to the left of the surgeon. The patient is aligned with the upper right corner of the table (*arrow*), with head turned slightly to the left. **(b)** The operating table is adjusted to a reclining lawn chair position, with the torso elevated 20° to 30° and the knees gently flexed. The dorsum of the nose is parallel to the walls of the room as well as the floor. (Adapted with permission from Jane JA, Thapar K, Kaptain GJ, Maartens N, Laws ER Jr. Pituitary surgery: transsphenoidal approach. Neurosurg 2002;51 (2):435–444.)

The surgical approach can be divided into three stages: nasal, sphenoidal, and sellar. In the nasal phase, the middle and inferior turbinates are deflected laterally to provide a working corridor for the introduction of instruments. Either an endonasal or a sublabial corridor may be made, with subperiosteal and perichondrial dissection to expose the posterior nasal septum and vomer. In pediatric patients with small nasal corridors, a sublabial submucosal transseptal approach may be favored. The degree of mucosal and nasal septum manipulation varies in extent, depending on the needs for exposure, the desire to preserve a pedicled nasoseptal flap, and the surgeon's preference. Nasal septal mucosa and its sphenopalatine or nasoseptal artery supply should be preserved if a high-flow CSF leak is anticipated. The sphenoid ostia are identified medial to underneath the superior turbinate and halfway up from the inferior tip of the middle turbinate, 1.5 cm above the arch of the choana, and the ostia are enlarged surgically for entry into the sphenoid sinus.

The bony face of the sphenoid sinus is opened widely to minimize obstruction to movement and the trajectory of instruments during tumor resection. Internal sphenoid sinus bony septations are removed, with attention to the fact that 20% of sphenoid septations lead to a carotid protuberance rather than the midline. Careful review of the preoperative imaging may help reduce the risk of complications in this setting, as well as liberal reassessment of location with stereotaxy during the approach. In a presellar or conchal sphenoid sinus, which is more frequently encountered in pediatric patients, excess bone may be removed using a drill or chisel under guidance of neuronavigation. The boundaries of the anterior sphenoidotomy are defined by the planum sphenoidale superiorly, and the floor of the sphenoid sinus inferiorly. Within the exposed sphenoid sinus, the sellar floor emerges into the center of view, flanked by the bulge of the carotid siphon bilaterally, the tuberculum and planum sphenoidale superiorly, the clivus inferiorly, the optic nerve canals superolaterally, and the opticocarotid recesses between the optic nerve and the carotid artery (▶ Fig. 18.2). Large macroadenomas extending to the suprasellar space may dictate an extended transsphenoidal exposure, with removal of the tuberculum sellae and the posterior planum sphenoidale as needed.[19] The sella floor can be carefully opened using a chisel, blunt nerve hook, or drill, after verification of the midline.

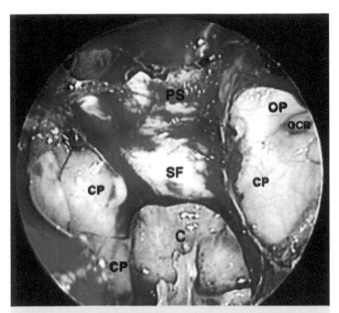

Fig. 18.2 Intraoperative image of the exposed sphenoid sinus, demonstrating the sellar floor in the center, the planum sphenoidale superiorly, the rostral clivus inferiorly, the wings of the optic nerves coursing superolaterally with respect to the sella, the bulge of the internal carotid siphon immediately juxtaposed to the sella, and the opticocarotid recess in between the optic nerve and the carotid artery, which leads to the anterior clinoid process. (Adapted with permission from Dr. Paolo Cappabianca; previously published in Bi et al.[17])

Following a tailored bony exposure dictated by the size and extent of the tumor, the dura overlying the pituitary gland is opened after confirmation of the position of the cavernous carotid arteries with a microvascular Doppler probe. Macroadenomas may compress the superior and inferior intradural intercavernous venous plexuses sufficiently to allow for a relatively avascular dural opening. A vertical midline incision, with lateral expansion, is frequently pursued. Although extracapsular dissection of microadenomas is favored, large tumors are usually resected piecemeal, with sequential inspection of inferior, posterior, lateral, and superior margins. Removal of the inferior tumor allows the superior portions to descend into the field and avoids an early CSF leak from unintentional disruption of the diaphragm or an arachnoid diverticulum. Suprasellar tumors constrained by a narrow diaphragmatic window may be coaxed downward with a pulse of increased intracranial pressure, such as through a Valsalva maneuver, a bilateral jugular vein compression, or the injection of air or saline through a lumbar drain. Rarely, the approach to the tumor may be deliberately left open at the end of the case, especially for macroadenomas with significant extension into the anterior, middle, or posterior fossae; dumbbell-shaped tumors that span above and below the diaphragm; or recurrent adenomas with a known firm consistency.

After tumor resection, the surgical field is inspected for the presence of CSF leak, which presents as dark fluid against the background of venous bleeding. A Valsalva maneuver at the end of tumor resection may help elicit an occult leak. Small leaks may be effectively controlled by a combination of fat, fascia, or synthetic collagen. High-volume CSF leaks are most effectively tamponaded by a vascularized nasoseptal flap. Fat, when used,

is packed in moderation to avoid compression of the optic chiasm. The sellar floor can be reconstructed with a biosynthetic plate, such as the MEDPOR polyethylene graft (Stryker, Kalamazoo, MI) or the allograft nasal septal cartilage or bone, which ideally is placed in the intrasellar extradural space. Alternative reconstruction techniques include the gasket-seal method and the use of synthetic grafts.[20,21] At the end of surgery, dependent blood in the gastric cavity is suctioned out with an orogastric tube to decrease postoperative nausea. If there is need for a lumbar drain or if frequent postoperative laboratory testing is anticipated, placing a peripherally inserted central venous catheter (PICC) line at the end of the case under anesthesia may be a useful maneuver in younger children with limited IV access.

Operative Pearls and Pitfalls

In pediatric patients, the following operative nuances should be considered:

- The pyriform aperture can be enlarged through a sublabial approach if additional room is needed during the surgical exposure to the sellar region.
- In dealing with a partially pneumatized sella, remove the anterior wall of cortical bone using a drill or chisel; scoop out the soft medullary bone with a curette; apply bone wax to tamponade venous bleeding; and progress until the inner layer of cortical bone, which forms the face of the sella, can be removed as usual. Repeated locational assessment with frameless stereotaxy can help provide safe navigation during bony drilling with limited anatomic landmarks.
- Careful attention to preservation of the normal gland is critical to optimize chances for growth and puberty.

18.4 Illustrative Case

A 14-year-old girl presented with primary amenorrhea and a 1-year history of intermittent headaches. She was found to have a sellar and suprasellar mass, with left cavernous sinus invasion, on contrast-enhanced MRI (▶ Fig. 18.3). Laboratory evaluation demonstrated normal studies, including electrolytes, alpha-fetoprotein (AFP), beta-human chorionic gonadotropin (bHCG), and placental alkaline phosphatase (PLAP); her endocrine panel was normal except for a serum prolactin of 97 ng/mL. Her neuro-ophthalmologic examination revealed subtle left abduction impairment with preserved visual acuity and normal visual fields.

An endoscopic endonasal approach was pursued for resection of the pituitary mass, employing a two-surgeon, three-handed technique as described earlier. The diaphragm was observed to descend at the end of tumor removal, and no CSF leak was encountered. Pathological analysis was consistent with a null-cell pituitary adenoma. Postoperatively, the patient experienced transient diabetes insipidus, managed with hydration and vasopressin, and was discharged in stable condition on postoperative day 4 without a need for long-term desmopressin. At 3-month follow-up, the patient reported improvement in headaches, and MRI revealed no obvious residual tumor. She had developed menses and her prolactin level had decreased to normal at 20 ng/mL.

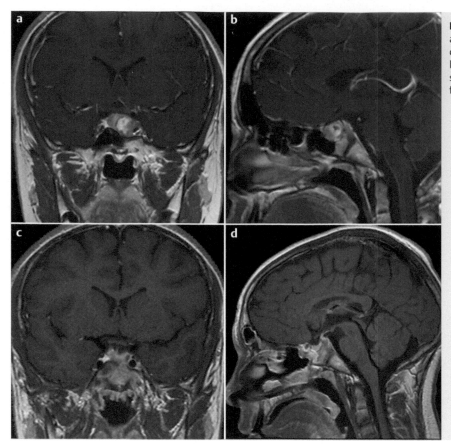

Fig. 18.3 Illustrative pituitary adenoma in an adolescent patient. Contrast-enhanced MRI demonstrates a sellar mass with suprasellar and left-cavernous sinus extension in the coronal and sagittal planes **(a,b)**, at presentation and **(c,d)** following endoscopic endonasal resection.

18.5 Conclusion

Endoscopic endonasal surgery for pituitary lesions has rapidly evolved in concept and utilization in recent decades. Relative barriers to the application of such techniques in the pediatric population are also diminishing with increased experience. Nonfunctional pituitary adenomas remain rare entities among children and may present as macroadenomas exerting mass effect. A multidisciplinary team approach and close patient monitoring will continue to promote increasingly safe and effective means to alleviate the tumor burden and improve neuroendocrinologic function with endoscopic endonasal surgery.

References

[1] Kane LA, Leinung MC, Scheithauer BW, et al. Pituitary adenomas in childhood and adolescence. J Clin Endocrinol Metab. 1994; 79(4):1135–1140

[2] Sinha S, Sarkari A, Mahapatra AK, Sharma BS. Pediatric giant pituitary adenomas: are they different from adults? A clinical analysis of a series of 12 patients. Childs Nerv Syst. 2014; 30(8):1405–1411

[3] Partington MD, Davis DH, Laws ER, Jr, Scheithauer BW. Pituitary adenomas in childhood and adolescence. Results of transsphenoidal surgery. J Neurosurg. 1994; 80(2):209–216

[4] Leinung MC, Kane LA, Scheithauer BW, Carpenter PC, Laws ER, Jr, Zimmerman D. Long term follow-up of transsphenoidal surgery for the treatment of Cushing's disease in childhood. J Clin Endocrinol Metab. 1995; 80(8):2475–2479

[5] Richmond IL, Wilson CB. Pituitary adenomas in childhood and adolescence. J Neurosurg. 1978; 49(2):163–168

[6] Cuny T, Pertuit M, Sahnoun-Fathallah M, et al. Genetic analysis in young patients with sporadic pituitary macroadenomas: besides AIP don't forget MEN1 genetic analysis. Eur J Endocrinol. 2013; 168(4):533–541

[7] Kirschner LS, Carney JA, Pack SD, et al. Mutations of the gene encoding the protein kinase A type I-alpha regulatory subunit in patients with the Carney complex. Nat Genet. 2000; 26(1):89–92

[8] Marx SJ. Molecular genetics of multiple endocrine neoplasia types 1 and 2. Nat Rev Cancer. 2005; 5(5):367–375

[9] Vierimaa O, Georgitsi M, Lehtonen R, et al. Pituitary adenoma predisposition caused by germline mutations in the AIP gene. Science. 2006; 312(5777): 1228–1230

[10] Tichomirowa MA, Lee M, Barlier A, et al. Cyclin-dependent kinase inhibitor 1B (CDKN1B) gene variants in AIP mutation-negative familial isolated pituitary adenoma kindreds. Endocr Relat Cancer. 2012; 19(3):233–241

[11] Thapar K, Kovacs K, Laws ER. The classification and molecular biology of pituitary adenomas. Adv Tech Stand Neurosurg. 1995; 22:3–53

[12] Lopes MBS. The 2017 World Health Organization classification of tumors of the pituitary gland: a summary. Acta Neuropathol. 2017; 134:521-535

[13] Laws ER, Jr, Vance ML. Radiosurgery for pituitary tumors and craniopharyngiomas. Neurosurg Clin N Am. 1999; 10(2):327–336

[14] Snead FE, Amdur RJ, Morris CG, Mendenhall WM. Long-term outcomes of radiotherapy for pituitary adenomas. Int J Radiat Oncol Biol Phys. 2008; 71 (4):994–998

[15] Colao A, Pivonello R, Di Somma C, Savastano S, Grasso LF, Lombardi G. Medical therapy of pituitary adenomas: effects on tumor shrinkage. Rev Endocr Metab Disord. 2009; 10(2):111–123

[16] de Divitiis E, Laws ER, Jr. The transnasal versus transcranial approach to lesions of the anterior skull base. World Neurosurg. 2013; 80(6):728–731

[17] Yonetsu K, Watanabe M, Nakamura T. Age-related expansion and reduction in aeration of the sphenoid sinus: volume assessment by helical CT scanning. AJNR Am J Neuroradiol. 2000; 21(1):179–182

[18] Bi WL, Dunn IF, Laws ER Jr. Pituitary surgery. In: Jameson JL, De Groot LJ, eds. Endocrinology: Adult and Pediatric. Philadelphia, PA: Elsevier Saunders; 2015

[19] Zada G, Du R, Laws ER, Jr. Defining the "edge of the envelope": patient selection in treating complex sellar-based neoplasms via transsphenoidal versus open craniotomy. J Neurosurg. 2011; 114(2):286–300

[20] Leng LZ, Brown S, Anand VK, Schwartz TH. "Gasket-seal" watertight closure in minimal-access endoscopic cranial base surgery. Neurosurgery. 2008; 62 (5) Suppl 2:E342–E343, discussion E343

[21] Kassam A, Carrau RL, Snyderman CH, Gardner P, Mintz A. Evolution of reconstructive techniques following endoscopic expanded endonasal approaches. Neurosurg Focus. 2005; 19(1):E8

19 Epidermoid and Dermoid Tumors

Amanda L. Stapleton, Elizabeth C. Tyler-Kabara, Juan C. Fernandez-Miranda, Eric W. Wang, Paul A. Gardner, and Carl H. Snyderman

Abstract

Dermoid and epidermoid tumors are rare congenital non-neoplastic conditions that often present in pediatric patients. Dermoid cysts are most commonly located along the midline of the neuraxis, while epidermoid cysts are more commonly found laterally within the cerebellopontine angle and parasellar cisterns. Due to the slow growth of the cysts, presenting symptoms can be vague and diverse. Headaches are the most common presenting symptom. Seizures, unilateral hearing loss, cranial nerve deficits, vision changes/loss, and behavioral changes have all been reported. Posterior fossa tumors present with cranial nerve involvement and cerebellar dysfunction. The diagnosis can usually be confirmed with imaging, with characteristic findings on MRI. Complete surgical excision is the treatment of choice. Endoscopic endonasal surgery is well suited for many of these tumors and avoids the morbidity of transcranial approaches. In the sagittal plane, transfrontal, transcribriform, transplanum, transsellar, and transclival approaches can be used to access and resect midline tumors with some lateral extension. For laterally-based lesions, the transpterygoid, transmaxillary, and transpetrous approaches can help resect tumors in the coronal plane. If the tumor is intracranial, reconstruction of the dural defect is an important part of the surgery. This is best accomplished with a multilayer reconstruction of inlay and onlay fascial grafts and a vascularized nasoseptal flap.

Keywords: dermoid, endoscopic endonasal approach, endoscopic endonasal surgery, epidermoid, transclival approach

19.1 Introduction

Dermoid and epidermoid tumors are rare congenital non-neoplastic lesions. They are comprised of a capsule made of epidermal and dermal elements with an internal cystic component. The cyst slowly enlarges over time as the desquamated cellular debris from the capsular cells accumulates internally within the cyst. Dermoid and epidermoid cysts are believed to originate from totipotent ectodermal cells remaining in the developing neural tube. They are believed to be due to a defective closure of the neural tube between the third and fifth weeks of gestation.

Epidermoid cysts originate from primitive ectodermal elements. They have a smooth capsule composed of stratified squamous epithelium surrounded by an outer layer of collagenous tissue.[1] The cysts are filled with soft, waxy, yellow material that is generated by the epithelial lining of the cyst. They are rare and make up 1% of all intracranial tumors and 7% to 9% of cerebellopontine angle (CPA) tumors.[2]

Dermoid cysts originate from ectodermal and mesenchymal elements. They have a thick capsule that can present with many different dermal derivatives. Hair follicles, squamous debris, sebaceous, and sweat glands can all be found within a dermoid cyst. Dermoid cysts are most commonly located along the midline of the neuraxis, while epidermoid cysts are more commonly found laterally within the CPA and parasellar cisterns. However, both cysts can occur anywhere along the craniospinal axis.

Dermoid cysts are frequently midline and often present with an associated dermal sinus tract. This is most commonly found at the glabella or rhinion of the nasal dorsum. However, the sinus tract can also be located at the occipital or spinal level. The cutaneous opening is often present with a tuft of hair or a history of drainage. Yellow, clear, or purulent fluid is often expressed from the cutaneous opening, and patients may have a history of infection. Some patients have a cutaneous angioma beneath the skin marking the location of the sinus tract.

Epidermoid cysts are typically located laterally. Their most common location is the CPA and the parasellar cisterns.[1] As the otic and optic vesicles develop later in early gestation, the ectodermal cells of the future epidermoid cyst are pushed laterally, which may explain their typical lateral location.

Dermoid and epidermoid cysts are characterized by their slow growth rate as the desquamated debris gradually accumulates. Malignant degeneration is extremely rare.[3] Due to their location, they are often associated with compression of the surrounding neural and vascular structures. They can lead to hydrocephalus, infection, aseptic meningitis, and intracranial hypertension. They most frequently present in the third decade of life as their size slowly grows from birth until detection. Epidermoids tend to grow along the cisterns of the CPA and can cause a chronic inflammatory response. This chronic inflammatory reaction may explain epidermoids' dense adherence to surrounding vessels and nerves found during surgical resection. Dermoid cysts are reported more frequently in childhood. Identification of the associated dermal sinus tract may explain why these lesions are recognized earlier in life than intracranial epidermoid cysts.

Due to the slow growth of the cysts, presenting symptoms can be vague and diverse. Headaches are the most common presenting symptom. Seizures, unilateral hearing loss, cranial nerve deficits, vision changes/loss, and behavioral changes have all been reported. Posterior fossa tumors present with cranial nerve involvement and cerebellar dysfunction. Hydrocephalus and meningitis are also presenting signs in some patients once the tumor has reached a size large enough to cause compression and obstruction of the cisterns.

Epidermoid tumors of the CPA or internal auditory canal typically present with unilateral hearing loss and headaches. In a recent pediatric series of CPA tumors, only 5% were epidermoid lesions and presented with a mean age of 12.8 years.[4] CPA tumors can also present with imbalance, vertigo, tinnitus, facial nerve paresis, otalgia, facial pain, or hypoglossal paresis.

On CT imaging, epidermoids and dermoids typically appear as a round/lobulated mass with a density similar to cerebrospinal fluid (CSF; ▶ Fig. 19.1). They are low-density masses that have no enhancement with contrast due to their low vascularity. Ten percent of intracranial epidermoids have calcifications.

On MRI, epidermoids will typically be hypointense on T1 and hyperintense on T2, with restricted diffusion (▶ Fig. 19.2). Internal heterogeneities seen on proton density and fluid-attenuated inversion recovery (FLAIR) images can help distinguish these cysts from arachnoid cysts.[5] They can be differentiated from arachnoid cysts on diffusion-weighted images because the epidermoid will appear bright (restricted diffusion) on these sequences (▶ Fig. 19.3). They do not unusually enhance with contrast imaging.

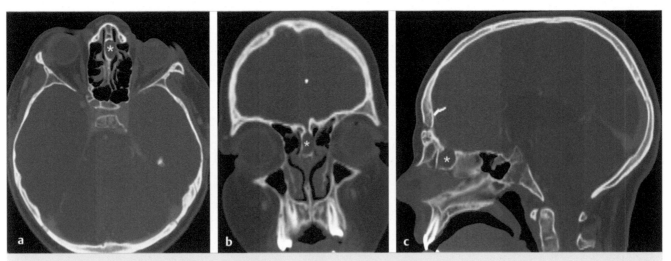

Fig. 19.1 Preoperative axial **(a)**, coronal **(b)**, and sagittal **(c)** CT images demonstrate an expansive lesion of the superior nasal septum with extension to the skull base.

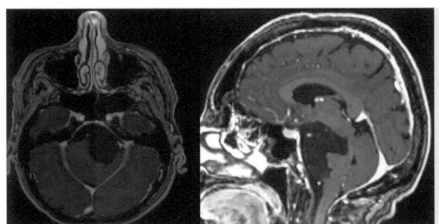

Fig. 19.2 Preoperative MRI (axial and sagittal T1-weighted images) demonstrates a low-signal-intensity mass of the posterior fossa with compression of the brainstem. It extends the full length of the clivus.

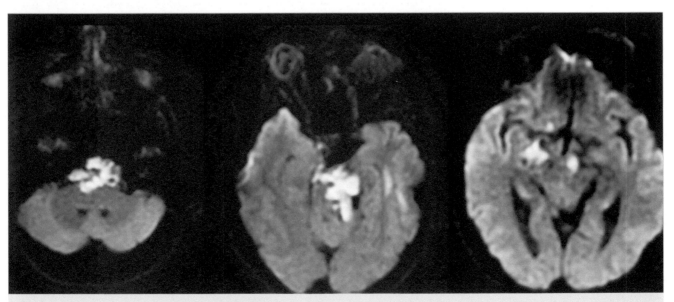

Fig. 19.3 The posterior fossa mass has extremely high-signal intensity on diffusion-weighted images, which is characteristic of an epidermoid.

19.2 Management Options: Medical, Surgical, and Adjuvant

Surgical excision has historically been the mainstay of treatment for dermoid and epidermoid cysts. These cysts are benign intracranial lesions that lack radio sensitivity, and therefore surgical resection is the only viable treatment option. Complete resection of the cyst and cyst wall with no damage to vital neurovascular structures is the goal of surgery to avoid local regrowth of the lesion. However, radical resection is not always possible if the cystic capsule is adherent to surrounding nerves, vessels, or brain parenchyma and cannot safely be removed without extensive collateral damage. If complete removal of the capsule wall is not possible due to adherence, then opening of the cyst wall with the removal of its contents must be approached with caution. Surgeons must be attentive to prevent spillage of the cystic material into the subarachnoid spaces. This can lead to aseptic meningitis in the postoperative period. Subtotal resection must be followed with scans for regrowth of the lesion.

The surgical technique for intracranial epidermoid tumors starts with internal debulking (two-handed suction dissection technique) and decompression of the lesion. This provides improved access to the bulk of the tumor with collapse of the tumor capsule. The margin can then be dissected circumferentially from the surrounding structures. Epidermoid tumors tend to expand into the subarachnoid spaces and therefore create a surgical channel that can allow surgical access from one intracranial compartment to another.

Anterior cranial fossa dermoid lesions with intradural extension have traditionally been approached by a frontolateral/unilateral or a subfrontal approach utilizing a bicoronal incision. Transfacial approaches have also been used in the past to resect the cutaneous tract and the intracranial lesion as one specimen.

A retrosigmoid/lateral suboccipital approach has long been used to provide visualization and resection of epidermoid tumors of the CPA. It allows good access in most cases without excessive cerebellar retraction. A translabyrinthine approach can also be used if the patient has severe, unilateral, irreversible sensorineural hearing loss. This approach allows access to the ventral aspect of the posterior fossa, where epidermoid lesions tend to occur. The subtemporal approach has also been described for tumors that extend supratentorially into the middle cranial fossa, but there is an increased risk of temporal lobe damage with this approach.[6] With the advent of the endoscope, endoscopic-assisted microsurgery was introduced in the late 1990s to provide improved visualization and resection of these lesions. The endoscope can provide angled views of the tumor and help ensure complete resection of the lesion without the collateral damage caused by excessive neurovascular retraction and manipulation.

Tumor recurrence typically happens over a prolonged period. Since the cysts are made of epithelial cells, they grow at a steady rate of one generation per month. Therefore, symptom recurrence can take 6 to 9 months to occur and is frequently longer than that. Close neuroradiology imaging at 3- to 6-month intervals for the first 2 years is recommended. If there is no substantial growth within that window, imaging can progress to every 12- to 24-month examinations.

Complications related to surgical resection can range from mild to severe. Injury to surrounding cranial nerves, vascular injury (venous or arterial), aseptic meningitis, and CSF leaks can have devastating consequences to the patient. Hypopituitarism, vision loss, and ataxia can also result from radical resection, depending upon the size and local of the tumor. Communicating hydrocephalus can develop postoperatively. Sinus thrombus requiring anticoagulation therapy has also been reported. Minimizing these complications and providing a safe and effective means of resection is the goal of endoscopic endonasal surgery.

19.3 Role of Endoscopic Endonasal Surgery

Endoscopic endonasal surgery allows excellent visualization of epidermoid and dermoid tumors without any retraction of neurovascular or intracranial structures. It provides superior visualization for some tumors and may decrease risk of morbidity. There are no external incisions, and it allows for a faster recovery time.[7]

The endoscopic endonasal approach provides direct access to dermoid tumors that are located midline in the anterior skull base. The endoscope allows excellent visualization of these midline tumors, and the lesion can be removed piecemeal without spillage into the subarachnoid space, thus preventing postoperative chemical meningitis.

The endoscopic endonasal technique can be used to work along multiple planes. In the sagittal plane, transfrontal, transcribriform, transplanum, transsellar, and transclival approaches can be used to access and resect midline tumors with some lateral extension. For laterally-based lesions, the transpterygoid, transmaxillary, and transpetrous approaches can help resect tumors in the coronal plane.[8]

The endonasal transclival approach allows the surgeon to approach and resect epidermoid tumors ventral to the brainstem. The surgical corridor consists of opening the sphenoid sinus, drilling the sella and the clivus, and providing direct visualization of the clival dura. Opening of the clival dura and the arachnoid membranes provides direct access to the tumor.

Reconstruction of the skull base is a key part of the endoscopic endonasal approach. The reconstructive options have continued to evolve over the past 15 years. Inlay and onlay grafts as well as vascularized tissue flaps have decreased the rate of postoperative CSF leaks. The use of collagen matrix to close the dural defect space and then placement of an onlay graft followed by vascularized nasal flaps with an outer layer of sealant are the mainstays of skull base reconstruction. Free middle turbinate mucosa grafts can be used as onlay grafts for small defects. Larger defects require a multilayer repair with vascularized tissue. Fascia lata is an excellent choice for either an inlay or an onlay graft to repair a large dural defect. The workhorse of vascularized reconstruction is the nasoseptal flap. This can be rotated to provide coverage from the anterior cranial fossa to the clivus. The use of the nasoseptal flap has been well documented in the pediatric population as a reliable source of vascularized tissue for reconstruction.[9,10,11] A vascularized pericranial flap or lateral nasal wall flap can also be used if there is no tissue available for a nasoseptal flap due to tumor involvement or previous surgery. The placement of an abdominal fat graft between the fascia lata onlay graft and vascularized flap to fill the dead space created by a transclival approach has also been described to decrease the rate of postoperative CSF leaks and minimize the risk of pontine herniation.[12,13]

19.4 Case Examples

19.4.1 Intracranial Epidermoid

Description of Endoscopic Skull Base Approach

The endonasal approach depends on the location of the intracranial epidermoid. An epidermoid of the anterior cranial fossa requires a transcribriform/transplanum approach, whereas an epidermoid of the posterior cranial fossa requires a transclival approach.

Transcribriform/Transplanum Approach

A nasoseptal flap is elevated at the beginning of surgery in anticipation of reconstruction. A bilateral sphenoethmoidectomy is performed to expose the bone of the anterior cranial base beyond the limits of the tumor. The anterior and posterior ethmoidal arteries are cauterized at the junction of the ethmoid roof and medial orbit as necessary. The superior attachment of the nasal septum is resected to provide binarial exposure. The bone of the anterior cranial base is thinned with a 4-mm coarse diamond drill bit and carefully elevated to expose the dura. Depending on the size and location of the epidermoid, it may be necessary to sacrifice olfaction on one or both sides. The olfactory fibers are cauterized with bipolar electrocautery. The dura is incised and resected to the margins of the tumor. Bimanual suction dissection of the epidermoid is performed with central debulking followed by peripheral dissection of the capsule and careful stripping of epithelium from the cortical vessels and pia mater. Reconstruction consists of an inlay collagen or fascia lata graft followed by transposition of the nasoseptal flap. If the nasoseptal flap does not provide adequate coverage, it is supplemented with an onlay fascial lata graft.

Transclival Approach

Bilateral sphenoidotomies are performed with removal of the sphenoid rostrum. The clivus is divided into thirds: superior, middle, and inferior. If the tumor is posterior to the dorsum sella, a pituitary transposition is performed. The sella is decompressed, and the dura of the cavernous sinus is incised bilaterally (▶ Fig. 19.4). Bleeding is controlled with infiltration of morselized oxidized cellulose (Floseal or Surgifoam). Intradural dissection of the sellar floor is performed, and the inferior hypophyseal arteries are cauterized and transected. The gland is elevated to provide access to the dorsum sella as high as the posterior clinoids. The bone is drilled in the midline and the clinoids are removed individually, taking care to avoid injury to the internal carotid artery (ICA; ▶ Fig. 19.5).

The middle clivus extends from the floor of the sella to the floor of the sphenoid sinus. The bone of the clival recess is drilled between the paraclival segments of the ICA. The abducens nerve enters Dorello's canal at the midpoint of the paraclival ICA and is susceptible to injury with drilling. If more lateral exposure is needed, the bone overlying the paraclival arteries can be removed to allow lateral displacement of the paraclival ICA (▶ Fig. 19.6). This provides access to the medial petrous apex.

Exposure of the lower clivus requires complete detachment of the nasal septum from the sphenoid rostrum. The mucosa between the Eustachian tubes is cauterized, and the underlying muscle (longus capitis) is resected to the underlying bone. The bone is drilled to the underlying dura, avoiding injury to the ICA at foramen lacerum. If more lateral exposure is needed, a transpterygoid approach provides access to the petrous ICA. Following a maxillary antrostomy, the sphenopalatine foramen is opened. The pterygopalatine space is exposed by removing the posterior wall of the maxillary sinus, and the contents are

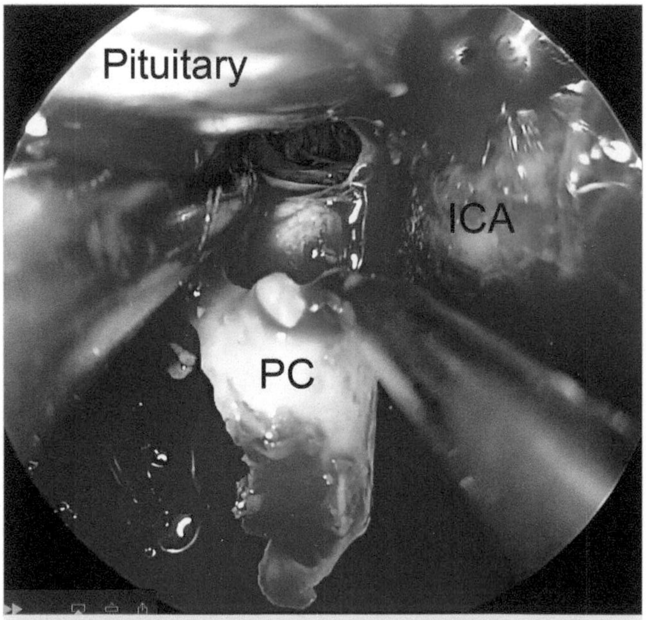

Fig. 19.4 Once the pituitary gland is mobilized superiorly, the posterior clinoid (PC) is mobilized on each side. Each PC is removed separately to avoid injury to the internal carotid artery (ICA).

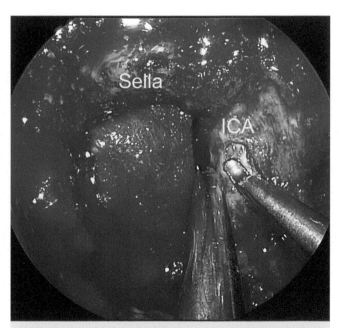

Fig. 19.5 The bone overlying the sella has been removed, and the central clivus has been drilled to the underlying dura. Here, the bone over the paraclival internal carotid artery (ICA) is carefully thinned with a drill and then elevated with Kerrison rongeurs.

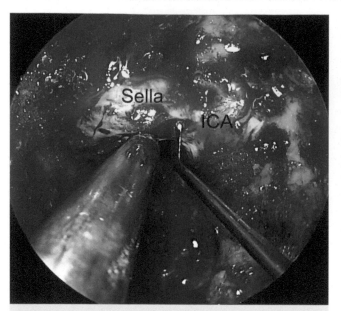

Fig. 19.6 The interdural space between the pituitary gland and the cavernous internal carotid artery (ICA) is opened with a hooked "featherblade" in order to perform a pituitary transposition.

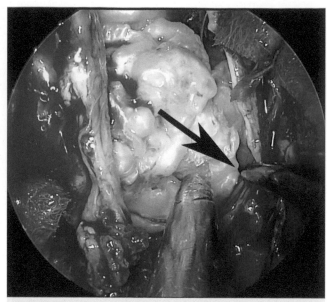

Fig. 19.7 The dura over the posterior fossa is incised distant from the basilar artery to expose the epidermoid tumor. A nerve stimulator is used to localize the abducens nerve in the midclival region (arrow).

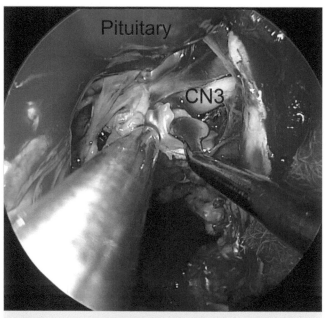

Fig. 19.8 Following identification of the oculomotor nerve (CN III) in the superior clival region, the epidermoid tumor is carefully dissected from the nerve using a sharp elevator or suction dissection.

displaced laterally. The vidian nerve is sacrificed, and the bone surrounding the pterygoid canal is drilled to the plane of the petrous ICA. Transection of the cartilaginous tissue of foramen lacerum separates the ICA from the Eustachian tube and provides lateral access inferior to the petrous ICA.

The outer layer of dura is incised, and bleeding from the basilar plexus is controlled with infusion of oxidized cellulose. The location of the basilar artery is determined using navigation and Doppler probe (if superficial). A nerve stimulator with neurophysiological electromyography monitoring is helpful in locating the abducens nerve deep to the dura prior to incision (▶ Fig. 19.7). Bimanual dissection is performed as described earlier with debulking of keratin debris, followed by careful extracapsular dissection of the cranial nerves (▶ Fig. 19.8) and the vascular structures (▶ Fig. 19.9).

Large transclival defects require a multilayer reconstruction consisting of inlay and onlay fascial grafts (fascia lata), adipose tissue graft to prevent pontine herniation, and a vascularized nasoseptal flap (▶ Fig. 19.10). Postoperative imaging demonstrates complete removal of the tumor with a well-vascularized nasoseptal flap (▶ Fig. 19.11).

Operative Pearls and Pitfalls

With a pituitary transposition, removal of the bone of the tuberculum provides room for superior displacement of the pituitary gland. The posterior clinoid should be removed carefully to avoid injury to the posterior surface of the ICA. If there is a complete dural ring of bone surrounding the ICA, it needs to be carefully drilled to detach the posterior clinoid.

The abducens nerve may be displaced by tumor and is easily injured. The position of the nerve should be confirmed with neurophysiological monitoring prior to incision of the dura. Drilling of bone of the petrous apex should be done carefully with frequent neurophysiological monitoring to avoid injury to the abducens nerve where it enters Dorello's canal.

19.4.2 Nasal Dermoid

Description of Endoscopic Skull Base Approach

A nasal dermoid has two components: extracranial and intracranial. The extracranial component includes both extranasal and intranasal disease and typically consists of a nasal pit and sinus tract that extends from the midline of the nasal dorsum

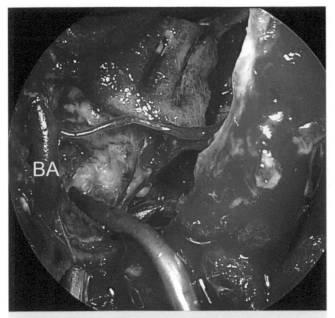

Fig. 19.9 A gentle two-suction dissection technique is preferred in order to avoid injury to branches of the basilar artery.

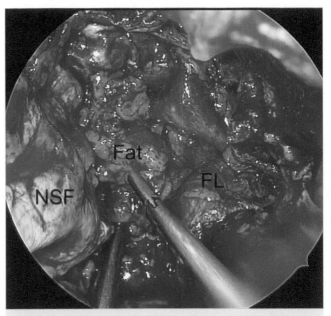

Fig. 19.10 Following removal of the epidermoid tumor, the transclival defect is reconstructed with an inlay collagen graft (not shown), onlay fascial lata (FL) graft, fat graft, and vascularized nasoseptal flap (NSF).

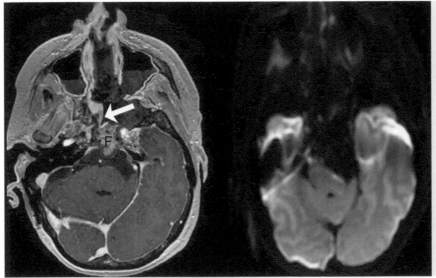

Fig. 19.11 Postoperative MRI (including diffusion-weighted image) demonstrates complete removal of the epidermoid tumor. The fat graft (F) is bright on the T1-weighted image and enhancement of the nasoseptal flap (arrow) confirms its vascularity.

between the nasal bones to the superior nasal septum. The intracranial component extends through foramen cecum to the surface of the dura. The extracranial component requires an external approach, either a vertical midline incision on the nasal dorsum or an external rhinoplasty approach. The nasal pit is excised along with the sinus tract to the defect between the nasal bones. Dissection of the sinus tract can be facilitated by injecting dye (methylene blue) into the tract or gently inserting a lacrimal probe.

The endonasal approach provides access to the intranasal and intracranial components of the dermoid.[14] Swelling of the superior septum is often evident. The overlying mucosa is removed, and the contents of the sinus tract are drained. The mucosa and cartilage/bone of the superior septum deep to the nasal bones

are resected to provide bilateral access and to connect to the extranasal part of the surgery (▶ Fig. 19.12). The contents of the cyst are removed to provide access to the expanded bone surrounding the cyst (▶ Fig. 19.13). If the frontal sinus is pneumatized, a Draf type III frontal sinusotomy is performed. Otherwise, the sinus tract can be followed to the skull base at the foramen cecum. The foramen cecum is anterior to the crista galli in the midline. Enlargement of the canal is evident, and the lining epithelium is dissected from the bone. The surrounding bone is drilled with a 3-mm coarse diamond drill bit to the plane of the dura (▶ Fig. 19.14). Enough bone is drilled to remove the intracranial/extradural component of the dermoid. Any attachments to the dura are cauterized using bipolar electrocautery (▶ Fig. 19.15). Reconstruction is not necessary if

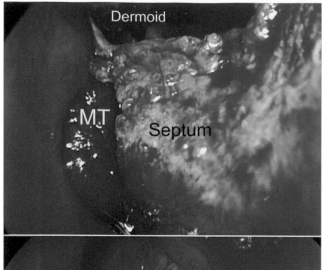

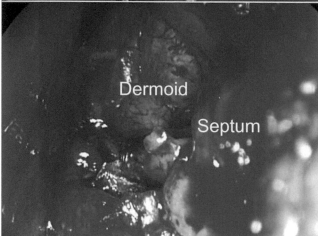

Fig. 19.12 (a) Endoscopic view of the right nasal cavity (0-degree endoscope) demonstrates a superior nasal defect anterior to the attachment of the middle turbinate (MT). (b) Septal bone has been removed to expose the dermoid cyst.

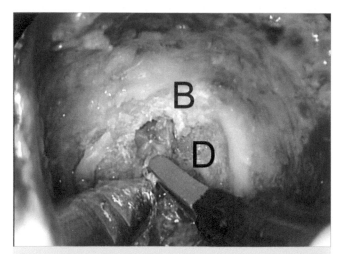

Fig. 19.15 The bone (B) at the skull base is drilled to expose the dura (D), and the last attachment of the dermoid to the dura is cauterized with bipolar electrocautery.

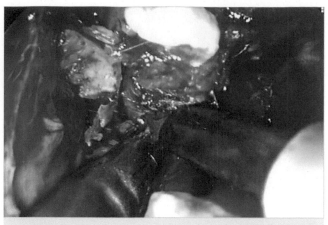

Fig. 19.13 Endonasal view of nasal dermoid with characteristic dermal contents (sebum and hair). The superior septum has been resected to expose the dermoid.

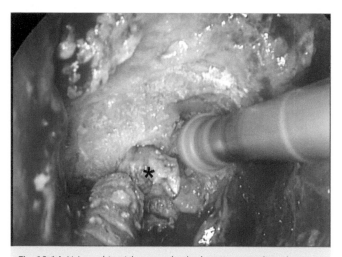

Fig. 19.14 Using a binarial approach, the bone surrounding the dermoid remnant (asterisk) is drilled until the dural margin is exposed.

there is no injury to the dura; the exposed dura is covered with fibrin glue.

Operative Pearls and Pitfalls

If the nasal pit is at the level of the nasion, a small drill bit (2-mm coarse diamond) can be used through the external incision to drill the bone surrounding the sinus tract. Creation of a superior septal defect provides added room for instrumentation. Endoscopic visualization is usually from the right side, while the drill is inserted through the left nasal cavity. Limiting the septal defect deep to the nasal bones prevents a saddle nose deformity. The creation of a superior septal defect also provides marsupialization in case all epithelial remnants are not removed.

19.5 Conclusion

Endoscopic endonasal surgery for the resection of dermoid and epidermoid tumors allows excellent visualization and access to midline and lateral lesions. Advantages include improved visualization and less manipulation of neurovascular structures. This technique can be used along many surgical planes to facilitate gross total resection without spillage of tumor into the subarachnoid spaces. Reconstructive principles used in endoscopic endonasal surgery help minimize the risk of a postoperative CSF leak.

References

[1] Caldarelli M, Massimi L, Kondageski C, Di Rocco C. Intracranial midline dermoid and epidermoid cysts in children. J Neurosurg. 2004; 100(5) Suppl pediatrics:473–480

[2] Ahmed I, Auguste KI, Vachhrajani S, Dirks PB, Drake JM, Rutka JT. Neurosurgical management of intracranial epidermoid tumors in children. Clinical article. J Neurosurg Pediatr. 2009; 4(2):91–96

[3] Link MJ, Cohen PL, Breneman JC, Tew JM, Jr. Malignant squamous degeneration of a cerebellopontine angle epidermoid tumor. Case report. J Neurosurg. 2002; 97(5):1237–1243

[4] Holman MA, Schmitt WR, Carlson ML, Driscoll CL, Beatty CW, Link MJ. Pediatric cerebellopontine angle and internal auditory canal tumors: clinical article. J Neurosurg Pediatr. 2013; 12(4):317–324

[5] Sirin S, Gonul E, Kahraman S, Timurkaynak E. Imaging of posterior fossa epidermoid tumors. Clin Neurol Neurosurg. 2005; 107(6):461–467

[6] Safavi-Abbasi S, Di Rocco F, Bambakidis N, et al. Has management of epidermoid tumors of the cerebellopontine angle improved? A surgical synopsis of the past and present. Skull Base. 2008; 18(2):85–98

[7] Kassam A, Thomas AJ, Snyderman C, et al. Fully endoscopic expanded endonasal approach treating skull base lesions in pediatric patients. J Neurosurg. 2007; 106(2) Suppl:75–86

[8] Chivukula S, Koutourousiou M, Snyderman CH, Fernandez-Miranda JC, Gardner PA, Tyler-Kabara EC. Endoscopic endonasal skull base surgery in the pediatric population. J Neurosurg Pediatr. 2013; 11(3):227–241

[9] Shah RN, Surowitz JB, Patel MR, et al. Endoscopic pedicled nasoseptal flap reconstruction for pediatric skull base defects. Laryngoscope. 2009; 119(6):1067–1075

[10] Purcell PL, Shinn JR, Otto RK, Davis GE, Parikh SR. Nasoseptal flap reconstruction of pediatric sellar defects: a radiographic feasibility study and case series. Otolaryngol Head Neck Surg. 2015; 152(4):746–751

[11] Giannoni CM, Whitehead WE. Use of endoscopic vascularized nasoseptal flap in children. Otolaryngol Head Neck Surg. 2013; 148(2):344–346

[12] Zanation AM, Carrau RL, Snyderman CH, et al. Nasoseptal flap reconstruction of high flow intraoperative cerebral spinal fluid leaks during endoscopic skull base surgery. Am J Rhinol Allergy. 2009; 23(5):518–521

[13] Koutourousiou M, Filho FV, Costacou T, et al. Pontine encephalocele and abnormalities of the posterior fossa following transclival endoscopic endonasal surgery. J Neurosurg. 2014; 121(2):359–366

[14] Pinheiro-Neto CD, Snyderman CH, Fernandez-Miranda J, Gardner PA. Endoscopic endonasal surgery for nasal dermoids. Otolaryngol Clin North Am. 2011; 44(4):981–987, ix

20 Juvenile Nasopharyngeal Angiofibroma

Tiruchy Narayanan Janakiram, Shilpee Bhatia Sharma, and Onkar K. Deshmukh

Abstract

Juvenile Nasopharyngeal Angiofibroma is a highly vascular, benign but locally aggressive neoplasm of the nasopharynx. It is the most common nasopharyngeal neoplasm constituting about 5 % of all the head and neck tumors. Its incidence is higher in the Indian subcontinent and Egypt as compared to the western world. Though multiple modalities have been employed to treat this tumor, surgical excision has proved to be the most promising. However these highly vascular tumors are notorious for intraoperative bleeding and post-operative recurrence. Based on his experience of endoscopically managing a large series of 242 primary JNA patients for over two decades, the author proposes an endoscopic classification system based on preoperative imaging, contrast enhanced CT (CECT). He proposes tailor made approaches and surgical steps for endoscopic excision of tumors in each stage in his classification system. This classification intends to establish a surgical protocol for excision of JNAs by endoscopic or endoscopic assisted approaches. The author has devised various techniques and surgical maneuvers that have significantly reduced intraoperative bleeding and reduced recurrence / residual tumor rates. Impetus has been laid to promote endoscopic management of JNA even for high staged tumors. For JNAs with massive parapharyngeal and intracranial extensions where a pure endoscopic approach is not adequate, the author recommends endoscopic assisted open approaches.

Keywords: JNA, endoscopic resection, Janakiram JNA staging

20.1 Introduction and Epidemiology

Juvenile nasopharyngeal angiofibroma (JNA) is a highly vascular, benign, yet locally aggressive tumor with a propensity toward skull base erosion and intracranial extension. Early description of this neoplasm was given by Hippocrates in the 4th century BC. In 1878, Bensch first elaborated the morphological and clinical features of JNA.[1] It was Chaveau in 1906 who suggested the term "juvenile nasopharyngeal angiofibroma."[2]

JNA is noted to be the most common benign tumor originating in the nasopharynx.[3] Biswas et al reported JNA as one of the most common benign otolaryngological tumors.[4] In accordance with available literature, JNA accounts for 0.05 to 0.5% of all head and neck neoplasms.[5,6] The incidence of JNA is approximately 1/150,000 and almost exclusively affects adolescent males between the ages of 10 and 25 years.[7,8] It is agreed that the incidence of JNA is higher in the Indian subcontinent and Egypt than in the United States and Europe. Furthermore, a study conducted by Mishra and Mishra states that India harbors the maximum burden of the disease, with a fourfold increase in incidence in the last decade.[9]

This chapter reviews the endoscopic approach to this formidable tumor and summarizes pertinent literature with respect to its evolving management. The approaches described in the chapter are based largely on the author's experience in managing an extensive series of nasal angiofibroma patients for more than two decades. The emphasis is on a thorough understanding of tumor extensions on imaging, pathways of spread, and endoscopic approaches to curtail perioperative mortality, as well as on achieving better surgical outcomes.

20.2 Natural History

It is proposed that after its intradiploic origin, JNA tends to spread submucosally along certain pathways. It is observed that the tumor commonly follows an anterolateral or less commonly, a posterior pathway. The anterior pathway of spread is from the nasopharynx to the sphenoid sinus superomedially and through the pterygopalatine fossa to the infratemporal fossa laterally. From here, the tumor takes multiple directions: superiorly to the temporal fossa, inferiorly to the parapharyngeal space, and laterally to the cheek (▶ Fig. 20.1a). In the less common posterior pathway, the tumor spreads to the quadrangular space extending to Meckel's cave and then to the cavernous sinus (▶ Fig. 20.1b). It is vital to extirpate the tumor surgically from all these extensions to avoid recurrence. Though spontaneous regression is noted in a few cases with postoperative residual tumors, the factors governing this behavior are still under investigation.

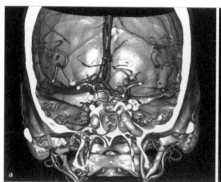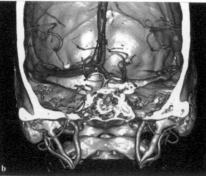

Fig. 20.1 (a) Anterior pathway of spread. Juvenile nasopharyngeal angiofibroma (JNA) is proposed to originate intradiploic at the pterygoid wedge bone (*circle*) to the sphenoid sinus superomedially (*red arrow*) nasopharynx (*yellow arrow*) and through the pterygoid palatine fossa to the infratemporal fossa along the anterolateral pathway (*blue arrow*). From here the tumor takes multiple directions: superiorly to the temporal fossa, inferiorly to the parapharyngeal space, and laterally to the cheek. (b) In the less common posterior pathway, the tumor spreads to the quadrangular space, extending to the Meckel cave and then to the cavernous sinus.

20.3 Clinical Assessment

Most commonly, JNA declares itself with gradually progressive painless nasal obstruction with intermittent unprovoked epistaxis. As a dictum, any adolescent male presenting with epistaxis should be subjected to endoscopic examination to rule out JNA.

Prolonged obstruction can cause sinusitis, headache, and hyposmia. Eustachian tube blockage by the mass can present with complaints of ear pain, effusion, and conductive hearing loss. The tumor may push the soft palate, protrude in the oral cavity, or extend into parapharyngeal space, causing difficulty in speech and swallowing.

Patients with advanced tumors extending posteriorly to the nasopharynx present with mouth breathing, snoring, and rhinolalia clausa (hypernasal speech).

The tumor extending anteriorly can obstruct the nasolacrimal duct and can cause dacryocystitis (infection of the lacrimal sac) and spread to the cheek, which can lead to a typical "frog face" facial deformity. Superior extension and invasion of the orbit lead to proptosis and diplopia in extreme gaze due to compromised space. Extension into the cavernous sinus can, albeit rarely, present with cranial nerve palsies (third to sixth cranial nerves).

A thorough general and otorhinolaryngological examination along with an examination of cranial nerves should be performed. On inspection of the face, swelling may be evident in the cheek or temporal fossa. The oral cavity should be examined for trismus or bulge in the soft palate. A 2.7-mm scope is preferred for nasal endoscopy in pediatric patients. It reveals a smooth, reddish, and lobulated mass in the nasopharynx. The patients should never be subjected to biopsy if JNA is suspected.

20.4 Imaging

Preoperative imaging is an integral part of workup for the diagnosis and management of JNA. Accurate preoperative imaging is essential for determining the extensions of the disease. CT scan forms the basis for the staging system of JNA and has prognostic significance. The osseous details, such as bone erosion and widening of foramen and fissures, are detected in CT scan bone windows. In the soft tissue and intermediate windows, contrast-enhancing extensions of the tumor should be studied at intervals as thin as 0.625 mm in both axial and coronal planes. Coronal CT images are preferred for evaluating the stage of the tumor, showing the relationship of the tumor to the vital structures, and choosing a surgical approach for providing adequate exposure.

A typical finding in a contrast-enhanced CT (CECT) scan is a lobulated nonencapsulated enhancing mass in nasopharynx and pterygopalatine fossa following administration of contrast. Lloyd et al[10] described the following three characteristic features suggesting a diagnosis of JNA:
- A soft-tissue mass in the nasopharynx and the nasal cavity.
- A mass in the pterygopalatine fossa.
- Erosion of the posterior osseous margin of the sphenopalatine foramen extending to the base of the medial pterygoid plate. The "Holman–Miller" sign represents

anterior bowing of posterior maxillary wall on axial CT sections.

20.4.1 Site of Origin

The site of origin and route of spread of JNA remains an enigma. The knowledge and recognition of tumor extent is essential for complete surgical extirpation, thus reducing residual and recurrent tumor. Currently, the accepted site of origin is in close proximity to the superior margin of sphenopalatine foramen, at the junction of attachment of the posterior part of the middle turbinate. Advances in imaging have highlighted new observations pertaining to the early phase of the tumor, thus providing new perspectives regarding the origin and behavior.

The current theory is being challenged by rare reported cases of JNA limited to the sphenoid.[11] Liu et al in a series of 46 male patients with histologically-proven JNA found the pterygoid canal involved in all cases with no involvement of pterygopalatine and infratemporal fossa.[12] The author reported three cases with a tumor limited to the sphenoid sinus and pterygoid wedge, even when other proposed sites of inception remained uninvolved. Further analyses of 242 cases revealed involvement of the pterygoid wedge without involvement of the vidian canal in 19% of cases. Thus, the author proposes it as a possible site of origin of JNA.

20.4.2 Significance of the Pterygoid Wedge

The pterygoid wedge is defined as a triangular area at the anterior junction of the lateral and the medial pterygoid plates. The involvement of the pterygoid wedge was observed in 99.1% of our preoperative images. The characteristic widening of the pterygoid wedge to a quadrangular appearance was observed in our cases consistently and was coined the "RAM HARAN" sign (▶ Fig. 20.2). In advanced cases and revision cases, this sign is not encountered due to bone destruction and surgical resection, respectively.

In the authors' series of 242 cases, it was observed that the average width of the pterygoid wedge of the involved side was approximately twice that of the uninvolved side. The pterygoid wedge was involved in 99.1% of our series, even in the earliest stages where other proposed sites of inception remained uninvolved. The pterygoid wedge was observed as the epicenter of the tumor.

At the authors' center, early postoperative evaluation included a CECT scan done after 36 hours of surgery to identify any residual tumor. It is of vital importance to assess any residual tumor in the soft-tissue window. Complete removal of the tumor is confirmed by the absence of enhancing areas in the sinonasal cavity or the nasopharynx. Another interesting finding seen in postoperative coronal scans was the typical appearance imparted by the interrelation of the medial and lateral pterygoid plates. Owing to complete removal of the pterygoid wedge, the pterygoid plates are seen as two parallel lines. This characteristic appearance was consistently noted by the authors in their series (▶ Fig. 20.3). Though MRI is superior in evaluating postoperative recurrence as it delineates soft tissues

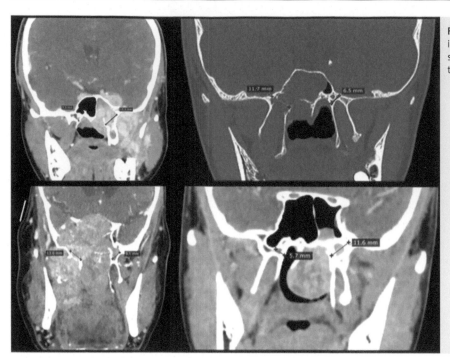

Fig. 20.2 Coronal contrast-enhanced CT scan images showing the contrast-enhancing mass seen widening the pterygoid wedge compared to the uninvolved side (the Ram Haran sign).

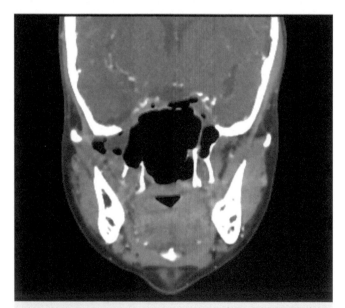

Fig. 20.3 Postoperative coronal CT section (postcontrast) showing medial and lateral pterygoid plates separately giving appearance of two parallel sticks, termed the "chop stick" sign.

better, it can sometimes be misleading, showing fibrosis as contrast enhancement, and is more prone to motion artifacts.

On MRI, the tumor shows a characteristic "salt and pepper" appearance, which is given by the tumor and the flow void areas, respectively. There can be several flow voids, owing to the tumor's highly vascular nature. The lesion characteristically shows low to intermediate signal intensity on T1-weighted images. On T2-weighted images, heterogeneous intermediate signal intensity is seen in the tumor mass, with flow voids appearing as dark areas, and in contrast-enhanced MR images, avid enhancement especially with T1-weighted images. MRI is

even more important postoperatively to show any residual or recurrent tumor and monitor the effects of radiotherapy.[13]

Digital subtraction angiography (DSA) is useful in defining both the feeding vessels and preoperative embolization. Residual tumor vascularity after embolization is employed as a criterion to stage JNAs in the University of Pennsylvania Medical Center (UPMC) classification system.[14] At our center, JNAs with feeders from the internal carotid artery (ICA) system are identified preoperatively. Such JNAs may have to be subjected to multiple-stage operations.

Preoperative embolization of JNA has shown to decrease intraoperative blood loss and operative time. Preoperative embolization is generally done 24 to 48 hours before the surgical procedure to avoid chances of revascularization. Even with newer agents, embolization is associated with risks like cranial nerve injuries, stroke, and blindness. The benefits of embolization should be gauged against risks of neurological complications.

20.5 Staging System

Staging is vital to describe the extent of tumor, facilitate decision-making regarding management protocol, and prognosticate outcome. An ideal staging system for JNA should provide information regarding prognosis, treatment options, anticipated blood loss, and possible complications that may ensue.

The first staging system for JNA was proposed by Sessions et al in 1981.[15] It was based on anatomical location and was similar to that used for nasopharyngeal carcinoma. Many modifications in classifications were described by Chandler et al,[16] Fisch,[17] Bremer et al,[18] and Andrews et al.[19] The most accepted classification was Radkowski et al's classification, which was a modification of Session's classification.[20] It described that the skull base extension was associated with higher levels of recurrence. It differentiated between minimal skull base erosion, minimal intracranial extension, and massive intracranial extension.

In the past decade, the endoscopic approach has emerged as an alternative to the external approach due to reduced morbidity and reduced recurrence rates. Based on advancement in imaging technology and expanded use of endoscopes, a new staging system was proposed by Onerci et al in 2006,[21] introducing endoscopes as a viable alternative. Snyderman et al[14] noted two important factors: route of skull base extension and residual vascularity after embolization to predict prognosis in angiofibroma patients, and proposed an endoscopic staging system for JNA. They noted that tumor size and extent of disease are less important in predicting complete tumor removal.

We have formulated a staging system that relies on tumor extensions on preoperative CECT imaging. This system emphasizes stratifying patients based on preoperative imaging into stages and proposes a tailor-made surgical approach for each stage (▶ Table 20.3). In our study, limits of the single-corridor, transnasal endoscopic approach were explored. In limited cases, an endoscopic multicorridor approach was employed to be minimally invasive. The tumors beyond that were managed by open approaches. The reproducibility of this staging system depends on the experience and skill of the surgeon. The various staging systems are elaborated in ▶ Table 20.1.

20.6 Endoscopic Approach

Different viewpoints about optimal surgical approaches are discussed in the literature. The very fact that numerous approaches were developed to access angiofibromas confirms the inaccessibility of this lesion. Moreover, JNA has a high propensity of postoperative recurrence, especially in areas that are surgically difficult to access. The introduction of endoscopes has improved visualization and surgical access in otorhinolaryngological disorders. The first endoscopic excision of JNA was performed by Reida Kamel in 1996. Since then, technical advancements and growing surgical expertise are constantly expanding the limits of endonasal endoscopic JNA surgery. Owing to better surgical outcomes, this corridor has now evolved as a preferred approach for small and medium-sized tumors.

20.7 Principles

Principles and philosophies of endoscopic approach should be followed to ensure better outcomes and results in comparison to conventional techniques.

20.7.1 Planning

Selecting a surgical approach and trajectory is based on preoperative imaging. It is a vital determinant of exposure for tumor excision and thereby surgical outcome. The preoperative imaging should be analyzed in detail for tumor extensions, the proximity of neurovascular structures, and vascular supply. Preoperative devascularization of the tumor via embolization aids in better visualization intraoperatively. On the basis of tumor extension, an intraoperative surgical trajectory is selected to provide maximal exposure while being minimally invasive. Based on the staging system, a tumor in difficult anatomical areas can be approached via multiple corridors as well as planned for staged resections.

20.7.2 Teamwork

Favorable outcomes depend not only on meticulous planning but also on collaborative teamwork. The coordinated effort by a multidisciplinary team comprising otorhinolaryngologists, neurosurgeons, and anesthesiologists is fundamental in providing effective surgical care. Detailed description of the endoscopic procedure with available benefits should be outlined with open procedures and other modalities as an alternative. Planning of the surgical approach and estimated blood loss should be discussed preoperatively. In patients with high risk of intraoperative bleeding and tumors in proximity to the ICA, the team should discuss staged surgery, less invasive options, and preoperative strategy for preventing and managing ICA injury.

20.7.3 Binostril Four-Handed Technique

A binostril, four-handed, two-surgeon technique allows the operating surgeon to use both hands for instrumentation. This increases surgical maneuverability, as well as the ability to identify the plane of dissection and maintain hemostasis. This collaborative effort is a prerequisite for endoscopic resection of angiofibroma. It allows for dynamic movements aiding in-depth perception, spatial orientation, and identification of landmarks. If this technique cannot be followed, surgery should be converted to the open approach.

20.7.4 Instrumentation

Intraoperative image guidance and navigation is essential to orient the surgeon and guide him or her through the intricate anatomy of the skull base. Specialized instruments improve the dexterity of a surgeon and translate to a successful outcome. Highly crafted, dedicated sets of instruments are required for tumor removal in narrow corridors in critical areas. High-speed, low-profile drills allow drilling of the thickest portion of the skull base precisely and facilitate safe drilling near neurovascular areas. Facilities to manage medical and anesthetic complications and massive hemorrhages, especially ICA injury, should be at hand while undertaking JNA surgery.

20.7.5 Centripetal Approach

The centripetal approach is adopted to expose the tumor prior to its handling. The wide exposure is obtained to visualize tumor extensions for excision under vision. A modified Denker approach and posterior septectomy improve access to the nasopharynx and skull base and also improve surgical maneuverability (▶ Fig. 20.4, ▶ Fig. 20.5, ▶ Fig. 20.6). The principle of devascularization of the tumor is crucial before attempting tumor resection. The feeder vessels based on the extension of the tumor are ligated to devascularize the tumor and decrease intraoperative blood loss. The supply from the external carotid system can be directly ligated during surgery. The feeders like the sphenopalatine artery (SPA), descending palatine artery (DPA), and internal maxillary artery (IMA) can be identified and ligated before tumor dissection (▶ Fig. 20.7, ▶ Fig. 20.8). The tumor receiving blood supply from the ICA system should be

Table 20.1 Various Classification Systems for JNA

	Sessions et al[15]	Chandler et al[16]	Andrews et al[19]	Radkowski et al[20]	Onerci et al[21]	Snyderman et al[14] (UPMC)	Janakiram et al[26]
Cases	12	13	14	23	36	35	242
Stage I	**Stage Ia** - limited to the nose and nasopharynx **Stage Ib** - extension into ≥ 1 sinus	Limited to the nasopharynx	Limited to the nasopharynx, bone destruction negligible or limited to sphenopalatine fossa	**Stage Ia** - limited to the nose or nasopharynx **Stage Ib** - as in **stage Ia** with extension into ≥ 1 sinus	Nose, nasopharynx, ethmoid, and sphenoid sinuses or minimal extension into pterygomaxillary fossa	Nasal cavity, pterygopalatine fossa	**Stage Ia** - the pterygoid wedge and/or paranasal sinus **Stage Ib** - with extension to the nasopharynx
Stage II	**Stage IIa** - minimal extension into the pterygomaxillary fossa **Stage IIb** - full occupation of the pterygomaxillary fossa with or without erosion of the orbit **Stage IIc** - infratemporal fossa with or without cheek extension	Extension into the nasal cavity or sphenoid sinus	Invading the pterygopalatine fossa or maxillary, ethmoid or Sphenoid sinus with bone destruction	**Stage IIa** - minimal extension through the sphenopalatine fossa and into the medial pterygomaxillary fossa, displacement of the posterior wall of maxilla forward, orbit erosion, displacement of the maxillary artery branches **Stage IIb** - infratemporal fossa, cheek, posterior to pterygoid plates	Maxillary sinus, full occupation of the pterygomaxillary fossa; limited extension to the infratemporal fossa	Paranasal sinuses, lateral pterygopalatine fossa, no residual vascularity	**Stage IIa** - with extension in the nasal cavity and/minimal involvement of the pterygopalatine fossa **Stage IIb** - involvement of the pterygopalatine fossa and infratemporal fossa **Stage IIc** - extending beyond ITF with involvement of check/pterygoid space/inferior orbital fissure/laterally along the greater wing of the sphenoid
Stage III	Intracranial extension	Tumor into the antrum, ethmoid sinus, pterygomaxillary fossa, infratemporal fossa, orbit and/or cheek	Invading infratemporal fossa or orbital region: **Stage IIIa** - no intracranial **Stage IIIb** - paraseller, (extradural) involvement	Erosion of skull base: **Stage IIIa** - minimal intracranial extension **Stage IIIb** - maximal intracranial extension cavernous sinus	Deep extension into cancellous bone at the pterygoid base or body and greater wing of the sphenoid. Significant lateral extension into the infratemporal fossa or pterygoid plates. Orbital, cavernous sinus obliteration	Skull base erosion orbit, infratemporal fossa, no residual vascularity	**Stage IIIa** - involvement of the quadrangular space/Meckel's space **Stage IIIb** - involvement of the cavernous sinus/ engulfing carotid artery
Stage IV	NA	Intracranial extension	Intracranial, intradural tumor **Stage IVa** with and **Stage IVb** without— cavernous sinus, pituitary or optic chiasm infiltration	NA	Intracranial extension between the pituitary gland and the internal carotid artery. Tumor localization lateral to the internal carotid artery. Middle fossa extension and extensive intracranial extension	Skull base erosion orbit, infratemporal fossa, residual vascularity	**Stage IVa** - Prestyloid, parapharyngeal extension **Stage IVb** - minimal intracranial extension
Stage V	NA	NA					

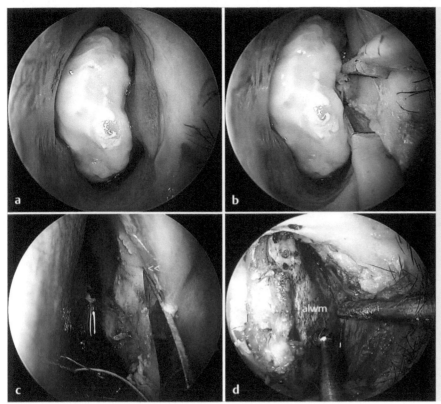

Fig. 20.4 **(a)** The tumor seen extending anteriorly toward the vestibule. **(b)** The inferior turbinate was cauterized. **(c)** Modified endoscopic Denker's procedure—using a knife, the anterior edge of the pyriform aperture is incised. **(d)** A Freer elevator is then used to elevate the subperiosteal plane to expose the anterolateral wall of the maxilla (ALWM).

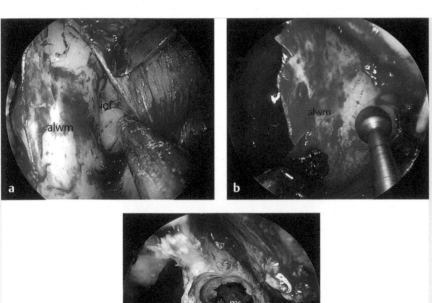

Fig. 20.5 **(a)** The superior limit of the exposure is the infraorbital nerve. Care is taken not to injure this nerve during the dissection. Iof, infraorbital fissure. **(b,c)** Using a mallet and gouge or a cutting burr, the anterolateral wall of the maxillary sinus is gouged or drilled away. The exposure of the anterolateral wall is done superiorly till the infraorbital nerve, laterally till the level of the zygomatic eminence, and inferiorly till the canine eminence. Using a Freer elevator, the mucosa of the lateral wall of the nose in the inferior meatus is elevated and debrided, thus exposing the bone. MS, maxillary sinus.

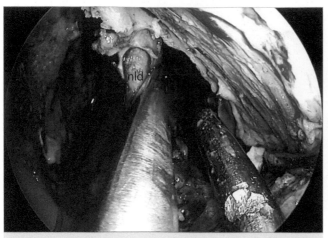

Fig. 20.6 The medial wall of the maxilla is then drilled anteriorly till the level of the nasolacrimal duct (nld), which is exposed and transected.

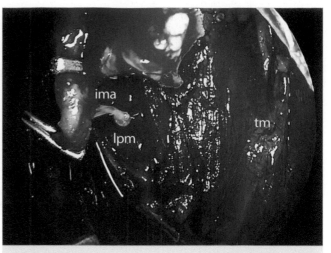

Fig. 20.8 Once the fat is removed, the internal maxillary artery (ima) is clipped. lpm, lateral pterygoid muscle; tm, temporalis muscle.

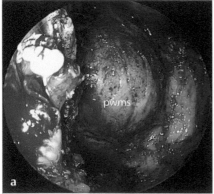

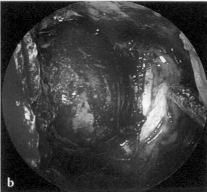

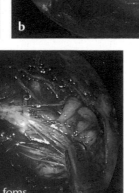

Fig. 20.7 **(a)** Posteriorly, bone is drilled up to the level of the junction of the palatine bone with the medial pterygoid plate, in which the descending palatine neurovascular bundle is seen and cauterized. **(b)** The posterior wall of the maxilla is drilled, and the bone is removed, exposing the periosteum. Exposure of the posterior wall of the maxillary sinus (pwms) extends far laterally up to the junction of the anterolateral wall with the posterior wall. Burrs cannot be used because the fat and the muscle in this area swirl around the burr, obviating its use; thus, Kerrison's rongeur is preferred. **(c)** The fat in the infratemporal fossa was removed to identify the internal maxillary artery. foms, floor of maxillary sinus.

staged on the basis of intraoperative blood loss, surgeon fatigue, and anesthetic complications.

Tumor dissection is done along the tumor bed, as a plane exists between the tumor and the neighboring structures. The magnified view of the endoscope helps visualization of the tumor's margins and ensures complete excision.

20.7.6 Segmental Resection

The principle of segmental resection is piecemeal resection of JNA at the level of the pterygoid wedge. The tumor posterior to the wedge receives blood supply from the ICA. The debulking of the tumor anterior to the pterygoid wedge is relatively blood-

less due to direct devascularization by ligation or embolization (▶ Fig. 20.9, ▶ Fig. 20.10). This also provides better visualization of the deeper location of the tumor with an improved degree of surgical freedom. The resection of this part can be staged depending upon blood loss and surgeon fatigue. The erosion of the cancellous bone can be visualized and drilled radically to avoid recurrence (▶ Fig. 20.11).

20.7.7 Hemostasis

Intraoperative hemostasis is of greatest concern for a surgeon performing the endoscopic excision of JNA. Meticulous intraoperative hemostasis is essential to ensure complete resection

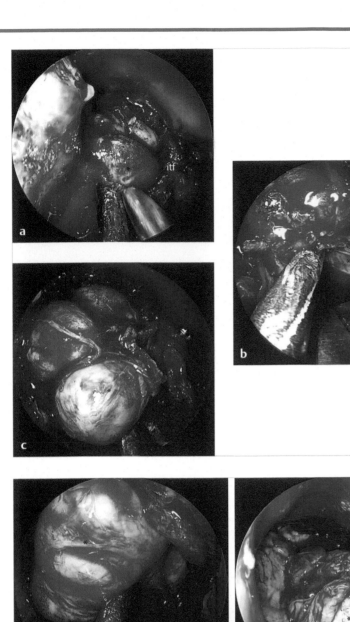

Fig. 20.9 (**a, b**) The tumor was dissected from the infratemporal fossa (ITF) and floor of the maxillary sinus (foms), and the part of the tumor in the cheek was delivered by gentle traction using a curved Luc's forceps. (**c**) The tumor was then dissected from its lateral and superior extensions.

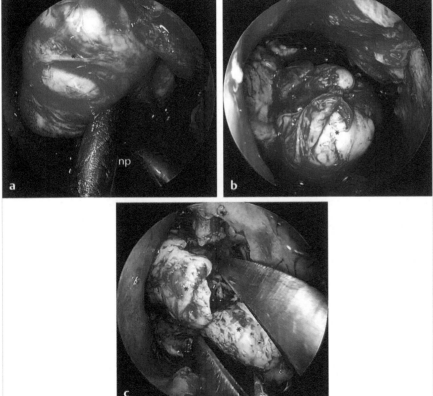

Fig. 20.10 (**a**) The tumor was then dissected from the nasopharynx (np). (**b**) The tumor was freed from all the attachments around. (**c**) Resection of the tumor was done at the level of the pterygoid wedge.

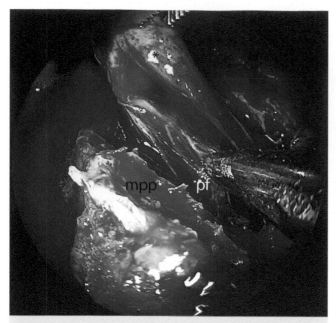

Fig. 20.11 The pterygoid wedge was drilled and the remnant tumor was removed. Medial pterygoid plate (mpp), Pterygoid fossa (pf).

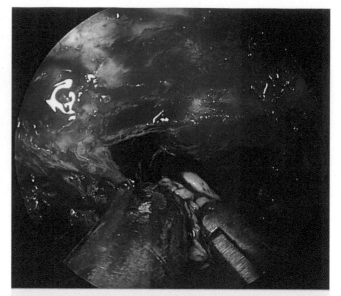

Fig. 20.12 Endoscopic excision of a juvenile nasopharyngeal angiofibroma from the wall of the cavernous sinus.

Table 20.2 Strategies for Homeostasis in JNA

Anesthetic strategies	
1. Preoperative evaluation	• Optimization of hemoglobin • Cessation of drugs acting on coagulation cascade[8]
2. Positioning	• Reverse Trendelenburg's position
3. Hypotensive anesthesia	• MABP 60–70 mm Hg; HR < 60 mm Hg • Maintain temperature
4. Replacement strategy	• Preoperative blood loss assessment
Surgical strategies	
1. Mechanical strategies	• Direct pressure • Ligaclips
2. Thermal strategies	• Bipolar cautery, e.g., Kassam bipolar • Warm saline irrigations
3. Chemical strategies	• Adrenaline soaked gauze packing • Hemostatic agents • Passive agents, e.g., cellulose • Active agents, e.g., thrombin products • Flowable agents, e.g., Floseal, Surgiflo • Fibrin Sealants, e.g., Duraseal, Tisseel
Source of bleeding	
1. Venous bleeding	• Diffuse mucosal: warm saline irrigations • Focal bleeding: hemostatic packing, e.g., thrombin soaked Gelfoam, bipolar cauterization
2. Arterial bleeding	• Low flow: bipolar cauterization, coblation • High flow: muscle patch

of this deep-seated vascular tumor. The role of the anesthesiologist is crucial in maintaining and monitoring the hemodynamic parameters of the patient and in providing a bloodless surgical field. The hemostasis can be achieved by thermal coagulation, laser, coblation, packing, and the use of hemostatic agents depending on the site and flow (▶ Table 20.2).

20.7.8 Advanced Tumors

The evolution of endoscopic skull base surgery with advancements in imaging and anesthesiology has led, in the past few years, to increased consideration of endoscopes for surgical resection in complex anatomical locations.

In advanced cases of JNA, the strategy is to devascularize and debulk the tumor anterior to the pterygoid wedge. In cases with involvement of ICA, cavernous sinus, and intracranial extension, we prefer to stage the surgery. The intraoperative blood loss, anesthetic complications, and surgeon fatigue are other deciding factors considered. This gives time to accommodate for blood loss and for stabilizing the patient.

The tumor engulfing the ICA is a surgical challenge. Thorough anatomical orientation of the complex 3D anatomy with intermittent use of navigation and carotid Doppler guides piecemeal resections. The endosteal layer of the ICA is identified from the uninvolved distal segment, and the tumor can be gently peeled away without causing traction on the vessel under increased magnification of the camera.

In the case of cavernous sinus involvement on MRI, it was noticed intraoperatively that in the majority of the cases, the tumor is pushing the sinus wall with intact layer of dura. Intraoperatively, it was possible to gently peel the tumor away from the sinus and leave the wall intact (▶ Fig. 20.12). This potential plane, which has been described previously, forms an endoscopic principle.

In our experience, a large number of intracranial extensions were found to be extradural in nature and thus resectable without additional craniotomy, thereby decreasing morbidity. Thus, a single endoscopic approach is preferred to a combined approach for minimal extradural components.

20.7.9 Surgical Training

The surgical expertise in endoscopic skull base surgery is a crucial factor for implementation of endoscopes in advanced cases. The long learning curve can be negotiated by repeated cadaver dissections to understand the complex 3D anatomy of the skull base. Repetitive stage-wise live surgery is required to get accustomed to distorted anatomy and learning to handle complications. Blood loss decreases with experience as surgery becomes familiar and faster, especially in advanced cases.

20.8 Approach

Based on the experience of endoscopic management of a large series of JNA patients, we have formulated some endoscopic surgical guidelines (▶ Table 20.3). The emphasis lies on adequate endoscopic approach to access the tumor to the extent that facilitates adequate vascular control and complete tumor removal.

20.9 Complications

The advancements in minimal-access approaches have decreased morbidity and improved cosmesis as compared to traditional approaches in complex sinonasal lesions extending to the skull base. Despite increased safety due to increases in skill and experience, complications do occur. Careful case selection, correct surgical approach, adequate surgical skill, and adherence to principles can avoid complications.

A rare anesthetic complication seen is the trigeminocardiac reflex (TCR). It is an established reflex that may occur following mechanical/electrical or any stimulation of the branches of the trigeminal nerve along its course.[22] We unexpectedly encountered the TCR in the transpterygoid approach during the removal of tumor from the infratemporal fossa, pterygopalatine fossa, quadrangular space, and greater wing of the sphenoid. Such an event is best managed by ceasing mechanical manipulation, application of a local anesthetic agent, and anticholinergics.

Surgical complications can be divided into intraoperative, early postoperative, and late postoperative. This has further been described in ▶ Table 20.4.

20.10 Postoperative Care and Surveillance

Depending on the blood loss, immediate postoperative care should be provided in the intensive care unit, with special emphasis on monitoring and maintaining the hemodynamic parameters. The nasal packs are removed after 3 to 5 days, followed by nasal saline irrigations to avoid crusting. Postoperative follow-up data included immediate CT scanning within 36 hours of surgery. Eventual follow-up includes a CT scan 6 months postoperatively as well as nasal endoscopic examinations every 3 months for the first year after surgery and every 6 months for the following 3 years, as well as a comprehensive clinical examination at each visit. Recurrent disease was defined as a new tumor seen during the follow-up observation period after an initially negative postoperative scan. A postoperative carotid angiogram should be performed if the ICA is handled or transposed intraoperatively.

20.11 Alternative Modalities

Radiotherapy is generally reserved for tumors with intracranial extension, unresectable tumors, and surgically unfit patients. Therapeutic results were appreciated with dose ranges between 30 and 46 Gy.[23] Amdur et al reported control rates up to 90%.[24] Potential long-term complications of radiotherapy of the head and neck region included ocular complications such as cataract, endophthalmitis, optic nerve atrophy, cranial nerve palsies, dental caries due to xerostomia, pan hypopituitarism, radionecrosis of the maxilla, and skull base osteomyelitis. Intensity-modulated radiotherapy (IMRT) precisely delivers radiation to the tumor, sparing the surrounding structures, thereby allowing larger cumulative doses of 45 Gy to be delivered. There are a few case reports of a cyber knife being used for the treatment of JNA; however, further studies are needed to establish effectiveness of this modality.

Chemotherapy has been investigated as a treatment option in cases of JNA that had recurred after surgery and radiation therapy (XRT), but a low therapeutic benefit coupled with poorly tolerated side effects has made this a rarely used endeavor.[25]

20.12 Conclusion

Introduction of endoscopic approaches has caused a paradigm shift in surgical management of JNA. Endoscopic approaches give superior surgical outcomes in terms of intraoperative blood loss, perioperative mortality, postoperative recurrence, and better cosmetic results. However, endoscopic JNA surgery is technically demanding and requires thorough understanding of skull base anatomy as well as surgical expertise. High-quality imaging and meticulous preoperative planning and implementation of principles are prerequisites for endonasal excision of JNA. The proposed staging system is based on one of the largest series of primary cases of JNA and classifies tumors based on CECT. Furthermore, it provides a comprehensive account of the surgical steps that we proposed for each stage in order to achieve superior surgical outcomes.[26] However, a multicentric trial is recommended for further validation of these surgical approaches.

Table 20.3 The Janakiram Classification for JNA

Stage	Extension on preoperative CT scan	Proposed endonasal endoscopic approaches and surgical guidelines
1a	Tumor limited to the pterygoid wedge with/without the sphenoid sinus	The exposure requires anterior and posterior ethmoidectomy with wide sphenoidotomy. The blood loss is controlled by cauterization of the posterior nasal branch of the sphenopalatine artery followed by tumor excision.
1b	Extension into the pterygoid wedge, sphenoid sinus with/without involvement of the nasopharynx	When the tumor extends to the nasopharynx, a middle meatal antrostomy is also essential for wide exposure. The tumor is devascularized by control of the sphenopalatine and descending palatine arteries and dissected off the nasopharynx and delivered.
2a	Tumor with minimal extension into the pterygopalatine fossa (PPF) with or without involvement of the nasal cavity	For a tumor extending into the pterygopalatine and further into the infratemporal fossa, stages 2a and b. Exposure is obtained by medial maxillectomy with removal of the medial part of posterior wall of maxillary sinus. A posterior septectomy/septal window is added to facilitate access with a four-handed binostril technique. Ligation of internal maxillary artery is done for devascularization. This vessel has to be carefully dissected out and identified lateral to the tumor margin. Up to this stage, it is prudent to drill away the pterygoid wedge after tumor resection and remove any tumor remnants in this area.
2b	Extension to the PPF/infratemporal fossa (ITF)	
2c	Involvement of ITF with/without further extension into the pterygoid space/inferior orbital fissure/laterally along the greater wing of sphenoid/cheek area	Transient clamping of the external carotid artery on the same side is recommended and carried out prior to starting the endoscopic procedure in order to control the blood loss. This is also done for all stages beyond stage 2c. In this setting, a modified endoscopic Denker approach is used to expose the angiofibroma at its most lateral extent before commencing the tumor dissection. Trigeminal branch V2 is identified and should be preserved, as it also serves as a landmark for inferior orbital fissure. In JNA cases with tumor extension into the inferior orbital fissure, the bony margins are drilled away with a 3-mm diamond drill burr to facilitate exposure and to allow extirpation of this part of the tumor. Any tumor anterior to the pterygoid wedge is debulked first to enable drilling of the involved cancellous bone.
3a	Involvement of the quadrangular space/Meckel's cave	Modified Denker's approach with clamping of external carotid artery is performed. The tumor is debulked first so that the pterygoid wedge can be accessed. The drilling of the greater sphenoid wing superiorly is important for better proximal exposure, which aids in removing the tumor from crevices in cancellous bone. It rarely extends laterally or superiorly to the anatomical path of V2. Further posterolateral extension beyond the pterygoid wedge is limited by middle cranial fossa dura. As the tumor respects the dura, it can be meticulously dissected away from it with gentle traction. The vidian nerve is then identified and can be freed by drilling out bone from the 6 to 9 o'clock position. The anterolateral wall of sphenoid is removed next. The paraclival internal carotid artery (ICA) is identified. The bone over the medial wall of the paraclival ICA is drilled away. The lingular process of the sphenoid bone is identified and also removed, which allows mobilization of the ICA. The paraclival ICA can now be gently transposed medially, which creates additional space to resect any tumor extending into Meckel's cave.
3b	Involvement of the cavernous sinus and/or engulfment of the carotid artery	The tumor is resected to the level of the pterygoid wedge. The tumor is carefully debulked in close proximity to the ICA. The microvascular Doppler probe can be used to identify the exact position of the ICA. Feeder vessels arising from the ICA supplying the tumor can be cauterized. The tumor around the ICA is carefully debulked in a piecemeal fashion. The position of the ICA needs to be confirmed as well, as its distance to the workspace that has been developed before opening the cavernous sinus. The tumor can now be gently dissected from the sinus wall while taking care not to injure cranial nerves.
4	Involvement of the prestyloid parapharyngeal space and/or with minimal intracranial extension lateral to the superior orbital fissure	In cases of such widespread tumor extension, we employed multiple corridors or changed our strategy to an endoscopic-assisted external approach. To this end, the surgical procedure can be divided into two steps, each tailored according to the tumor extension. For the transnasal corridor, again a modified Denker approach is used to expose the angiofibroma to its most lateral extent before tumor dissection is carried out. V2 is again identified and preserved. The tumor is cleared from the sinonasal corridor step by step as described earlier.
4a	Involvement of the prestyloid parapharyngeal space	In cases with parapharyngeal extension stage 4a, a transoral corridor should be adopted. In this approach, the tumor bulge is identified in the soft palate and an intraoral incision is made anterior to the anterior pillar. The mucosa, submucosa, and fibers of palatoglossus and superior constrictor pharynges are dissected to visualize and expose the tumor. With constant traction on the inferior part of the tumor, the mass is bluntly dissected along the tumor bed in the prestyloid space. It is then pushed superiorly to be delivered via the infratemporal fossa. The attachment of the tumor to any residual mass is now sharply cut near the foramen ovale. The intraoral part of the JNA, depending on its size, is delivered intraorally or through the nasal cavity. Hemostasis is performed and the incision is closed in a watertight fashion to prevent infection.
4b	Involvement of the prestyloid parapharyngeal space with minimal intracranial extension lateral to the superior orbital fissure	In cases with tumor extension through the superior orbital fissure into the intracranial compartment (middle cranial fossa and toward the temporal lobe), the tumor can best be accessed via a transorbital endoscopic approach. An incision at the level of the brow or inferiorly to it is made to enter the supraorbital area. The periorbita is moved and elevated away to allow drilling of greater wing of the sphenoid bone. This corridor is bounded laterally by the temporalis muscle, posteromedially by the superior orbital fissure, and superiorly by the dura of the anterior cranial fossa. Using this corridor, the tumor is exposed lateral to the superior orbital fissure, and microsurgical dissection is performed with regular cauterization of the blood vessels using bipolar cautery prior to delivery of the tumor mass.
5	Massive parapharyngeal, maximal intracranial extensions, and bilateral JNA	In cases with poststyloid parapharyngeal extension or bilateral JNAs, the author prefers an external approach to access the tumor. The external approach implemented by the author is a bilateral facial translocation approach as proposed by Ivo Janecka. However, the authors do not advocate any specific external approach. The choice of external approach is at the discretion of the provider.

Abbreviation: JNA, juvenile nasopharyngeal angiofibroma.

Table 20.4 Complications of JNA Surgery

Intraoperative	Early postoperative (1–30 d)	Late postoperative
1. Vascular	1. Erosion of nares	1. Alar collapse
a) ICA spasm b) Blood loss c) ICA Injury	2. Crusting synechiae	2. Caroticocavernous fistula
2. Neurological complication a) CSF leak b) Cranial nerve palsies	3. Orbital hematoma	3. Residual and recurrent tumors
	4. Infraorbital nerve paresthesia	
	5. Rhinosinusitis	

Abbreviations: CSF, cerebrospinal fluid; ICA, internal carotid artery.

References

[1] Bensch H. Beitrage zur Beurtheilung der Chirurgischen Behandlung der Nasenrachenopolypen. Breslau, Poland: E. Morgenstern; 1878

[2] Chaveau C. Histoire de Maladies du Pharynx. Vol. 5. Paris, France: J.B. Bailliere et fils; 1906

[3] Lee DA, Rao BR, Meyer JS, Prioleau PG, Bauer WC. Hormonal receptor determination in juvenile nasopharyngeal angiofibromas. Cancer. 1980; 46(3):547–551

[4] Biswas D, Saha S, Bera SP. Relative distribution of the tumours of ear, nose and throat in the paediatric patients. Int J Pediatr Otorhinolaryngol. 2007; 71 (5):801–805

[5] Schiff M. Juvenile nasopharyngeal angiofibroma. a theory of pathogenesis. Laryngoscope. 1959; 69:981–1016

[6] Batsakis JG. Tumors of head and neck. 2nd ed. Baltimore, MD. Williams and Wilkins; 1979:291–312

[7] Ungkanont K, Byers RM, Weber RS, Callender DL, Wolf PF, Goepfert H. Juvenile nasopharyngeal angiofibroma: an update of therapeutic management. Head Neck. 1996; 18(1):60–66

[8] Nicolai P, Berlucchi M, Tomenzoli D, et al. Endoscopic surgery for juvenile angiofibroma: when and how. Laryngoscope. 2003; 113(5):775–782

[9] Mishra A, Mishra SC. Time trends in recurrence of juvenile nasopharyngeal angiofibroma: experience of the past 4 decades. Am J Otolaryngol. 2016; 37 (3):265–271

[10] Lloyd G, Howard D, Lund VJ, Savy L. Imaging for juvenile angiofibroma. J Laryngol Otol. 2000; 114(9):727–730

[11] Davis KR. Embolization of epistaxis and juvenile nasopharyngeal angiofibromas. AJR Am J Roentgenol. 1987; 148(1):209–218

[12] Liu ZF, Wang DH, Sun XC, et al. The site of origin and expansive routes of juvenile nasopharyngeal angiofibroma (JNA). Int J Pediatr Otorhinolaryngol. 2011; 75(9):1088–1092

[13] Mishra S, Praveena NM, Panigrahi RG, Gupta YM. Imaging in the Diagnosis of Juvenile Nasopharyngeal Angiofibroma J Clin Imaging Sci.. 2013; 3:1

[14] Snyderman CH, Pant H, Carrau RL, Gardner P. A new endoscopic staging system for angiofibromas. Arch Otolaryngol Head Neck Surg. 2010; 136(6):588–594

[15] Sessions RB, Bryan RN, Naclerio RM, Alford BR. Radiographic staging of juvenile angiofibroma. Head Neck Surg. 1981; 3(4):279–283

[16] Chandler JR, Goulding R, Moskowitz L, Quencer RM. Nasopharyngeal angiofibromas: staging and management. Ann Otol Rhinol Laryngol. 1984; 93(4, pt 1):322–329

[17] Fisch U. The infratemporal fossa approach for nasopharyngeal tumors. Laryngoscope. 1983; 93(1):36–44

[18] Bremer JW, Neel HB, III, DeSanto LW, Jones GC. Angiofibroma: treatment trends in 150 patients during 40 years. Laryngoscope. 1986; 96(12):1321–1329

[19] Andrews JC, Fisch U, Valavanis A, Aeppli U, Makek MS. The surgical management of extensive nasopharyngeal angiofibromas with the infratemporal fossa approach. Laryngoscope. 1989; 99(4):429–437

[20] Radkowski D, McGill T, Healy GB, Ohlms L, Jones DT. Angiofibroma. Changes in staging and treatment. Arch Otolaryngol Head Neck Surg. 1996; 122(2): 122–129

[21] Onerci M, Oğretmenoğlu O, Yücel T. Juvenile nasopharyngeal angiofibroma: a revised staging system. Rhinology. 2006; 44(1):39–45

[22] Potti TA, Gemmete JJ, Pandey AS, Chaudhary N. Trigeminocardiac reflex during the percutaneous injection of ethylene vinyl alcohol copolymer (Onyx) into a juvenile nasopharyngeal angiofibroma: a report of two cases. J Neurointerv Surg. 2011; 3(3):263–265

[23] McAfee WJ, Morris CG, Amdur RJ, Werning JW, Mendenhall WM. Definitive radiotherapy for juvenile nasopharyngeal angiofibroma. Am J Clin Oncol. 2006; 29(2):168–170

[24] Amdur RJ, Yeung AR, Fitzgerald BM, Mancuso AA, Werning JW, Mendenhall WM. Radiotherapy for juvenile nasopharyngeal angiofibroma. Pract Radiat Oncol. 2011; 1(4):271–278

[25] Lee JT, Chen P, Safa A, Juillard G, Calcaterra TC. The role of radiation in the treatment of advanced juvenile angiofibroma. Laryngoscope. 2002; 112(7, pt 1):1213–1220

[26] Janakiram TN, Sharma SB, Kasper E, Deshmukh O, Cherian I. Comprehensive preoperative staging system for endoscopic single and multicorridor approaches to juvenile nasal angiofibromas. Surg Neurol Int. 2007; 8:55

21 Optic Pathway Glioma and Juvenile Pilocytic Astrocytoma

Neil Majmundar, John R.W. Kestle, Douglas L. Brockmeyer, Jean Anderson Eloy, and James K. Liu

Abstract

This chapter describes the prevalence, natural history, and management of optic pathway gliomas (OPGs) in the pediatric age group. The authors discuss the presentation of OPGs in both the general population and neurofibromatosis type 1 (NF1) patients. The various treatment modalities of observation, chemotherapy, radiation therapy, and surgery are discussed. The role of endoscopy for the treatment of these tumors is discussed, and two case examples are presented demonstrating the importance of multimodal therapy.

Keywords: optic pathway glioma, juvenile pilocytic astrocytoma, neurofibromatosis type 1, endoscopy

21.1 Introduction

Optic pathway gliomas (OPGs) are rare benign tumors that involve eloquent neurologic structures, such as the optic nerves, chiasm, tracts, radiations, and hypothalamus. This relatively rare tumor type accounts for approximately 2 to 7% of all pediatric brain tumors.[1,2] Approximately 60 to 65% of these tumors are diagnosed in children younger than 5 years of age and nearly 75% during the first decade of life.[1,2] Although they are typically found in a younger age group, with a mean age at presentation of 8 years, OPGs have been reported in patients up to the age of 79 years.[1,3] In the general population, they tend to present proportionately in men and women.[1]

The prevalence of OPGs is greater in patients with neurofibromatosis type 1 (NF1) when compared to sporadic cases in the general population, affecting approximately 11 to 30% of children with NF1.[1,4] More than half of all OPGs occur in patients with NF1. The diagnosis of NF1 has a large impact on the clinical presentation, natural history, and treatment paradigm in patients with OPGs. In these patients, OPGs generally have a more benign presentation and clinical course. They can also be bilateral, multifocal, and found within the optic nerves.[1] They are not typically found at the hypothalamus in patients with NF1. However, when they do occur at the hypothalamus, they can exhibit an aggressive clinical course, presenting with diencephalic syndrome resulting in cachexia and hypersomnia.[1] OPGs in patients with NF1 rarely progress after the patient reaches 6 years of age, significantly changing the manner in which this disease is treated when compared to patients with sporadic OPGs.[5] Although the pathologic and radiographic appearance of OPGs in patients both with and without NF1 may be similar, OPGs found in NF1 patients are noticeably less aggressive than sporadic cases in the general population.[6]

Histologically, the majority of OPGs are comprised of WHO grade I juvenile pilocytic astrocytomas (JPAs), while a smaller proportion are pilomyxoid astrocytomas. In rare instances, they can be WHO grade II astrocytomas. JPAs are most commonly found in the cerebellum (60%), followed by the optic pathway (optic nerve/chiasm, hypothalamus/third ventricle; 25–35%),

and finally the pons/medulla and tectum.[1] Because of their intimate involvement with critical neurovascular structures, such as the optic pathway and hypothalamus, the optimal treatment remains controversial. In this chapter, we discuss the clinical presentation, natural history, and multimodal management of OPGs.

21.2 Natural History and Clinical Presentation

The true prevalence and natural progression of OPGs is difficult to determine, as many of these patients only present once they become symptomatic. The natural history can vary greatly among patients, as it can depend upon the presence of NF1, age of onset, and location of the tumor. Generally, OPGs are low-grade lesions with a slow growth rate and good long-term patient survival.[1] However, their natural history can sometimes be unpredictable, with variable growth patterns ranging from extended periods of tumor stability to rapid progression, or they can have erratic growth patterns, with alternating periods of growth and stabilization.[7] Spontaneous regression of OPGs has also been reported in patients with close observation and serial imaging.[2]

While a proportion of patients with OPGs may be asymptomatic, many patients with OPGs can present with a variety of symptoms depending upon size and location of the tumor. Most frequently, patients with OPGs present with decreased visual acuity. However, if the tumor involves the intraorbital optic nerve, patients may present with proptosis, strabismus, and vision loss due to pressure upon the orbital contents and optic nerve.[5] OPGs isolated to the optic nerve do not generally infiltrate the eye, but cause extrinsic compression of the globe.[8] Patients with intracranial tumors may present with visual symptoms, which can range from impaired color vision, decreased visual acuity, visual field deficits, optic atrophy, and total blindness. Intracranial tumors may also present with hypothalamic and endocrine disturbances, such as precocious puberty, anterior pituitary dysfunction, obesity, and diencephalic syndrome, due to the relative proximity of the hypothalamic–pituitary axis. When OPGs obstruct the normal flow of cerebrospinal fluid (CSF), patients can develop obstructive hydrocephalus, often requiring surgical intervention, such as CSF shunting and/or tumor debulking.[1]

OPGs can be located anywhere along the optic pathway, including the optic discs, nerves, chiasm, tracts, and radiations. Approximately 25% of OPGs occur at the optic disc and nerves, and 40 to 75% occur at the chiasm.[1] About one-third to two-thirds of all chiasmatic OPGs can also involve the third ventricle or hypothalamus.[1]

The prognosis for OPGs varies with age and symptoms at presentation, preexisting diagnosis of NF1, and location. Typically, sporadic OPGs in children without NF1 are thought to be more aggressive and result in worse clinical outcomes.[8] In a recent series of 65 pediatric OPGs, the event-free survival rate at 4 years was higher in NF1 patients than in non-NF1 patients (72.9 vs. 48.4%, respectively), while the overall survival rate at 4 years was 90% for NF1 and 84.3% for non-NF1 patients.[7] When sporadic OPGs are diagnosed before the age of 5 years, a less favorable prognosis is expected.[1] Anteriorly located OPGs within the optic pathways, in the presence of NF1, have a more favorable prognosis. Tumors can either present in a perineural or an intraneural growth pattern. Patients with NF1 tend to have a perineural growth pattern, while sporadic cases generally exhibit an intraneural growth pattern. Patients with OPGs confined to the optic nerve have a higher rate of survival than patients with OPGs involving the optic chiasm/hypothalamus. Although progression- or event-free survival varies in many case series based upon OPG location, age at presentation, and treatment modality, the 5-year event-free survival rate ranges from 30 to 40%.[9]

Histologically, OPGs are low-grade gliomas that can manifest as pilocytic, fibrillary, or pilomyxoid astrocystomas.[1] Pilocytic astrocytomas comprise the majority of OPGs and express a biphasic pattern with Rosenthal fibers and eosinophilic granular bodies. The more aggressive pilomyxoid astrocytomas display piloid cells in a loose fibrillary and myxoid background, and, unlike the pilocytic subtype, they do not have Rosenthal fibers and rarely demonstrate eosinophilic granular bodies.[1] The pilomyxoid subtype also has a younger mean age at presentation (18 months), has a more aggressive clinical course, and is more likely to present with CSF dissemination.[1]

21.3 Management Options

The management of and treatment options for OPGs consist of observation with serial imaging, chemotherapy, radiotherapy, and surgery. An individualized tailored approach of management is recommended, with a multidisciplinary team of specialists consisting of neurosurgeons, neuro-ophthalmologists, neuro-oncologists, endocrinologists, radiation oncologists, and otolaryngologists.

21.3.1 Observation

Patients with small tumors that are confined to the optic nerves or chiasm with preserved visual function and non-obstructed CSF pathways can be carefully observed using a wait-and-scan strategy. As many as half of all OPGs have been reported to remain stable and require no intervention.[2] Patients with NF1, who tend typically to have a more benign course, with fewer patients needing intervention for tumor progression, typically undergo observation initially with a serial wait-and-scan approach, especially in the presence of stable radiographic disease or stable visual/neurologic status.[1,2] NF1 patients should have close follow-up with a neuro-ophthalmologist and undergo a complete ophthalmologic examination every year until they reach 8 years of age, and then every 2 years afterward.[1,8] The examination should include funduscopy, visual acuity, and visual field assessment. Spontaneous regression of OPGs has also been reported in patients with close observation and serial imaging.[2] This excludes patients who develop visual symptoms, obstructive hydrocephalus, or endocrine dysfunction from involvement of the hypothalamic–pituitary axis.

Interventional treatment (chemotherapy, radiation therapy, and surgery) is indicated in patients who exhibit radiographic tumor progression or become symptomatic from increased intracranial pressure (mass effect or obstructive hydrocephalus), visual worsening, or diencephalic syndrome. Treatment is individualized with the goal of reducing tumor mass effect and volume while preserving neurological function.

21.3.2 Chemotherapy

Chemotherapy is generally considered the first-line treatment in symptomatic OPGs causing visual loss, hypothalamic–pituitary axis dysfunction, and endocrine disturbances. Chemotherapy is well tolerated in younger children and is associated with lower rates of complications and adverse long-term effects when compared to radiation therapy and surgery. Because radiation has an increased risk of long-term cognitive deficits and growth hormone deficiency, chemotherapy is considered the primary treatment modality in children younger than 5 years of age who present with visual deterioration (▶ Fig. 21.1).[1,5] A variety of chemotherapeutic agents, including carboplatin, cisplatin, vincristine, vinblastine, actinomycin D, lomustine, thioguanine, procarbazine, etoposide, tamoxifen, and temozolomide, have been used as adjuvant or first-line chemotherapy treatment for OPGs.[1] However, the most optimal and effective agents have yet to be defined. The most widely used chemotherapy regimen is carboplatin and vincristine in a 10-week induction phase. This is then followed by carboplatin/vincristine-maintenance for 48 weeks, resulting in a progression-free survival of 50% at 5 years.[1] The combination of cisplatin and etoposide has also been shown to improve visual acuity.[10] Temozolomide, which has been shown to help stabilize progression, can be considered an option for patients in whom first-line therapy has failed.[1] Other combinations, such as a five-drug regimen utilized by Petronio et al, and another similar four-drug regimen, have been shown as reasonable first- and second-line treatments, respectively.[11,12]

21.3.3 Radiation Therapy

While an effective treatment for OPGs, the role for radiation therapy as a first-line therapy has diminished over the years due to its significant long-term side effects, which include the development of neurocognitive deficits, secondary neoplasms, neuroendocrine deficits (especially growth hormone deficiency), and moyamoya syndrome.[2,13] Therefore, radiation therapy is administered as adjuvant therapy rather than primary treatment for progression of disease after failure of other treatment modalities. Studies regarding radiation therapy have varied, with some demonstrating no benefit of radiation over surgery or observation, while others reporting good visual outcomes and tumor-free progression rates.[1] More recently developed modalities of radiation therapy, mainly proton beam radiotherapy, stereotactic radiosurgery, and intensity-modulated radiation therapy (IMRT), have demonstrated better results in terms of 5-year survival rates, with less neurocognitive decline and endocrine disturbances.[1] Currently, radiation therapy is generally avoided as first-line therapy in patients younger than 5 to 7 years. Radiation treatment is delayed as late as possible in order to avoid the devastating effects of neurocognitive deficits and growth hormone deficiency in children.[1,2,14,15]

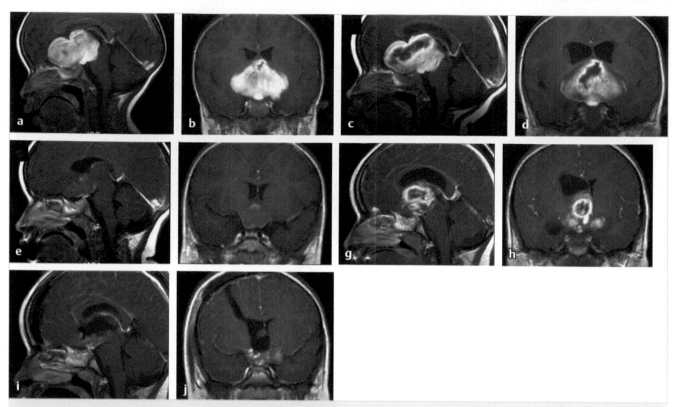

Fig. 21.1 This 19-month-old girl presented with failure to thrive and visual loss. **(a)** Sagittal and **(b)** coronal views of the initial postgadolinium T1-weighted MRI showed a large enhancing lesion in the suprasellar and third ventricular region. An endoscopic transventricular biopsy revealed a juvenile pilocytic astrocytoma. Chemotherapy was initiated and a follow-up MRI 3 months later showed decreased central enhancement but increased hydrocephalus: **(c)** sagittal and **(d)** coronal views. A ventriculoperitoneal shunt was placed and additional courses of chemotherapy were given. Follow-up MRI 1 year later showed significant shrinkage of the tumor: **(e)** sagittal and **(f)** coronal views. Two years after chemotherapy treatment, tumor growth progressed within the third ventricle with a trapped right lateral ventricle: **(g)** sagittal and **(h)** coronal views. Tumor debulking was performed via a right transcortical transventricular transforaminal approach. Residual tumor was left adherent to the walls of the hypothalamus and cerebrospinal fluid pathways were opened up without requirement of an additional shunt: **(i)** sagittal and **(j)** coronal views.

21.3.4 Surgery

The role of surgery in the treatment of OPGs has been a controversial and much-debated topic. While gross total resection of OPGs is not feasible or recommended in the vast majority of cases due to its involvement of vital critical structures (optic nerves, hypothalamus), the role of surgery has generally been limited to tissue biopsy for pathologic diagnosis, and tumor debulking to relieve mass effect from tumor progression.[4,7] Shunt surgery may also be required for CSF diversion in patients who develop hydrocephalus. If a tumor involving the third ventricle is obstructing both foramen of Monro, an endoscopic septum pellucidum fenestration can be considered at the time of unilateral shunt placement to avoid bilateral shunt placement.

Biopsy is generally not performed in NF1 patients who exhibit nonprogressive tumors with classical radiological and clinical features. While biopsy of OPGs prior to initiating chemotherapy or radiation is not required, in some cases with atypical radiographic features, it can provide a more accurate histopathologic diagnosis as well as molecular characterization for prognosis assessment and for guidance of therapeutic options in some clinical trials.[4] It may be important to distinguish pathology types between pilocytic astrocytoma and pilomyxoid astrocytoma, as these two tumors have different clinical courses and prognosis. The indication for biopsy in cases of OPG is institution-dependent and, therefore, can vary across centers. In a large series of 65 pediatric OPGs in Egypt, a more conservative approach was taken, where the aim of surgery was primarily for biopsy and tissue diagnosis, followed by adjuvant chemotherapy.[7] Only four patients received debulking surgery. The 4-year overall survival rate was 86.3%, which suggests that more radical surgical debulking may not be indicated. Surgical approaches for biopsy of OPGs depend largely upon tumor location, as well as surgical risks associated with the selected approach. Biopsy can be performed via stereotactic needle biopsy, or under direct vision using the endoscopic endonasal approach (EEA), endoscopic transventricular approach, or open craniotomy.

Because of the intimate involvement with eloquent neurovascular structures, gross total resection is avoided, as this results in devastating hypothalamic injury, as well as endocrine and visual deficits. The role of surgical resection remains controversial, as there is a lack of consensus and paucity of literature supporting this strategy. However, it is generally accepted that surgery can play a role in surgical debulking in select patients who exhibit tumor progression and/or symptomatic mass effect after failed chemotherapy or radiation therapy. The primary goals of surgical debulking in OPGs are to delay tumor

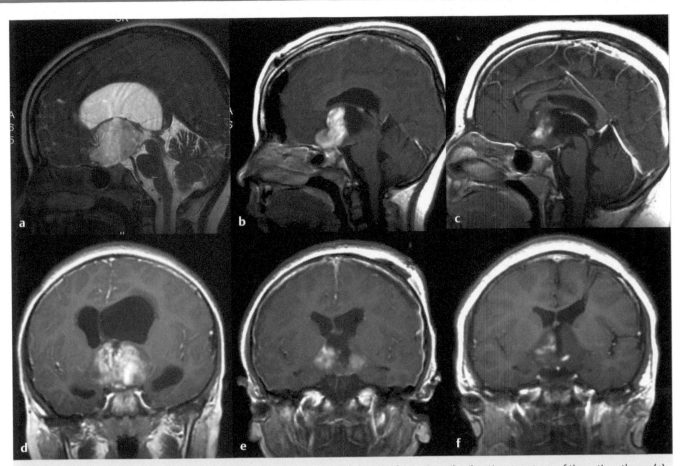

Fig. 21.2 A 5-year-old girl presented with headaches, visual loss, nausea, and vomiting from a juvenile pilocytic astrocytoma of the optic pathway. **(a)** T2 sagittal and **(d)** T1 postgadolinium coronal views of the initial MRI demonstrated an enhancing mass in the third ventricle and suprasellar region with obstructive hydrocephalus. After an initial endoscopic biopsy, septal fenestration, and external ventricular drain placement, a more definitive surgical debulking was performed through a left transcortical transventricular transforaminal corridor 1 week later. **(b)** Sagittal and **(e)** coronal views of the postoperative T1-weighted postgadolinium MRI showed decompression of the cerebrospinal fluid pathways with residual tumor that was adherent to the walls of the third ventricle and hypothalamus. The external ventricular drain was removed and a permanent shunt was not required. Postoperatively, the patient underwent adjuvant carboplatin and vincristine chemotherapy. **(c)** Sagittal and **(f)** coronal views of the MRI at 9 months after surgery demonstrated further decrease in size and enhancement of the residual tumor.

progression in patients who have failed other therapies and to relieve mass effect resulting in neurological impairment or obstructive hydrocephalus. Operative risks can be minimized or avoided by central debulking of the exophytic component of the tumor and leaving a rim of tumor around the base and sides near the hypothalamus (▶ Fig. 21.1). While tumor debulking is not ideal for a large portion of patients, there are select patients who may benefit from debulking of OPGs. In cases where there is an exophytic or cystic component extending into the third ventricle causing obstructive hydrocephalus or symptomatic compression of the optic chiasm and nerves, surgical debulking or cystic drainage may be indicated to help relieve mass effect from the visual apparatus. In a recent study by Goodden et al,[2] where seven patients underwent salvage surgical debulking for tumor progression after failed nonsurgical treatments (chemotherapy and/or radiation therapy), surgery resulted in stable disease without further progression in six patients (85.7%) with a median follow-up of 24.3 months.

The same authors have advocated early surgery (primary surgical debulking) at the time of presentation and diagnosis before initiating chemotherapy in select cases (▶ Fig. 21.2).[2] Patient selection for this strategy included those who had progressive symptoms attributable to the tumor at presentation, a large exophytic midline tumor growing superiorly into the third ventricle resulting in obstructive hydrocephalus, or a large exophytic or cystic extension causing symptomatic compression and mass effect. In their study, 10 patients underwent primary surgical debulking followed by a period of observation. Seven patients (70%) remained stable without progression with a median follow-up of 66.9 months, while tumor progression was seen in three patients (30%) at a median interval of 4.3 months, thus requiring further multimodal adjuvant treatment. Four patients underwent primary surgical debulking followed by planned chemotherapy. One of these patients received additional concurrent radiation therapy. All four patients have remained stable without progression with a median follow-up of 44.6 months. The overall survival in their series was 92.9%, with tumor control in 81%, with a median follow-up period of 6.4 years.[2] In some instances, spontaneous tumor regression of residual disease as well as tumor stabilization can occur after significant tumor debulking.

It is important to note that visual deterioration alone is not an appropriate indication for surgical intervention in all cases, since visual loss can occur from tumor infiltration of the optic apparatus. However, extrinsic compression on the optic apparatus from an enlarging cyst can be considered an indication for surgery.[2] Other studies have shown mixed results for the role of debulking in terms of tumor progression, but as the approaches and patient selection criteria continue to be refined, careful surgical debulking along with radiation and/or chemotherapy can provide favorable tumor control in select patients.[1,2]

The management of pure optic nerve tumors without chiasmatic involvement has varied over the years. A study by Jenkin et al reported 92% survival at 15 years after gross total resection of OPGs in NF1 patients involving solely a unilateral optic nerve.[16] On the other hand, some authors have recommended against surgical excision or debulking in patients with OPGs purely involving the intraorbital optic nerve unless there is significant concern for cosmetic deformity, particularly in patients who still have useful visual function. This philosophy is largely based upon the relatively benign behavior of OPGs that are confined to a unilateral optic nerve, which rarely progress or become infiltrative lesions. Patients presenting with OPGs confined to one optic nerve must be managed on an individual basis, as decision for treatment can vary on a number of factors, and complete resection in patients who already have irrecoverable vision loss can provide a curative option with excellent long-term prognosis.[1]

Because of the complex behavior of OPGs and their treatment strategies, it is not uncommon for patients to undergo cycles of treatment (surgery or chemotherapy) during episodes of tumor progression followed by an interval of observation during periods of tumor stability. This cycle can be repeated as necessary, with treatment tailored to the individual's needs.[2]

21.4 Surgical Approaches

The surgical approaches used for biopsy or surgical debulking of OPGs largely depend on the location of the mass and the goals of surgery. The approaches that are typically performed include the midline interhemispheric transcallosal, the transcortical transventricular (open or endoscopic), frontotemporal (pterional or modified orbitozygomatic), and the EEA.

The midline transcallosal approach or transcortical transventricular approach is effective for exophytic tumors confined within the third ventricle. It is important to keep tumor debulking in the central portion while leaving a thin rim of tumor laterally and inferiorly to protect the hypothalamus, as the tumor tends to invade hypothalamic tissue. This strategy also allows one to open up CSF pathways to avoid the need for a permanent shunt if hydrocephalus is present (▶ Fig. 21.1).

The frontotemporal approach (pterional or orbitozygomatic) is favored if there is significant lateral extension of the tumor or if there is an exophytic and cystic component compressing the optic apparatus. Optic canal unroofing for nerve decompression can also be performed in this approach. It is important to preserve visual and hypothalamic function, since the anatomy can be distorted and difficult to discern normal anatomic structures. The optic nerves and chiasm can often be swollen and infiltrated with the tumor, thereby prohibiting safe removal. Therefore, it may be more prudent to limit surgery to decompression of any enlarging cyst instead of tumor removal to avoid resection of vital visual fibers in these instances.

The role of the EEA is not well defined due to the paucity of its use in the literature. It may be considered an approach for a biopsy if there is a component of the tumor that can be safely accessible in the infrachiasmatic area via the transplanum transtuberculum or transsellar corridor. Surgical debulking can be considered cautiously if there is exophytic tumor or a cystic component that presents itself to the infrachiasmatic and retrochiasmatic space extending upward into the third ventricle. If, however, the pituitary function is normal, there can be a high rate of postoperative anterior hypopituitarism and diabetes insipidus. Again, one should be judicious in the aggressivity in tumor debulking via the EEA because of the risk to the optic apparatus as well as incurring hypothalamic injury and postoperative endocrine dysfunction. Although the endoscopic endonasal transplanum transtuberculum approach is favorable for retrochiasmatic craniopharyngiomas, its application to hypothalamic OPGs is more limited because of the high possibility of an intraneural growth pattern. In these instances, the tumor is intertwined with normal functioning neural tissue, and resection can result in injury to the hypothalamus and optic apparatus. In addition, a tumor in the infrachiasmatic region can also share the blood supply to the normal chiasm. As such, tumor biopsy or debulking can result in potential visual impairment and even blindness.[8] Therefore, careful study of the preoperative scan and intraoperative inspection is paramount before removing tumor tissue. If removal or biopsy of tumor is not deemed feasible, it may be more prudent to come from an approach from above, such as the transcallosal interforniceal approach to the third ventricle, as mentioned previously. Also, if hydrocephalus is present without a preexisting shunt, it may not be favorable to approach the tumor from an EEA since the presence of increased intracranial pressure will increase the risk of postoperative CSF leakage (▶ Fig. 21.3). However, in the absence of hydrocephalus, meticulous multilayered reconstruction of the skull base defect with a vascularized pedicled nasoseptal flap is critical in minimizing postoperative CSF leakage. Although the role for endoscopy via the endonasal route is limited, the use of endoscopy is more readily applied for transventricular biopsy, septum pellucidum fenestration, and guidance for shunt placement.

21.5 Case Example 1

A 19-month-old girl was admitted to the pediatric service for failure to thrive and weight loss in the prior 2 months. When she was less than a year of age, she was strong, healthy, and bigger than other children her age. On neurological examination, the patient was awake and alert, pupils were equal and reactive to light, and she was moving all extremities well with excellent strength. Formal neuro-ophthalmological examination showed severe optic nerve pallor without papilledema and horizontal rotatory and pendular nystagmus. MRI demonstrated a large symmetric and enhancing suprasellar lesion with third ventricular involvement (▶ Fig. 21.1a, b).

A stereotactic biopsy was performed, and the pathologic result was JPA. The patient was started on carboplatin and vincristine chemotherapy. Although the tumor decreased in size initially, it grew back about 3 months later with symptomatic hydrocephalus (▶ Fig. 21.1c, d). An endoscopic septal fenestration and

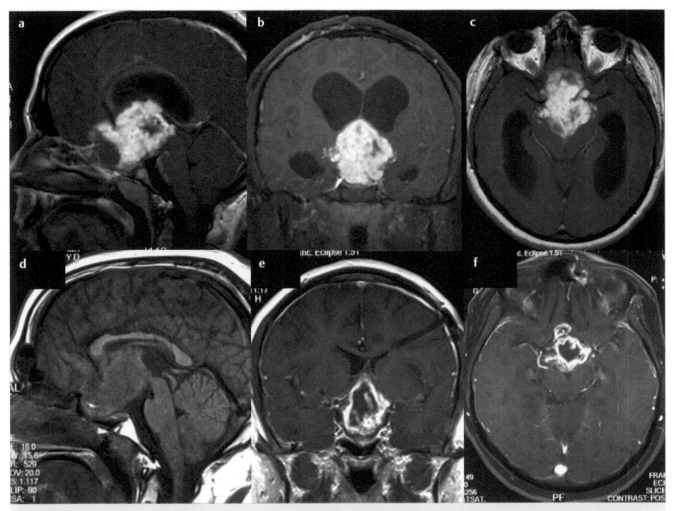

Fig. 21.3 This 5-year-old boy presented with progressive visual loss and hydrocephalus. **(a)** Sagittal, **(b)** coronal, and **(c)** axial views of the initial postgadolinium T1-weighted MRI demonstrated an enhancing suprasellar mass involving the optic chiasm and hypothalamus with extension into the third ventricle. Although an endoscopic endonasal biopsy can be considered based on the anatomic location of this tumor, there is a significant risk of postoperative cerebrospinal fluid rhinorrhea because of the presence of florid hydrocephalus. Instead, the patient was shunted, and an open biopsy via a pterional approach revealed a juvenile pilocytic astrocytoma. Chemotherapy was initiated and **(d)** T1-weighted sagittal, **(e)** postgadolinium coronal, and **(f)** postgadolinium axial **(f)** views of follow-up MRI at 15 months after treatment demonstrated decrease in tumor size and central enhancement.

endoscopic left-sided ventriculoperitoneal shunt was performed. Adjuvant chemotherapy was restarted with two additional cycles. MRI at 1 year after shunting demonstrated further decrease in size and enhancement of the tumor (▶ Fig. 21.1e, f).

At 5 years of age, the patient presented with progressive headaches, worsening vision, and vomiting in the mornings. MRI showed progression of the tumor within the third ventricle with obstructive hydrocephalus with a trapped right lateral ventricle (▶ Fig. 21.1g, h). The patient underwent a right transcortical transventricular approach for tumor debulking to open up CSF pathways and to avoid a second shunt. Intraoperatively, the septum pellucidum was fenestrated widely. Residual tumor was left adherent to the walls of the hypothalamus inferiorly to avoid hypothalamic complications.

Postoperatively, the patient was neurologically stable without motor deficits and had stable vision, and the patient did not require a second shunt. Postoperative MRI demonstrated excellent debulking of the third ventricular tumor with subsequent

decompression of the previously obstructed CSF pathways (▶ Fig. 21.1i, j).

21.6 Case Example 2

A 5-year-old girl presented with headaches, visual loss, nausea, and vomiting. An MRI demonstrated an enhancing mass in the third ventricle and suprasellar region (▶ Fig. 21.2a, d). Using a left transcortical transventricular route, an initial endoscopic biopsy and endoscopic septal fenestration was performed, with placement of an external ventricular drain to relieve the hydrocephalus. Pathologic examination revealed a pilocytic astrocytoma.

One week later, the third ventricular tumor was debulked through the left transcortical transventricular transforaminal corridor. The posterior component of the tumor had a clear plane of dissection from the third ventricular walls, while the more anterior component was more adherent and blended with the walls of the third ventricle. The cerebral aqueduct was decompressed, and the CSF pathways were adequately opened to avoid a permanent ventriculoperitoneal shunt, which was confirmed on an immediate postoperative MRI (▶ Fig. 21.2b, e).

Postoperatively, the patient underwent adjuvant carboplatin and vincristine chemotherapy. An MRI at 9 months after surgery demonstrated further decrease in size and enhancement of the residual tumor. She remained neurologically intact with stable vision (▶ Fig. 21.2c, f).

21.7 Conclusion

OPGs are predominantly pediatric tumors that can be found anywhere along the optic pathway. Involvement of the optic chiasm and hypothalamus is common, and larger tumors can extend into the third ventricle resulting in obstructive hydrocephalus. Chemotherapy is generally the first line of treatment, although primary surgical debulking can be considered in select cases. Salvage debulking in cases of tumor progression after initial chemotherapy can be considered to relieve mass effect and to open CSF pathways. The role for surgery via EEA remains limited; however, endoscopy is readily used for transventricular biopsy, septum pellucidum fenestration, and guidance for shunt placement. Radiation therapy is delayed as long as possible in children and can be used in cases of tumor progression after failed chemotherapy and surgery. A multidisciplinary team approach tailored to the individual is critical in managing this complex disease.

References

[1] Binning MJ, Liu JK, Kestle JR, Brockmeyer DL, Walker ML. Optic pathway gliomas: a review. Neurosurg Focus. 2007; 23(5):E2

[2] Goodden J, Pizer B, Pettorini B, et al. The role of surgery in optic pathway/hypothalamic gliomas in children. J Neurosurg Pediatr. 2014; 13(1):1–12

[3] Bessero AC, Fraser C, Acheson J, Davagnanam I. Management options for visual pathway compression from optic gliomas. Postgrad Med J. 2013; 89(1047):47–51

[4] Walker DA, Liu J, Kieran M, et al. CPN Paris 2011 Conference Consensus Group. A multi-disciplinary consensus statement concerning surgical approaches to low-grade, high-grade astrocytomas and diffuse intrinsic pontine gliomas in childhood (CPN Paris 2011) using the Delphi method. Neuro-oncol. 2013; 15(4):462–468

[5] Jahraus CD, Tarbell NJ. Optic pathway gliomas. Pediatr Blood Cancer. 2006; 46 (5):586–596

[6] Tow SL, Chandela S, Miller NR, Avellino AM. Long-term outcome in children with gliomas of the anterior visual pathway. Pediatr Neurol. 2003; 28(4):262–270

[7] El Beltagy MA, Reda M, Enayet A, et al. Treatment and Outcome in 65 Children with Optic Pathway Gliomas. World Neurosurg. 2016; 89:525–534

[8] Avery RA, Myseros JS, Packer RJ. Optic/visual pathway gliomas. In: Keating RF, Goodrich JT, Packer RJ, eds. Tumors of the Pediatric Central Nervous System. 2nd ed. New York, NY: Thieme; 2013:188–196

[9] Fried I, Tabori U, Tihan T, Reginald A, Bouffet E. Optic pathway gliomas: a review. CNS Oncol. 2013; 2(2):143–159

[10] Massimino M, Spreafico F, Cefalo G, et al. High response rate to cisplatin/etoposide regimen in childhood low-grade glioma. J Clin Oncol. 2002; 20(20): 4209–4216

[11] Petronio J, Edwards MS, Prados M, et al. Management of chiasmal and hypothalamic gliomas of infancy and childhood with chemotherapy. J Neurosurg. 1991; 74(5):701–708

[12] Lancaster DL, Hoddes JA, Michalski A. Tolerance of nitrosurea-based multi-agent chemotherapy regime for low-grade pediatric gliomas. J Neurooncol. 2003; 63(3):289–294

[13] Fouladi M, Wallace D, Langston JW, et al. Survival and functional outcome of children with hypothalamic/chiasmatic tumors. Cancer. 2003; 97(4):1084–1092

[14] Listernick R, Ferner RE, Liu GT, Gutmann DH. Optic pathway gliomas in neurofibromatosis-1: controversies and recommendations. Ann Neurol. 2007; 61 (3):189–198

[15] Walker D. Recent advances in optic nerve glioma with a focus on the young patient. Curr Opin Neurol. 2003; 16(6):657–664

[16] Jenkin D, Angyalfi S, Becker L, et al. Optic glioma in children: surveillance, resection, or irradiation? Int J Radiat Oncol Biol Phys. 1993; 25(2):215–225

22 Germ Cell Tumors

Domenico Solari, Gianpiero Iannuzzo, Maria Laura Del Basso De Caro, Luigi Maria Cavallo, Michelangelo Gangemi, and Paolo Cappabianca

Abstract

Germ cell tumors (GCTs) of the central nervous system (CNS) are a heterogeneous group of tumors, which primarily occur in childhood, arising predominantly at midline and involving areas such as the pineal and suprasellar regions. The diagnosis of CNS GCTs is based on clinical symptoms and signs, cerebrospinal fluid (CSF) and serum tumor markers, neuroimaging characteristics, and cytologic (CSF) and histologic assessments; however, biopsy of the tumor is required for diagnosis. All GCTs present a certain degree of radiosensitivity, and most of them are chemosensitive. However, the possibility of achieving surgical access to intracerebral GCTs is of utmost importance in order to obtain tissue sampling, eventually perform CSF diversion, and decompress vital neurovascular structures with cytoreduction. Surgical approach to GCTs located in the suprasellar area utilized different transcranial and transfacial routes in the past. Nowadays, endoscopic endonasal techniques can be considered a viable surgical option for the management of GCTs, providing the possibility of achieving either tissue sampling via a minimally invasive biopsy or decompression of neurovascular structures. In this regard, first-line surgery with the aim of a conspicuous mass reduction helps increase the effectiveness and safety of radiochemotherapy, which can be addressed on a more affordable target.

Keywords: germ cell tumors, endoscopic endonasal surgery, radiotherapy, cerebrospinal fluid, suprasellar area, pineal region, brain tumors, sellar region

22.1 Introduction

Germ cell tumors (GCTs) of the central nervous system (CNS) are a heterogeneous group of tumors that primarily occur in childhood, arising predominantly at midline and involving areas such as the pineal and suprasellar regions.

These tumors are morphologic, immunophenotypic, and genetic homologs of gonadal and other extraneuraxial germ cell neoplasms. CNS GCTs are divided into germinomas, the most frequent form, and nongerminomatous GCTs. The current World Health Organization (WHO) classification of CNS GCTs identifies the following major forms, according to histologic elements:

- Germinoma: pure and with syncytiotrophoblasts.
- Nongerminomatous GCTs:
  - Teratoma: mature, immature, and exhibiting malignant transformation.
  - Yolk sac tumor.
  - Embryonal carcinoma.
  - Choriocarcinoma.

Neoplasms harboring multiple histologic types are called mixed GCTs; CNS GCTs are also classified according to the secretion of tumor marker. Blood and CSF levels of α-fetoprotein (αFP) and β-human chorionic gonadotropin (βHCG) could be considered as important factors to be ruled out in the diagnostic workup. αFP elevation is associated with yolk sac tumor, dysgerminoma or seminoma, embryonal carcinoma, and immature teratoma. β-human chorionic gonadotropin (βHCG), normally secreted by placental trophoblastic tissue, is elevated in choriocarcinoma or embryonal carcinoma. Secreting tumors present CSF αFP level greater than 10 ng/mL (or a level higher than the institutional normal) and/or CSF β-HCG level greater than 50 IU/L (or a level higher than the institutional normal).[1] Germinomas are frequently positive for placental alkaline phosphatase (PLAP), optical coherence tomography 4 (OCT-4) and c-kit. Pure germinomas usually do not secrete appreciable tumor markers.

22.2 Epidemiology

CNS GSTs account for 3 to 4% of brain tumors in the first two decades, with a peak of incidence reported around the time of puberty. Nongerminomatous GCTs are more frequently diagnosed earlier in life, while germinomas are usually diagnosed between 10 and 21 years of age; an overall male preponderance is described.[2]

Gender is predictive of tumor localization: the pineal region accounts for the great majority of this tumors in males, while suprasellar lesions occur predominantly in females.[3]

22.3 Etiology

The issue of histogenesis of CNS GCTs is controversial. It is assumed that CNS GCTs arise from nests of primordial germ cells, migrated aberrantly during embryonic development and subsequently undergone malignant transformation. They either differentiate into a germinoma, mismigrational pluripotent embryonic cells, or give rise to other types of GCTs.[4] Current studies show matches in messenger RNA (mRNA) profiles of GCTs and pluripotent embryonic stem cells. This may confirm that GCTs originate from primordial germ cells.[5,6] GCTs that arise from gonadal and extragonadal sites are histologically, clinically, and genetically similar. Chromosomal comparative genomic hybridization analysis suggests that genomic alterations in CNS GCTs are almost indistinguishable from their extracranial counterparts.[7]

CNS GCTs arising after early childhood show characteristically aneuploid profiles and complex chromosomal anomalies. Cytogenetic abnormalities include loss of 1p and 6q, increased copies of the X chromosome, and rarely abnormalities in 12p.[8] Gain of an extra X chromosome is a frequent genotype abnormality. Individuals with Klinefelter's syndrome (XXY) are prone to develop intracranial GCTs, as are those with Down's syndrome and those with neurofibromatosis type 1.[9]

The most common abnormality in adult-onset CNS GCTs is duplication of the short arm of chromosome 12 due to isochromosome (i(12p)) formation.[10] c-kit mutations and increased kit expression have been seen in 23 to 25% of intracranial germinomas, and somatic mutations in AKT/mTOR pathway were found in 19% of patients. C-myc and N-myc amplifications were found in a minority of tumors. Distinct mRNA and micro-RNA profiles revealed with genomic analysis may be correlated with histologic differentiation and clinical outcome and, in the future, serve as novel therapeutic targets.[11,12]Otherwise, pure intracranial teratomas presenting as congenital or infantile growth have a typically diploid status and a general chromosomal integrity, and resemble teratomas of infant testis.

22.4 Clinical Features

The great majority of CNS GCTs arise along a midline axis extending from the pineal gland (the most common site) to the suprasellar region (the second most common site), where tumors originate from the neurohypophyseal infundibular region. Intraventricular, diffuse periventricular, thalamostriate, cerebral hemispheric, cerebellar, bulbar, intramedullary, and intrasellar localizations have been described. Multifocal CNS GCTs usually involve the pineal and suprasellar regions, either simultaneously or sequentially. The significance of these lesions is controversial; actually, it is debated if they are synchronous lesions or metastasis. The bifocal presentation of these tumors may be a poor prognostic sign and should alert clinicians to the possibility of a disseminated disease.[13] The initial clinical presentation in CNS GCTs is dependent upon the patient's age, tumor location, tumor size, and disease duration.

Congenital tumors, often teratomas, detectable by ultrasound as a heterogeneous echogenic mass with cystic and solid components, can produce polyhydramnios and obstructive hydrocephalus. CNS GCTs in young infants can cause irritability, listlessness, failure to thrive, macrocephaly, and bulging fontanelle; teratoma and choriocarcinoma are the most common CNS GCTs in this age group. Beyond infancy, clinical presentation depends on tumor location.

22.4.1 Pineal Region Tumor

Lesions in the pineal region compress and obstruct the cerebral aqueduct, resulting in progressive hydrocephalus and intracranial hypertension. Symptoms include headache, nausea and vomiting, papilledema, somnolence, ataxia, seizures, and behavioral abnormalities. Compression and invasion of the tectum cause Parinaud's syndrome, seen at presentation in up to 50% of pineal GCTs and characterized by paralysis of upward gaze, loss of light perception and accommodation, nystagmus, and failure of convergence. Endocrinopathies and disturbances in sexual development are less common in patients with isolated pineal region tumors.

22.4.2 Suprasellar Region Tumors

GCTs of the suprasellar region usually cause hypothalamic/pituitary axis dysfunction: diabetes insipidus and enuresis and anterior hypopituitarism, with thyroid and/or cortisol deficiency, growth failure, delayed puberty, regression of sexual development, or sexual dysfunction. Tumors secreting β-HCG may cause precocious puberty due to increase in testosterone production (isosexual pseudoprecocity in boys). Optic chiasm impingement can cause visual field defects, bilateral temporal hemianopia overall, diplopia, blurred vision, and vision loss.

22.4.3 Rare Presentation

Psychiatric abnormalities such as psychosis and behavioral changes are atypical presentations in patients with multiple lesions or GCTs in the pineal gland. Midbrain outflow tremor (Holmes' tremor) has been reported in patients with germinoma. It is a hyperkinetic movement disorder that presents as mild to severe tremors, dystonia, and cerebellar deficits.

22.5 Diagnosis

The diagnosis of CNS GCTs is based on clinical symptoms and signs, CSF and serum tumor markers, neuroimaging characteristics, cytologic CSF, and histologic assessments. Both CT and MRI are very sensitive in detecting suprasellar and pineal region masses, but the radiographic characteristics are very similar in all GCTs, limiting their usefulness in determining the exact histology of these tumors. Therefore, biopsy of the tumor is required for diagnosis, unless characteristic serum or CSF tumor marker elevation coexists.

22.6 Management Options

All GCTs present a certain degree of radiosensitivity, and most of them are chemosensitive. However, the possibility of achieving surgical access to intracerebral GCTs is of utmost importance in order to obtain tissue sampling, eventually perform CSF diversion, and decompress vital neurovascular structures with cytoreduction.

It should be said that the definition of the histologic subtype is crucial to define the most appropriate therapeutic strategy, because sensitivity to radiation and/or chemotherapy varies among different histotypes.

In addition, GCTs have a significant risk of spreading throughout the CNS, so the investigation of the entire neuroaxis, eventually by means of MRI, is mandatory for treatment planning and prognostic purposes. Patients with confined disease and negative CSF cytology are considered to be metastatic negative; patients with positive CSF cytology or patients with drop metastases are considered to be metastatic positive. Appropriate staging is crucial because patients with metastatic disease may receive higher total doses of radiation and more extended radiation fields.

Therefore, in patients with marker-positive GCTs, measurement trends of the markers can also be useful to monitor therapeutic response and as a sensitive early sign of tumor recurrence.

22.6.1 Radiotherapy

Patients with malignant GCTs require radiation therapy. The recommended radiation strategy delivers daily doses to the whole ventricular system and an additional boost to the tumor bed.[14] Craniospinal irradiation is controversial, and the current trend is to reserve it to tumors with documented spinal seeding. Pediatric patients are particularly vulnerable to adverse radiation effects. In order to reduce radiation-related toxicity, recent therapeutic strategies combine reduced radiation doses with chemotherapy. Germinomas are highly sensitive to both radiotherapy and chemotherapy and have an excellent prognosis, with an overall survival of 90% at 10 years.[15]

In contrast, nongerminomatous germ cell tumors (NGGCTs) are less responsive to radiation, with 5-year overall survival rates of 30 to 50%.[1]

22.6.2 Chemotherapy

Most of the germ cell chemotherapy regimens have been extrapolated from experience with treating extracranial GCTs, in which success has been remarkable. Currently, a regimen with etoposide and carboplatin or cisplatin is the most widely used. Chemotherapy has been explored for germinomas in an effort to reduce radiation therapy doses and associated neurodevelopmental morbidity. Patients affected by NGGCTs have an inferior outcome compared with patients affected by germinomas; therefore, chemotherapy is typically used with radiation to improve prognosis, resulting in reasonable expectation for long-term survival.[16]

22.6.3 Surgery: The Role of Endoscopic Endonasal Surgery

Surgical approach to GCTs located at the suprasellar area relied mostly on different transcranial and transfacial routes. Nowadays, the evolution of endoscopic endonasal techniques has permitted the extension of the indications to a variety of lesions involving the suprasellar area[17,18,19] in pediatric patients.[20,21]

We have been employing the endoscopic endonasal technique since 1997 on more than 2,000 patients aiming to remove, first, different sellar lesions and, then, lesions involving the surrounding skull base areas. In fact, the endonasal corridor provides a direct, multiangled, and close-up view of the inferior aspects of the suprasellar neurovascular structures without any brain retraction.[17,19,21] Early devascularization of the tumor can be obtained, thus limiting intraoperative blood loss and the risk of postoperative visual loss, which is strictly related to the integrity of the vascularization of the optic chiasm. Further-

more, the endoscopic approach permits a clear visualization of the pituitary gland and stalk, thereby reducing the risks of harming endocrine and hypothalamic functions, which is of utmost importance in the pediatric population.[20,21]

Remarkably, when dealing with GCTs at the suprasellar area, first-line surgery via the endoscopic endonasal approach increases the effectiveness and safety of radiochemotherapy via cytoreduction and a lower target volume.[22,23,24,25,26]

However, in most cases tumors are not treated surgically, so this approach represents a viable and easy technique to achieve tissue sampling with minimal morbidity. In this chapter, we present a case of a pediatric patient affected by a large, intra- and suprasellar mixed GCT which was removed via a transplanum/transtuberculum endoscopic endonasal approach.

22.7 Case Example

A 12-year-old girl was admitted to our hospital with a few months' history of polyuria, polydipsia, and secondary amenorrhea; amaurosis in the left eye and temporal hemianopsia in the right eye were disclosed. MRI results revealed a large intra-suprasellar mass compressing the optic chiasm and extending into the third ventricle (▶ Fig. 22.1).

According to clinical conditions—particularly, a progressive visual impairment and lesion features—surgical treatment via endoscopic endonasal transtuberculum/transplanum was indicated. The procedure is performed with a rigid endoscope (0 degrees) 18 cm in length and 4 mm in diameter (Karl Storz & Co, Tuttlingen, Germany) as the sole visualizing tool during the entire procedure.

After creating an adequate nasosphenoidal surgical corridor, a middle turbinate is displaced laterally on one side, and the contralateral one is removed and tailored bilateral ethmoidectomy and wide sphenoidotomy are completed; bone is then removed off the superior half of the sella and the planum sphenoidale under image guidance.

Dural opening led to the identification of a greenish-yellow mass (▶ Fig. 22.2a, b). According to conventional microsurgical

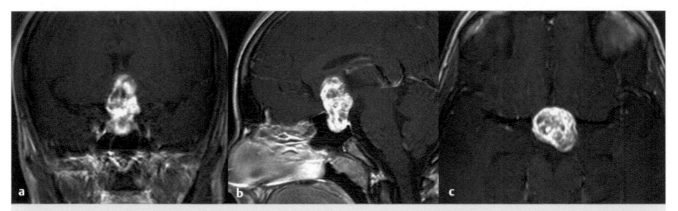

Fig. 22.1 T1-weighted magnetic resonance imaging with contrast. Preoperative coronal (a), sagittal (b), and axial (c) scans show a large intra- and suprasellar mass compressing the optic chiasm and extending into the third ventricle with strong and heterogeneous contrast enhancement. (Adapted from Somma et al.[22])

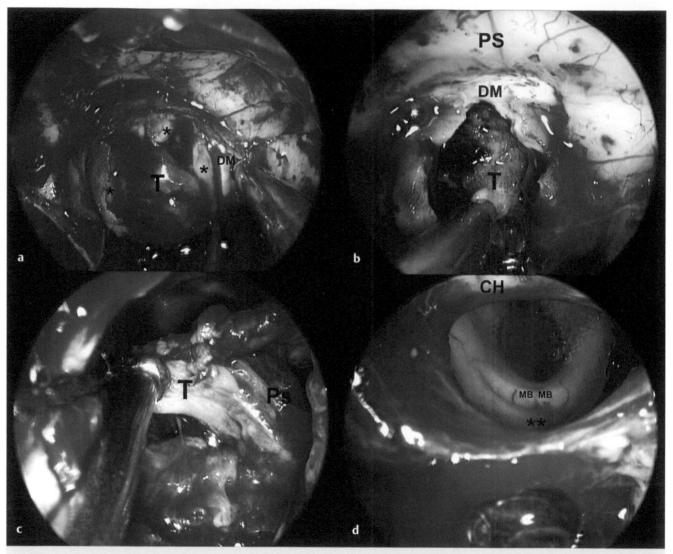

Fig. 22.2 (a) Upon dural opening, the lesion appears splitting the pituitary gland in several parts. **(b)** intracapsular debulking of the tumor with the aid of the Cavitron ultrasonic aspirator (CUSA) in order to remove the intrasellar component. **(c)** identification of the pituitary stalk: a little tumor fragment close to it and the infundibulum is intentionally left in place. **(d)** close-up view of the floor of the third ventricle. T, tumor; *, pituitary gland; PS, planum sphenoidale; DM, dura mater; Ps, pituitary stalk; CH, optic chiasm; MB, mammillary bodies; **, tuber cinereum. (Adapted from Somma et al.[22])

paradigm, intracapsular debulking of the tumor, followed by fine extracapsular dissection under direct endoscopic visualization was performed. Finally, the tumor capsule was peeled off the infundibular recess of the third ventricle and the pituitary stalk; however, a little tumor fragment tightly attached to the infundibulum was intentionally left in place (▶ Fig. 22.2c). It is advisable "not to force" resection in order to achieve "maximum allowed" surgical outcome and above all maintain tissue integrity and function.

After lesion removal, skull base defect reconstruction has been accomplished according to the so-called sandwich technique. Vascularized Hadad-pedicled flap was placed over the posterior wall of the sphenoid sinus with fibrin glue and oxidized cellulose to ease adherence and hold the material in place.[27]

The postoperative course was marked by a conspicuous improvement of temporal hemianopsia in the right eye, and light perception was reported in the left eye. One-month postoperative MRI confirmed near-total tumor removal (▶ Fig. 22.3), and adjuvant chemotherapy and radiation therapy treatment were administered.

22.8 Conclusion

Endoscopic endonasal approach is a viable surgical option for the management of germ cell lesions, providing the possibility of achieving either tissue sampling via a straight, minimally invasive biopsy or decompression of neurovascular structures. Therefore, first-line surgery with the aim of a conspicuous mass reduction increases the effectiveness and safety of radiochemotherapy, which can then be addressed on a more affordable target.

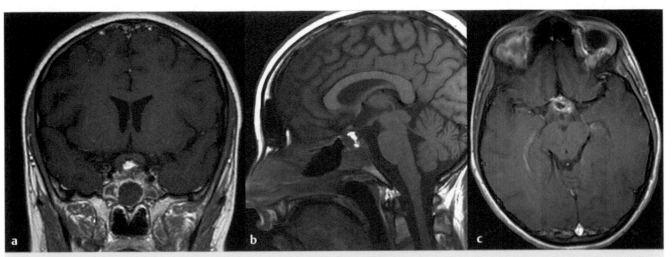

Fig. 22.3 T1-weighted MRI with contrast postoperative. Coronal (**a**), sagittal (**b**), and axial (**c**) scans demonstrate the near-total removal of the lesion. The autologous fat (hyperintensity), used for reconstruction, fills the surgical cavity. (Adapted from Somma et al.[22])

References

[1] Echevarría ME, Fangusaro J, Goldman S. Pediatric central nervous system germ cell tumors: a review. Oncologist. 2008; 13(6):690–699

[2] McCarthy BJ, Shibui S, Kayama T, et al. Primary CNS germ cell tumors in Japan and the United States: an analysis of 4 tumor registries. Neuro-oncol. 2012; 14(9):1194–1200

[3] Goodwin TL, Sainani K, Fisher PG. Incidence patterns of central nervous system germ cell tumors: a SEER Study. J Pediatr Hematol Oncol. 2009; 31(8):541–544

[4] Packer RJ, Cohen BH, Cooney K. Intracranial germ cell tumors. Oncologist. 2000; 5(4):312–320

[5] Wang HW, Wu YH, Hsieh JY, et al. Pediatric primary central nervous system germ cell tumors of different prognosis groups show characteristic miRNome traits and chromosome copy number variations. BMC Genomics. 2010; 11:132

[6] Sperger JM, Chen X, Draper JS, et al. Gene expression patterns in human embryonic stem cells and human pluripotent germ cell tumors. Proc Natl Acad Sci U S A. 2003; 100(23):13350–13355

[7] Schneider DT, Zahn S, Sievers S, et al. Molecular genetic analysis of central nervous system germ cell tumors with comparative genomic hybridization. Mod Pathol. 2006; 19(6):864–873

[8] Palmer RD, Foster NA, Vowler SL, et al. Malignant germ cell tumours of childhood: new associations of genomic imbalance. Br J Cancer. 2007; 96(4):667–676

[9] Sato K, Takeuchi H, Kubota T. Pathology of intracranial germ cell tumors. Prog Neurol Surg. 2009; 23:59–75

[10] Looijenga LH, Zafarana G, Grygalewicz B, et al. Role of gain of 12p in germ cell tumour development. APMIS. 2003; 111(1):161–171, discussion 172–173

[11] Kamakura Y, Hasegawa M, Minamoto T, Yamashita J, Fujisawa H. C-kit gene mutation: common and widely distributed in intracranial germinomas. J Neurosurg. 2006; 104(3) Suppl:173–180

[12] Wang L, Yamaguchi S, Burstein MD, et al. Novel somatic and germline mutations in intracranial germ cell tumours. Nature. 2014; 511(7508):241–245

[13] Phi JH, Kim SK, Lee J, et al. The enigma of bifocal germ cell tumors in the suprasellar and pineal regions: synchronous lesions or metastasis? J Neurosurg Pediatr. 2013; 11(2):107–114

[14] Kyritsis AP. Management of primary intracranial germ cell tumors. J Neurooncol. 2010; 96(2):143–149

[15] Bamberg M, Kortmann RD, Calaminus G, et al. Radiation therapy for intracranial germinoma: results of the German cooperative prospective trials MAKEI 83/86/89. J Clin Oncol. 1999; 17(8):2585–2592

[16] Calaminus G, Bamberg M, Jürgens H, et al. Impact of surgery, chemotherapy and irradiation on long term outcome of intracranial malignant non-germinomatous germ cell tumors: results of the German Cooperative Trial MAKEI 89. Klin Padiatr. 2004; 216(3):141–149

[17] Cappabianca P, Cavallo LM, Esposito F, de Divitiis O, Messina A, de Divitiis E. Extended endoscopic endonasal approach to the midline skull base: the evolving role of transsphenoidal surgery. In: Pickard JD, Akalan N, Rocco C, et al., eds. Advances and Technical Standards in Neurosurgery. New York, NY: Springer; 2008:152–199

[18] de Divitiis E, Cavallo LM, Cappabianca P, Esposito F. Extended endoscopic endonasal transsphenoidal approach for the removal of suprasellar tumors: part 2. Neurosurgery. 2007; 60(1):46–58, discussion–58–59

[19] Kassam A, Snyderman CH, Mintz A, Gardner P, Carrau RL. Expanded endonasal approach: the rostrocaudal axis. Part I. Crista galli to the sella turcica. Neurosurg Focus. 2005; 19(1):E3

[20] de Divitiis E, Cappabianca P, Gangemi M, Cavallo LM. The role of the endoscopic transsphenoidal approach in pediatric neurosurgery. Childs Nerv Syst. 2000; 16(10–11):692–696

[21] Kassam A, Thomas AJ, Snyderman C, et al. Fully endoscopic expanded endonasal approach treating skull base lesions in pediatric patients. J Neurosurg. 2007; 106(2) Suppl:75–86

[22] Somma AD, Bronzoni C, Guadagno E, et al. The "extended" endoscopic endonasal approach for the removal of a mixed intrasuprasellar germinoma: Technical case report. Surg Neurol Int. 2014; 5:14

[23] Hardenbergh PH, Golden J, Billet A, et al. Intracranial germinoma: the case for lower dose radiation therapy. Int J Radiat Oncol Biol Phys. 1997; 39(2):419–426

[24] Matsutani M, Sano K, Takakura K, et al. Primary intracranial germ cell tumors: a clinical analysis of 153 histologically verified cases. J Neurosurg. 1997; 86(3):446–455

[25] Oka H, Kawano N, Tanaka T, et al. Long-term functional outcome of suprasellar germinomas: usefulness and limitations of radiotherapy. J Neurooncol. 1998; 40(2):185–190

[26] Saeki N, Murai H, Kubota M, Fujimoto N, Yamaura A. Long-term Karnofsky performance status and neurological outcome in patients with neurohypophyseal germinomas. Br J Neurosurg. 2001; 15(5):402–408

[27] Hadad G, Bassagasteguy L, Carrau RL, et al. A novel reconstructive technique after endoscopic expanded endonasal approaches: vascular pedicle nasoseptal flap. Laryngoscope. 2006; 116(10):1882–1886

23 Chordoma

Moujahed Labidi, Shunya Hanakita, Kentaro Watanabe, Vincent Couloigner, Bernard George, and Sébastien Froelich

Abstract

Chordomas are rare benign lesions arising from notochordal remnants in the skull base region and the spine. The majority of pediatric chordomas are located in the spheno-occipital region. Within the pediatric population, the location of chordomas is dependent on age. Cranial chordomas are almost exclusively seen in very young patients, while the sacrococcygeal forms are seen in older adolescents. This chapter explores chordomas, their malignant clinical behavior and surgical removal as the foundation of treatment.

Keywords: chordoma, tuberous sclerosis, reconstruction, intradural dissection, nasoseptal flap, pediatric, bony osteolysis

23.1 Epidemiology

Chordomas are benign lesions arising from notochordal remnants in the skull base region and the spine. Their prevalence is low, especially in pediatric patients, as they represent less than 1% of intracranial tumors in this population (with an estimated annual incidence of < 1 in 1,000,000 children aged ≤ 10 years).[1,2,3] In a large surveillance, epidemiology, and end result (SEER) database study, only 6.3% of all chordomas affected patients younger than 20 years.[4] In chordomas affecting the skull base, the mean age of presentation is 8.8 years.[1] The majority of pediatric chordomas are located in the spheno-occipital region (~50–60% of children with chordomas), while they are more evenly distributed in adult patients between the sacrococcygeal, mobile spine, and skull base regions.[4,5] Even in the subgroup of pediatric patients, the location of chordomas seems to be age dependent, with the very young patients presenting almost exclusively with cranial chordomas, while the sacrococcygeal forms are only seen in older adolescents.[2]

23.2 Familial Forms

The majority of chordoma cases are sporadic, but, in some rare cases, their occurrence has been linked to tuberous sclerosis complex or familial forms of chordoma.[2] These rare associations, which are overrepresented in the pediatric age group, might provide clues as to the pathophysiology and molecular biology of these tumors.

23.3 Clinical Presentation and Natural History

Cranial chordomas usually present as well-delineated multilobulated lesions of the midline cranial base. They are typically T2-hyperintense, and contrast enhancement is heterogeneous.

Notwithstanding their "benign" histology, these lesions tend to grow on follow-up, with resulting osteolysis of the cancellous bone in which they are embedded. Eventually, they break through the cortical bone and invade the surrounding structures and the intradural compartment. Clinically, children with cranial chordomas most frequently present with a cranial nerve palsy (60% of children), usually a sixth nerve palsy, while headaches (40%) and other symptoms of intracranial hypertension (28%) are also common complaints at presentation.[1,6] Pediatric chordomas more often present with distant metastasis than adults, especially for those younger than 5 years, although distant metastases were also more associated with sacrococcygeal locations.[3,4] Prolonged survival can be achieved in the majority of the patients, with an overall survival (OS) of 63% at 15 years in a combined series of patients from Hôpital Lariboisière and Hôpital Necker – Enfants Malades.[1] However, patients younger than 5 years seem to have a worse prognosis.[6]

23.4 Management Options: Medical, Surgical, and Adjuvant

The mainstay of treatment of pediatric cranial chordomas is surgical resection. Gross total resection (GTR) with preservation of neurological function must be the goal of surgeons undertaking resection of these lesions. In a recent meta-analysis of adult chordoma cases, we found a clinically and statistically significant difference in tumor control between GTR and subtotal or partial resections.[7] In a cohort of 610 patients with skull base and clivus chordomas, recurrences were less frequent in complete resections than incomplete resections (24.3 vs. 55.0%, $p < 0.0001$) with an odds ratio of 0.289 (95% confidence interval [CI]: 0.184 –0.453) of having a recurrence for patients who had a GTR compared with incomplete resections. In the largest pediatric chordoma series, George et al and Ridenour et al also reported a survival advantage when GTR was achieved, although this association between increased survival and GTR did not reach statistical significance.[1,5]

Another important prognostic factor to take into consideration is the quality of the resection at first attempt. In fact, in most surgical series, GTR appears harder to achieve in residual and recurrent diseases than during the first surgical attempt. In chordomas, more than in any other skull base lesions, we very frequently combine different surgical approaches and stages to obtain the desired resection and resulting progression-free survival (PFS) and OS advantages. In our systematic review and meta-analysis of the literature, we found a statistically significant relationship between the rate of multiple surgeries undertaken for chordoma resection and the GTR rate achieved ($p < 0.0001$). This correlation confirms that in many cases, a GTR or maximally safe resection cannot be achieved through only one corridor.

There is a lack of data specific to the pediatric population regarding the role of radiation therapy in skull base chordomas. However, most authors agree that high-dose irradiation is indicated in all cases where a partial resection was undertaken. After GTR, the role of adjuvant radiation therapy is controversial.[3,8] Chordomas are relatively radio-resistant tumors, and high doses of radiation are required to achieve adequate local control rates (in the 65–75 Gy range). In this context, charged particle radiation therapy (e.g., protons or carbon ions) appear ideally suited, with their steep dose falloff beyond the target that allows high doses to be delivered to the tumor and minimization of toxicity to the surrounding critical structures.[9] Even with these highly specialized techniques, late complications of radiation therapy are not uncommon, including partial or complete pituitary insufficiency, visual toxicity, and hearing loss.

Even if significant investigative efforts are engaged in developing new drug therapy for chordomas, none have so far been able to demonstrate a clear benefit in OS and PFS. Novel molecular markers associated with chordoma cells have been identified, and a number of targeted-therapy protocols are currently in trial.[10]

23.5 The Role of Endoscopic Endonasal Surgery

23.5.1 Rationale and Surgical Corridor Selection

To achieve an optimal resection in chordoma surgery, it is fundamental to choose the most appropriate surgical corridor for each lesion treated. Although chordomas preferentially affect the midline skull base region, they also have the a tendency to extend locally and invade different compartments and anatomical structures around the skull base. An experienced multidisciplinary skull base team should carry out a careful examination of the preoperative CT scan and MRI to precisely delineate and record all extensions of the lesion to be resected. Compartments of the chordoma that are out of reach for radiation therapy, such as those in close proximity to the brainstem, optic apparatus, or metallic reconstruction material, should be considered important surgical targets. Larger compartments of the tumor or those causing severe compression of neurological structures or which are responsible for neurological deficits should also be resected. As mentioned previously, staged surgeries and combined approaches are often required to achieve maximal safe resection.

The role of the endoscopic endonasal approach (EEA) in chordoma surgery has increased significantly in the last decade, and the rationale for this approach is solid in many of these lesions. In addition to the fact that they frequently originate from midline bony structures and that cranial nerves need not to crossed to access the tumor through an EEA, these lesions are often soft and easily aspirated, with no brain retraction required. A few studies have compared surgical results between EEA and "classic" posterolateral approaches in adult patients, although selection bias greatly limits interpretation of such data.[7,11] Unfortunately, there are no equivalent data in the pediatric population. However, in a systematic review of the adult literature, we observed significant differences in the rate of GTR obtained in series reporting on chordomas operated exclusively though the endoscopic midline corridor from that obtained in series also including resections through posterolateral approaches (60.7 vs. 42.0%, respectively, $p = 0.02$). There were also notable differences in postoperative complications between these two groups. As expected, there was a higher number of postoperative cerebrospinal fluid (CSF) leaks in series including endoscopic midlines cases only (22.1 vs. 9.5%, $p = 0.06$). The opposite was observed with CNS infection (1.9 vs. 6.1%, $p = 0.09$); however, these differences did not reach statistical significance. There was a trend toward a higher number of de novo postoperative cranial nerve deficits in the series including posterolateral techniques in the surgical armamentarium (16.1 vs. 7.7% in pure endoscopic midlines series, $p = 0.10$).[7] Nevertheless, it is our opinion that these different techniques should not be viewed as competing but as complementary.

The availability of vascularized mucosa and soft tissues for reconstruction needs to be part of the preoperative planning. In fact, these lesions tend to recur, and many patients require multiple surgeries, and a well-vascularized nasoseptal flap (NSF), generally used as first-line reconstruction material, may have already been used or compromised. In children younger than 10 years, septal development may be incomplete, and the surface the septal mucosa can eventually cover may be limited.[12] Still, its length and surface may be sufficient to cover correspondingly smaller defects in children.[13] It is therefore important to pay particular attention to this element when considering the preoperative CT scan and to consider an alternate graft, if necessary. In some cases, when we deem the CSF leak risk too high or expect difficult dissection planes from the brainstem or neurovascular structures, we prefer leaving the intradural component of the chordoma for a second surgical stage through a posterolateral corridor. The use of endoscopic assistance has also proven to be an invaluable tool to increase the reach of these approaches (far lateral, lateral cervical, etc.).

When considering an EEA in a child, three particularly important anatomical limitations must be considered before surgery: the anterior nasal aperture (piriform aperture), the degree of sphenoid sinus pneumatization, and the localization of the internal carotid artery (ICA) within the sphenoid sinus. The piriform aperture is rarely an obstacle in children ≥ 3 years. As for the sphenoid sinus, pneumatization begins at 2 years, and a sellar-type pneumatization is usually reached between the ages of 6 and 13 years. With adequate preoperative imaging and intraoperative image guidance, the remainder of non-pneumatized sinus can usually be safely drilled away. Although there is only slight variation of the intercarotid distance, especially at the superior clivus, the degree of pneumatization of the carotid prominences should be carefully assessed, as it varies greatly depending on patient age.[14]

23.5.2 Operative Setup

In all EEA cases, we use surgical navigation with both MRI (T2-weighted or CISS/FIESTA and T1-weighted with gadolinium) and CT imaging fusion. The microvascular ultrasound Doppler probe is used systematically to localize the internal carotid and sphenopalatine arteries. Another technological adjunct that has proven useful in EEA is electromyographic monitoring of cranial nerves. In chordoma cases, we usually monitor both 6th nerves and the 5th nerve on the side of a transpterygoid approach, as well as the 12th nerve and lower cranial nerves (10th and 11th), depending on the tumor extensions and planned surgical exposure.

The head is positioned in a fixed head holder in children ≥ 2 years. The head is flexed, rotated, and tilted toward the side of the surgical team. To improve venous outflow, we usually elevate the head and thorax, in addition to a slight reverse Trendelenburg positioning of the surgical table. The abdomen and/or anterolateral thigh are prepared for harvesting a fat and/or fascia lata graft to repair the bony and dural defects.

23.5.3 Surgical Technique

When fine intradural dissection is required, a two-surgeon, four-hand technique is employed. A binostril access and wide septectomy and sphenoidotomy are required to gain adequate maneuverability for both surgeons. However, we now strive to minimize resection of endonasal mucosa and structures (turbinates and septum) to reduce the short- and long-term morbidity associated with their resection. We have therefore used a uninarial access in many, if not the majority, of our most recent endonasal clival chordoma cases.

Exposure

The first step is to identify key landmarks, including the choanal arches, the middle and inferior turbinates, and sphenoid ostia. A middle turbinectomy is usually required on one side. This is followed by a posterior ethmoidectomy that gives increased space for the endoscope and suction. In very young children, care should be taken at this stage, as the roof of the ethmoid can be ossified only partially. The bulla ethmoidalis is followed posteriorly and the basal lamella of the middle turbinate is opened to gain access to the posterior ethmoid. The lamina papyracea serves as the lateral limit of the posterior ethmoidectomy and demarcates the orbit. The sphenoid ostium is a valuable landmark to locate and preserve the posterior septal artery (PSA) when resecting the basal lamella, as the PSA travels below the level of the ostium. A wide sphenoidotomy is then made to expose widely the upper and middle thirds of the clivus. If there is significant lateral extension of the chordoma, a maxillary antrostomy, transpterygoid approach, and dissection of the Vidian nerve can help gain the lateral visualization required to expose the tumor and, more importantly, better define its relationship with the ICA. The maxillary sinus may be very small in younger patients, with the top of the inferior turbinate being often at the level of the floor of the orbit with a risk of orbital penetration when opening the maxillary sinus. An inferior turbinectomy may be required for a proper opening of the maxillary sinus.

Certain simple maneuvers, such as outfracturing the inferior turbinates and putting retraction on a stitch placed in the soft palate, increase exposure of the lower third of the clivus and upper cervical region. When approaching the lower third of the clivus, an important bony landmark is the supracondylar groove, which marks the height of the hypoglossal canal. Drilling the anteromedial aspect of the condyle and thus skeletonizing the hypoglossal canal leads to inferior delineation of the jugular tubercle, which separates the hypoglossal canal from the jugular foramen. Lateral limits to bone drilling and intradural exposure are the inferior petrosal sinus that courses along the intracranial aspect of the petroclival fissure, and the vertebral artery when the drilling involves C1 and C2. Opinions differ between authors as to the maximal amount of occipital condyle that can be resected before craniocervical instability is encountered. In a cadaveric study, Perez-Orribo et al have suggested that a threshold of 75% anterior condylectomy may be associated with clinical significant hypermobility.[15]

Chordoma Resection

In most cases, chordomas are soft, easily aspirated lobulated tumors. The use of an ultrasonic aspirator is often not neces-

sary, although a rotating angled aspirator tip may be useful under angled endoscopic visualization to reach otherwise blind spots. There is no "true" tumor capsule in most chordomas, and piecemeal resection often allows safer tumor removal without compromising GTR. The pseudocapsule that is sometimes identified is a conjunctive inflammatory reaction around the tumor that can be aspirated along with the tumor. In the rare occurrences that the chordoma is found to be fibrous, we have found that GTR is hard to achieve safely, since these lesions are also more adherent to the ICA and cranial nerves. Very often, chordomas present multiple separated lobules disseminated in and adherent to pharyngeal muscles (longus capitis and rectus capitis anterior muscles). If it allows for an increased extent of resection, these muscles can be partially resected safely.

During tumor resection, every precaution should be taken to limit tumor seeding in the surgical corridor and CSF. As a rule, intratumoral debulking must be maximized before intradural exploration. We also try to limit irrigation when dealing with the intradural compartments of the lesion. As for surgical corridor dissemination, it can probably be minimized by careful inspection and abundant irrigation at the end of the case. Likewise, in order to reduce the occurrence of avoidable tumor seeding, biopsy of clivus lesions, when imaging features are highly evocative of chordoma, should be avoided in most cases.

Since chordomas arise from notochordal remnants in the cancellous bone of the clivus, it is important to resect as much of the involved bone as possible. It is reasonable to assume that delayed recurrences after GTR are due to chordoma cells left in the cancellous bone surrounding the macroscopic tumor resected during the initial surgery.

Reconstruction

Harvesting the NSF is done in a standard fashion, with care taken to preserve the olfactory mucosa.[12] We perform the septal mucosa cuts in order for the flap to be tailored to the expected dural defect and structures to be covered. In larger dural defects, including the nasal floor mucosa can extend the NSF or a contralateral NSF flap can be raised concomitantly. We usually use a combination of fascia lata, Tachosil©, and fibrin glue as a first reconstructive layer. In the clival area, a fat graft is placed in the vast majority of cases to fill the void left by the clival drilling. In pediatric cases, postoperative synechia are frequent in the endonasal cavity. We use a Silastic sheet that is positioned between the septum and turbinates and stitched to the nasal septum to prevent their occurrence.

23.6 Case Example

A 15-year-old male patient presented with palsy of the right oculomotor and abducens nerves. On CT and MRI (▶ Fig. 23.1), a lesion centered on the right posterior clinoid was found. This lesion, highly evocative of clival chordoma, was hyperintense on T2 and presented a heterogeneous aspect on CT, with areas of osteolysis and calcifications. With the right cavernous carotid pushed laterally by the tumor, the endoscopic endonasal route was deemed to be the most effective surgical strategy (▶ Fig. 23.2). A contralateral uninarial approach was used to improve the working angle. Following the completion of a wide

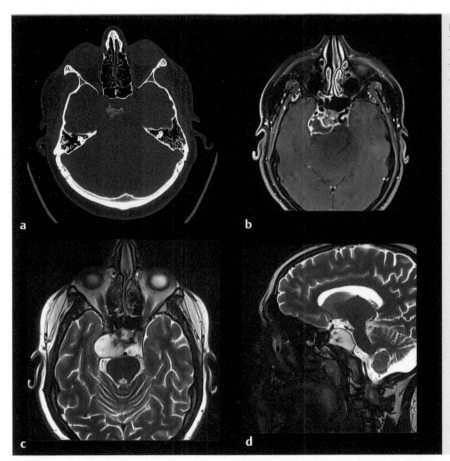

Fig. 23.1 Preoperative **(a)** axial CT scan, **(b)** axial T1 with gadolinium, **(c)** axial T2, and **(d)** sagittal T2 images of a chordoma of the upper third of the clivus. The lesion is centered on the posterior clinoid and extends into the right petrous apex.

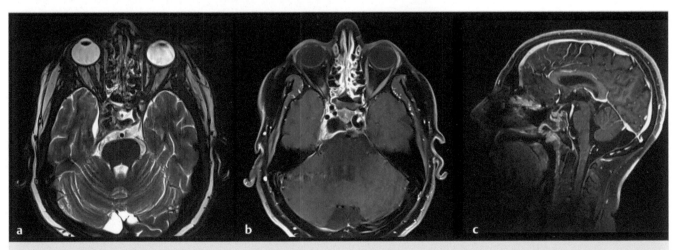

Fig. 23.2 Postoperative MRI **(a)** axial T2, **(b)** axial T1 with gadolinium, and **(c)** sagittal T1 with gadolinium images of an endoscopic endonasal resection of a chordoma of the upper third of the clivus and right petrous apex. Gross total resection was achieved through a contralateral left uninarial approach with preservation of all turbinates and the nasal mucosa on the left side.

sphenoidotomy and exposure of the parasellar (cavernous) ICA, the medial wall of the cavernous sinus, and the dura of the posterior fossa in the clival recess, a posterior clinoidectomy was completed. Tumor resection was facilitated by the use of a malleable suction tip and angled endoscopes. A free fat graft and an NSF were used for reconstruction. Even if the resection was purely extradural with no intraoperative CSF leakage, a vascularized mucosal graft was used to provide coverage for the exposed ICA. MRI done in the immediate postoperative period demonstrated GTR (▶ Fig. 23.3).

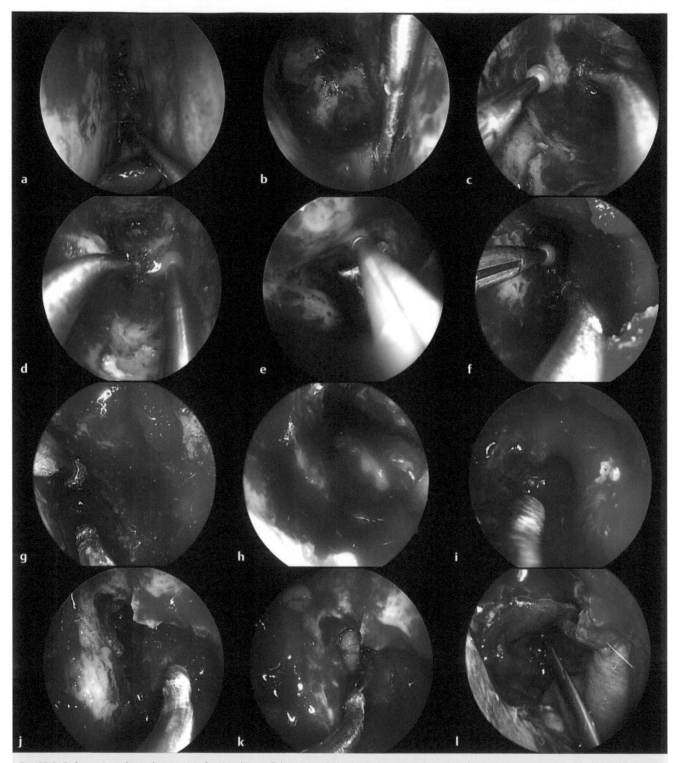

Fig. 23.3 Endoscopic endonasal resection of a chordoma of the upper clivus. A 15-year-old male with a clival chordoma (see Fig. 23.1) that presented with third and sixth nerve palsies. Step-by-step description of the endoscopic endonasal exposure and resection of the tumor through a uninarial corridor. **(a)** After identification of the endonasal anatomy, the middle turbinate is outfractured and kept and a nasoseptal flap (NSF) is harvested. **(b)** A wide sphenoidotomy is undertaken with the drill and rongeurs. **(c)** The right parasellar internal carotid artery (ICA) is unroofed. **(d)** Drilling of the clival recess; control of the bleeding arising from the clival plexus is obtained with injectable hemostatic agents. **(e)** Exposure of the dura mater on the right side of the sella turcica. **(f)** The medial wall of the cavernous sinus is exposed, completing the removal of the three pillars of the posterior clinoid process. **(g)** The posterior clinoid is first hollowed out and then **(h)** dissected from its ligamentous attachment and removed. **(i)** Tumor resection is done with a malleable suction tip and angled endoscopes. **(j)** The resection bed after tumor removal. **(k)** A fat graft if placed to fill the petrous apex and upper right clival space. **(l)** The NSF that was initially harvested is placed over the fat graft and, most importantly, the exposed right ICA and supplemented with fibrin glue.

23.7 Operative Pearls and Pitfalls

- Careful preoperative planning and detailed study of the MRI and CT scans allow for safer and more radical tumor resections.
- In the pediatric population, particular attention should be paid to the level of maturation of the septum (for the NSF), the degree of sphenoid sinus pneumatization and anatomy, and the course of ICAs.
- In many clival chordomas, a uninarial access is sufficient to gain exposure on and resect the tumor, thus minimizing the surgical trauma to the turbinates and nasal mucosa.

23.8 Conclusion

Pediatric skull base chordomas are rare bony tumors that present with malignant clinical behavior. The surgical removal of these lesions is the cornerstone of treatment, and safe maximal resection should be sought. The EEA is an essential element of the surgical armamentarium when dealing with these tumors. It is often used as a complementary technique to other approaches.

References

[1] George B, Bresson D, Bouazza S, et al. Les chordomes. Neurochirurgie. 2014; 60(3):63–140
[2] McMaster ML, Goldstein AM, Parry DM. Clinical features distinguish childhood chordoma associated with tuberous sclerosis complex (TSC) from chordoma in the general paediatric population. J Med Genet. 2011; 48(7):444–449
[3] Beccaria K, Sainte-Rose C, Zerah M, Puget S. Paediatric chordomas. Orphanet J Rare Dis. 2015; 10:116
[4] Lau CSM, Mahendraraj K, Ward A, Chamberlain RS. Pediatric chordomas: a population-based clinical outcome study involving 86 patients from the Surveillance, Epidemiology, and End Result (SEER) Database (1973–2011). Pediatr Neurosurg. 2016; 51(3):127–136
[5] Ridenour RV, III, Ahrens WA, Folpe AL, Miller DV. Clinical and histopathologic features of chordomas in children and young adults. Pediatr Dev Pathol. 2010; 13(1):9–17
[6] Borba LA, Al-Mefty O, Mrak RE, Suen J. Cranial chordomas in children and adolescents. J Neurosurg. 1996; 84(4):584–591
[7] Labidi M, Watanabe K, Bouazza S, et al. Clivus chordomas: a systematic review and meta-analysis of contemporary surgical management. J Neurosurg Sci. 2016; 60(4):476–484
[8] Chivukula S, Koutourousiou M, Snyderman CH, Fernandez-Miranda JC, Gardner PA, Tyler-Kabara EC. Endoscopic endonasal skull base surgery in the pediatric population. J Neurosurg Pediatr. 2013; 11(3):227–241
[9] Habrand J-L, Schneider R, Alapetite C, et al. Proton therapy in pediatric skull base and cervical canal low-grade bone malignancies. Int J Radiat Oncol Biol Phys. 2008; 71(3):672–675
[10] Stacchiotti S, Sommer J, Chordoma Global Consensus Group. Building a global consensus approach to chordoma: a position paper from the medical and patient community. Lancet Oncol. 2015; 16(2):e71–e83
[11] Komotar RJ, Starke RM, Raper DMS, Anand VK, Schwartz TH. The endoscope-assisted ventral approach compared with open microscope-assisted surgery for clival chordomas. World Neurosurg. 2011; 76(3–4):318–327, discussion 259–262
[12] Shah RN, Surowitz JB, Patel MR, et al. Endoscopic pedicled nasoseptal flap reconstruction for pediatric skull base defects. Laryngoscope. 2009; 119(6): 1067–1075
[13] Purcell PL, Shinn JR, Otto RK, Davis GE, Parikh SR. Nasoseptal flap reconstruction of pediatric sellar defects: a radiographic feasibility study and case series. Otolaryngol Head Neck Surg. 2015; 152(4):746–751
[14] Tatreau JR, Patel MR, Shah RN, et al. Anatomical considerations for endoscopic endonasal skull base surgery in pediatric patients. Laryngoscope. 2010; 120 (9):1730–1737
[15] Perez-Orribo L, Little AS, Lefevre RD, et al. Biomechanical evaluation of the craniovertebral junction after anterior unilateral condylectomy: implications for endoscopic endonasal approaches to the cranial base. Neurosurgery. 2013; 72(6):1021–1029, discussion 1029–1030

24 Chondrosarcomas

Daniel M. Prevedello, Ricardo L. Carrau, Camila S. Dassi, and Ana B. Melgarejo

Abstract

Pediatric chondrosarcomas of the skull base are extremely rare malignant tumors. They are indolent but have a propensity for recurrence if inadequately treated. The best treatment plan is still a subject of discussion. Total or near-total surgical resection followed by radiotherapy seems to be the option with the best outcomes. The approach is usually selected based on the involvement of cranial nerves, the location of the tumor, and the surgeon's experience. The endoscopic endonasal approach using the ventral transnasal corridor is an effective approach for their surgical management since it provides a direct exposure of the petroclival synchondrosis.

Keywords: chondrosarcoma, pediatric, skull base surgery, endoscopy, endonasal

24.1 Introduction

Sinonasal and skull base lesions in childhood have distinct clinical presentations and outcomes depending on the child's age, tumor's location, and lesion's pathology.[1]

Chondrosarcomas are infrequent lesions with predilection for long bones and pelvis, with only 10% occurring in the head and neck.[2] They represent 6% of skull base lesions and 0.15% of all intracranial tumors.[3]

Pediatric chondrosarcomas of the skull base are extremely rare malignant tumors with a challenging treatment because of their location. They are indolent but have a propensity for recurrence if inadequately treated.[3]

Chondrosarcomas arise from cells of chondroid origin and can be composed of myxoid cartilage, hyaline cartilage, or a combination of both of these matrices.[4] They commonly originate from the petroclival synchondroses. Unlike chordomas, which tend to be midline, chondrosarcomas usually arise in a paramedian location.[5] In the skull base, more than half of chondrosarcomas arise in the middle fossa, 14% involve both middle and posterior fossae, 14% occur in the anterior fossa, and 7% originate in the posterior fossa.[5]

The histological classification of chondrosarcomas is divided into four groups: conventional (majority), mesenchymal (< 10%), clear cell, and dedifferentiated. The major histological differential diagnosis is chondroid chordoma, which has the presence of notochordal elements.[6] The prognosis is determined primarily by its World Health Organization (WHO) histological grade. By the analyses of histological features, such as cellularity, nuclear size, mitotic rate, and frequency of lacunae with multiple nuclei, this grading system includes three categories: grade I (well differentiated), grade II (moderately differentiated), and grade III (poorly differentiated).[3]

Imaging studies, such as computed axial tomography scan (CT) and MRI, are important for diagnosis and planning the surgical approach. Bony destruction of the skull base lateral to the midline is usually found on CT. MRI is useful to evaluate tumor involvement of neural and vascular structures. Chondrosarcomas have low-to-intermediate signal intensity on T1-weighted images and high signal intensity on T2-weighted images. Heterogenous enhancement is usually seen following administration of contrast material.[5]

Symptoms most commonly arise from cranial nerve or brainstem compression: diplopia, hoarseness, dysphasia, facial dysesthesia, hearing loss, headache, and gait disturbances.[5] An important factor in approach selection for these tumors is the presence of particular cranial nerve deficits at presentation.[4]

24.2 Management Options

The differentiation between chordomas and chondrosarcomas of the skull base is necessary to define final treatment. Both lesions have very similar appearances and radiological characteristics, making imaging alone not reliable to differentiate them.[7]

The prognosis of chondrosarcomas is grounded on three pillars. The first is extent of tumor resection. The second pillar is the tumor histological grade. Grade III tumors have worse prognosis than grade I and II tumors. Adjuvant radiotherapy treatment is the third pillar, and it seems to improve survival rates. The best treatment plan is still controversial. Most treatment regimens with the best outcomes involve total or near-total surgical resection followed by radiotherapy.[7]

24.2.1 Surgical Resection

Surgical resection of the tumor is necessary to obtain a definitive tissue diagnosis. Maximal safe surgical resection is the primary consensus for initial treatment of chondrosarcoma. The main goals of surgical treatment are decompression of neurovascular structures and removal of the tumor near important neural structures like the brainstem in order to allow safe high-dose radiotherapy.[6]

The approach is usually selected based on the involvement of cranial nerves and tumor location. Chondrosarcomas often destroy the pericranial layer of the dura, and they often only displace the meningeal layer of dura instead of transgressing it. Consequently, cranial chondrosarcomas are generally located completely extradurally, with origin on the petroclival synchondrosis, and with potential extension to the middle fossa, posterior fossa, and superior cervical space around the jugular foramen. Because of these characteristics, the ventral transnasal corridor is the most direct and effective extradural approach for their surgical management.[8]

Extensive skull base chondrosarcomas may have higher morbidity related to radical surgery, which leads some surgeons to advocate for a less radical resection as the surgical goal. A safe cytoreduction followed by radiotherapy to residual tumor would result in lower morbidity, and therefore better quality of life. Radical excision or cytoreduction with adjuvant radiotherapy seems to offer similar 5-year tumor recurrence rates of 70 to 80% and overall survival rates of 80 to 90%.[4] We believe, however, that radical resection should always be the primary goal of the surgical strategy, and the decision to leave residual should be an exception based on intraoperative detection of potential morbidity related to its resection.

24.2.2 Radiotherapy

Radiotherapy as an adjuvant treatment for chondrosarcomas has been increasingly accepted to improve both tumor-free survival and overall survival.[2] The proximity to important structures such as the brainstem, cranial nerves, optic pathway, and temporal lobes, along with the fact that skull base tumors require high-radiation doses, are important considerations in choosing the adjuvant therapy.[9] Conventional fractionated photon radiotherapy, stereotactic radiosurgery, and proton therapy are the most used methods to administrate radiation to the skull base.[7] The true concern over radiation on infant patients with chondrosarcoma is the fact they would live to experience the side effects from radiotherapy.

Proton therapy has physical properties that spare normal tissues and reduce the integral dose, making it increasingly recognized as the preferred treatment for childhood cancer.[9] Numerous short follow-up clinical studies involving small numbers of patients have suggested a satisfactory clinical outcome using protons on children with chondrosarcoma. Proton therapy has been correlated with less complications compared to other radiotherapy modalities.[4]

24.2.3 Chemotherapy

Chemotherapy has not been an effective option for the treatment of chondrosarcomas. It can be used with a very limited proven efficacy in patients with advanced chondrosarcoma, such as mesenchymal grade III tumors.[10]

24.3 The Role of Endoscopic Endonasal Surgery

The main challenges of endoscopic endonasal surgery in the pediatric population are small working spaces and the possibility of lack of pneumatization. Neuronavigation is very helpful to allow for safer access in the absence of key landmarks.[1] The team should have experience with skull base pathologies and pediatric care.

Endoscopic endonasal approaches (EEA) provide the most direct access to the ventral skull base. Chondrosarcomas usually originate in the petroclival region and tend to displace neurovascular elements laterally, superiorly, and posteriorly. For that reason, we advocate the use of EEA as the initial surgical corridor.[6] In a single procedure, EEA allows access to multiple skull base compartments, avoiding extensive retraction of neurovascular structures. It also allows extensive drilling of the clivus, sphenoid bone, and petrous portions of the temporal bone, which are frequently invaded by tumors.[8]

For lesions located in the upper petroclival region, cavernous sinus, and middle cranial fossa, the transsphenoidal approach, with removal of the sphenoid and temporal bony encasement is indicated. Tumors extending into the middle third of the clivus can be approached through a transsphenoidal approach along with clivectomy and petrosectomy. Lesions in the lower clivus and infratemporal fossa require a transpterygoid approach.[6]

24.3.1 Surgical Technique

The surgery is performed under general anesthesia with orotracheal intubation. Prophylactic antibiotics are given. The patient is positioned supine, with the head fixed on the Mayfield head holder. The neck is slightly extended and the head turned to the right and tilted to the left. Nasal irrigation with oxymetazoline hydrochloride solution and facial/nasal decontamination with iodine solution is performed. The abdomen and the right thigh are also prepped in case fat or muscle grafts are necessary.

The surgical approach is initially comprised of right middle turbinectomy, bilateral posterior ethmoidectomies, elevation of the nasoseptal flap (NSF),[11] and posterior septectomy. Reverse flap (incision and rotation of the now-exposed contralateral septal mucosa to cover the denuded septum) is usually performed.[12] A large sphenoidotomy by drilling of the sphenoid floor until it is flush with the clivus is the next step. In order to access the pterygopalatine fossa, the removal of the posterior wall of the maxillary sinus is necessary and allows identification of the infraorbital and vidian nerve. The vidian nerve may be spared or sacrificed by drilling of the vidian canal, which is also a landmark for the foramen lacerum (▶ Fig. 24.1).[13] In sequence, the drilling of the clivus is performed, and it needs to be taken into account that massive venous bleeding from the basilar plexus can occur. It can be managed using direct infusion of hemostatic products. The petrous apex drilling and the skeletonization of the internal carotid artery (ICA) must be done (▶ Fig. 24.2).[8]

Depending on the location of the tumor, some other steps may be necessary. Tumors located inferior to the petrous apex may require removal or mobilization of the Eustachian tube.[8] The infratemporal fossa can be accessed by removing the pterygoid processes and adjacent musculature. In order to gain

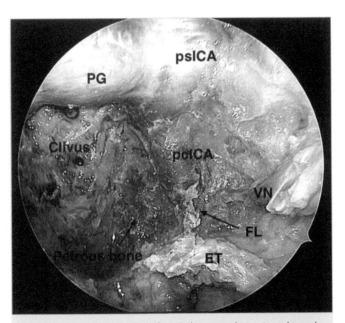

Fig. 24.1 Anatomical image under 45-degree endoscopic endonasal view of the left petroclival region. ET, Eustachian tube; FL, foramen lacerum; pcICA, paraclival internal carotid artery; PG, pituitary gland; psICA, parasellar ICA; VN, vidian nerve.

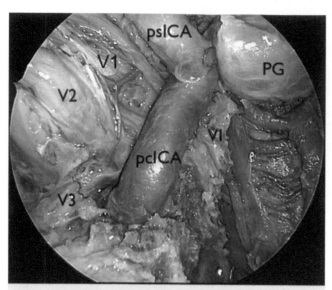

Fig. 24.2 Exposure of the right medial middle cranial fossa and Meckel's cave. PG, pituitary gland; pcICA, paraclival internal carotid artery (ICA); psICA, parasellar ICA; V1, ophthalmic nerve; V2, maxillary nerve; V3, mandibular nerve; VI, abducens nerve.

access to the anterior portion of Meckel's cave and the medial middle cranial fossa, the lateral sphenoid recess must be accessed.[14]

Chondrosarcomas are often soft; however, sometimes they can be hard and very calcified. Usually, the tumor's resection starts within the petrous apex. Lateralization of the ICA allows the removal of the tumor located on the petroclival synchondrosis. Dissection within the cavernous sinus, jugular foramen, infratemporal fossa, and high cervical region is performed using stimulating dissectors to prevent cranial nerve injuries. The presence or absence of a cerebrospinal fluid (CSF) leak guides the type of skull base reconstruction. If present, the dural defect is plugged with a partial inlay/onlay sheet of collagen matrix and covered with the NSF. In the absence of CSF leak, the flap is positioned over the exposed ICA for protection.[8]

24.3.2 Operative Pearls and Pitfalls

- EEA provides direct ventral access to the petroclival synchondrosis, where chondrosarcomas usually originate. For that reason, we advocate this approach as the initial corridor.
- EEA facilitates removal of large segments of diseased and infiltrated bone without the need for manipulation of neurovascular structures. Chondrosarcomas tend to displace neurovascular elements laterally, superiorly, and posteriorly.
- Dissection within the cavernous sinus, jugular foramen, infratemporal fossa, and high cervical region is also performed with stimulating dissectors to prevent cranial nerve injuries.
- Closure is performed based on the presence or absence of a CSF leak. NSF is always used to cover the dural defect and for protection over the skeletonized ICA.

24.3.3 Preoperative Evaluation and Postoperative Care

Preoperative neuroimaging is indispensable. The fusion of previously performed MRI of the brain and computed axial tomography scan is used for intraoperative navigation.

Otolaryngology evaluation is recommended in order to detect sinonasal abnormalities and signs of infection. Cases of jugular foramen involvement must have swallowing evaluation. Audiological examination needs to be performed in patients whose tumors involve the cerebellopontine angle and/or internal acoustic canal.

All patients must have postoperative care in the intensive care unit. Administration of prophylactic IV antibiotics starts preoperatively and is suspended in 24 hours. Oral antibiotics are continued while there is packing in place and usually are discontinued around the fifth postoperative day. A noncontrast head computed axial tomography scan is performed to ensure that there are no immediate complications and to determine the extent of bone removal. A brain MRI is also necessary to determine the extent of resection.

The patient is usually discharged on the second postoperative day. After the pathology results confirm the tumor as chondrosarcoma, most patients are referred for adjuvant radiation. Follow-up is determined by histologic type and extent of resection.

24.3.4 Complications and Management

The main complication is postoperative CSF leakage, which requires a second surgery for flap repositioning or fat graft augmentation. Meningitis is extremely rare, even in the setting of a CSF leak. Sinonasal infection and scarring are uncommon. Cranial neuropathies that are present preoperatively may be exacerbated; this is usually transient, and most patients experience recovery. Permanent postoperative cranial nerve dysfunction is extremely rare, since the cranial nerves are pushed to the periphery of the tumor, and the EEA allows removal of the tumor from the center primarily.

Chondroid tumors are most frequently associated with carotid injuries. In the event of an ICA rupture, intraoperative management is based on direct compression with a muscle graft. Angiography should be performed to investigate the presence of a pseudoaneurysm at the site of the vascular injury. ICA endovascular stenting should then be considered to facilitate endothelial healing and complement the repair.

Resection of the cartilaginous portions of the Eustachian tube may result in a serous middle ear effusion that can be treated with a tympanostomy tube.

24.4 Case Example

A young female patient presented with nasal congestion and difficulty breathing (antrochoanal polyp). She had no other neurological deficits during physical examination. MRI showed a large enhancing mass in the petrous apex, right clivus, and sphenoid sinus with bone erosion and destruction (▶ Fig. 24.3).

An expanded endonasal transpterygoid approach with resection of middle cranial and posterior fossa extradural tumor was performed. Skull base reconstruction was performed using a matrix collagen inlay, fat graft, and NSF (▶ Fig. 24.4). Postoperative CT scan and MRI demonstrate complete resection and no complications (▶ Fig. 24.5 and ▶ Fig. 24.6).

24.5 Conclusion

Pediatric population can develop chondrosarcomas; however, they are extremely rare at the skull base location. The standard treatment for chondrosarcomas of the skull base is resection followed by radiation therapy, which demonstrated

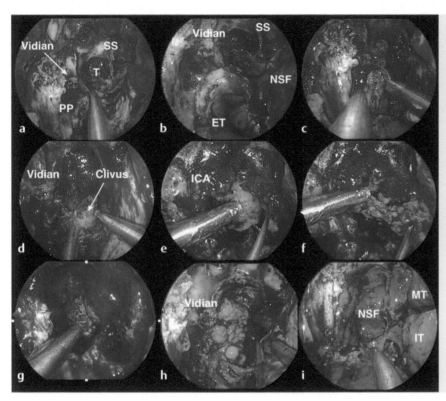

Fig. 24.3 Intraoperative endoscopic endonasal view showing the resection of right side chondrosarcoma. (a) Right transpterygoid approach. (b) NSF in the left choana, elevated in the beginning of the procedure. Tumor in the right petroclival synchondrosis. (c) Removal of the ET allows complete visualization of the entire petroclival mass. (d) Exposure of vidian nerve to localize ICA and drilling of the clivus to remove tumor. (e,f) Removing the tumor by suction and dissection while visualizing the plane with the healthy dura. (g) Operative site after complete resection. (h;i) Reconstruction with fat graft and nasoseptal flap. ET, Eustachian tube; ICA, internal carotid artery; IT, inferior turbine; MT, middle turbine; NSF, nasoseptal flap; SS, sphenoid sinus; PP, pterygoid plate.

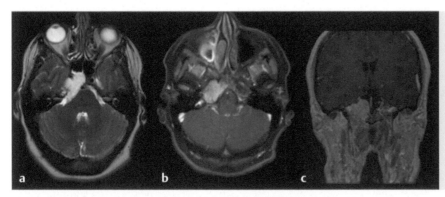

Fig. 24.4 Preoperative imaging. (a) Axial T2-weighted MR showing hyperintense lesion. (b,c) Preoperative axial and coronal, gadolinium enhanced T1-weighted MR images revealing enhancing mass in the right petrous apex, clivus, and sphenoid sinus.

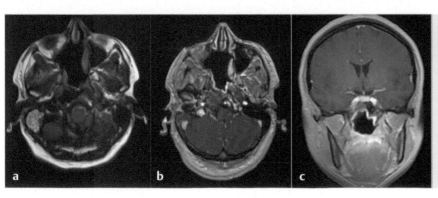

Fig. 24.5 (a–c) Postoperative MR images showing gross total resection and no evidence of recurrence (1-year follow-up).

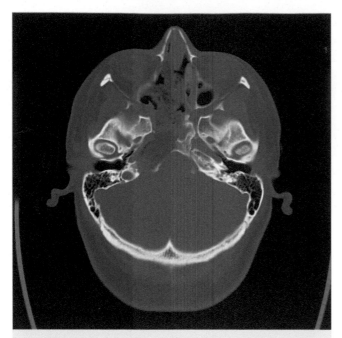

Fig. 24.6 Postoperative CT showing extent of bone resection.

an overall good prognosis. EEA appears to be a safe and appropriate technique, capable of achieving total or near-total removal in most cases with low complication rates. Inadequate pneumatization of air sinuses in younger patients can be overcome with neuronavigation, anatomical knowledge, and experience.

References

[1] Rastatter JC, Snyderman CH, Gardner PA, Alden TD, Tyler-Kabara E. Endoscopic endonasal surgery for sinonasal and skull base lesions in the pediatric population. Otolaryngol Clin North Am. 2015; 48(1):79–99

[2] Rombi B, Ares C, Hug EB, et al. Spot-scanning proton radiation therapy for pediatric chordoma and chondrosarcoma: clinical outcome of 26 patients treated at Paul Scherrer institute. Int J Radiat Oncol Biol Phys. 2013; 86(3):578–584

[3] Bloch OG, Jian BJ, Yang I, et al. A systematic review of intracranial chondrosarcoma and survival. J Clin Neurosci. 2009; 16(12):1547–1551

[4] Bloch O, Parsa AT. Skull base chondrosarcoma: evidence-based treatment paradigms. Neurosurg Clin N Am. 2013; 24(1):89–96

[5] Brackmann DE, Teufert KB. Chondrosarcoma of the skull base: long-term follow-up. Otol Neurotol. 2006; 27(7):981–991

[6] Mesquita Filho PM, Ditzel Filho LF, Prevedello DM, et al. Endoscopic endonasal surgical management of chondrosarcomas with cerebellopontine angle extension. Neurosurg Focus. 2014; 37(4):E13

[7] Awad M, Gogos AJ, Kaye AH. Skull base chondrosarcoma. J Clin Neurosci. 2016; 24:1–5

[8] Ditzel Filho LF, Prevedello DM, Dolci RL, et al. The endoscopic endonasal approach for removal of petroclival chondrosarcomas. Neurosurg Clin N Am. 2015; 26(3):453–462

[9] Leroy R, Benahmed N, Hulstaert F, Van Damme N, De Ruysscher D. Proton therapy in children: a systematic review of clinical effectiveness in 15 pediatric cancers. Int J Radiat Oncol Biol Phys. 2016; 95(1):267–278

[10] Italiano A, Mir O, Cioffi A, et al. Advanced chondrosarcomas: role of chemotherapy and survival. Ann Oncol. 2013; 24(11):2916–2922

[11] Kassam AB, Thomas A, Carrau RL, et al. Endoscopic reconstruction of the cranial base using a pedicled nasoseptal flap. Neurosurgery. 2008; 63(1) Suppl 1:44–52, discussion 52–53

[12] Kasemsiri P, Carrau RL, Otto BA, et al. Reconstruction of the pedicled nasoseptal flap donor site with a contralateral reverse rotation flap: technical modifications and outcomes. Laryngoscope. 2013; 123(11):2601–2604

[13] Prevedello DM, Pinheiro-Neto CD, Fernandez-Miranda JC, et al. Vidian nerve transposition for endoscopic endonasal middle fossa approaches. Neurosurgery. 2010; 67(2) Suppl operative:478–484

[14] Kassam AB, Prevedello DM, Carrau RL, et al. The front door to meckel's cave: an anteromedial corridor via expanded endoscopic endonasal approach-technical considerations and clinical series. Neurosurgery. 2009; 64(3) Suppl: 71–82, discussion 82–83

25 Malignant Skull Base Tumors

Paolo Castelnuovo, Apostolos Karligkiotis, Muaid I. Aziz Baban, Paolo Battaglia, and Mario Turri-Zanoni

Abstract

Malignant tumors involving the skull base are exceedingly rare in the pediatric population, representing less than 0.9% of all the head and neck cancers. Rhabdomyosarcoma is the most common sinonasal malignancy in children, followed by sarcoma, lymphoma, and olfactory neuroblastoma. Management of these tumors requires a team approach of medical and surgical services with extensive training and experience, including otorhinolaryngologists, neurosurgeons, radiologists, pathologists, radiation oncologists, and pediatric oncologists. Treatment is generally tailored according to the age of the patient, extent of the disease, and histologic subtype. Surgery is performed in both curative and palliative settings and it is usually associated with different protocols of chemotherapy and radiotherapy. External transfacial approaches have been largely used in the past to manage such complex tumors, entailing non-negligible rates of complications, especially disturbing and potentially dangerous in children. The endoscopic endonasal approach is well established in the management of inflammatory conditions and benign lesions in the pediatric population; it can also be applied in well-selected cases of sinonasal and skull base malignancies. Data currently available are encouraging, with overall survival rates comparable to those of traditional external surgery, while morbidity and complication rates are reduced. Absence of facial incisions or the need for osteotomies, absence of retraction of the brain, absence of impairments in the growing craniofacial skeleton, less postoperative pain, decreased hospitalization time, and reduced mortality rates are the major advantages of endoscopic endonasal surgery.

Keywords: rhabdomyosarcoma, lymphoma, endoscopic transnasal craniectomy, pediatric skull base disease, sinonasal tumor, multidisciplinary approach, radiochemotherapy

25.1 Introduction

Pediatric sinonasal lesions can arise from a number of congenital, developmental, or neoplastic processes. Fortunately, less than 2% of all paranasal masses diagnosed in children are malignant. Pediatric sinonasal and skull base cancers include a wide range of histologies with various symptoms of presentation, depending on the child's age, location of the lesion, and disease-specific characteristics.[1] The diagnosis and management of these lesions can be complex and demand an understanding of sinonasal and skull base embryology, developmental anatomy, location-specific symptoms, and disease-specific behavior. The management of these tumors requires a team approach of medical and surgical services with extensive training and experience, including otorhinolaryngologist, neurosurgeon, radiologist, pathologist, radiation oncologist, and pediatric oncologist.[2] In particular, surgical management demands extensive clinical training supplemented by cadaveric dissection to gain the required knowledge of 3D anatomy, specialized instrumentation, and teamwork necessary for optimal outcomes and safety. The resection of malignant tumors via conventional approaches (e.g., craniofacial surgery) harbors difficulties because of the important structures involved and the complexity of the anatomical sites. Needless to say, these external approaches carry considerable risks, which may give rise to many complications, such as intracranial, orbital, neural, cutaneous, and others.[3,4] Not less important, especially in the pediatric population, is the concern regarding the future skeletal development of the child; this can be significantly impaired in cases of disruption of the craniofacial complex growth centers.[5] Better understanding of the skull base anatomy, improved anesthesiological techniques, and the greatly enhanced visualization provided by endoscopes have led to a tremendous evolution of the endonasal approaches. At present, the endoscopic endonasal surgery is well established in the management of inflammatory conditions and benign lesions in the pediatric population, and it is also applied with satisfactory oncological outcomes for sinonasal and skull base malignancies in well-selected cases.[2]

25.2 Epidemiology and Pathology

Malignancies of the paranasal sinuses and nasal cavities are rare in the adult population, accounting for approximately 3% of all head and neck cancer. Paranasal sinus malignancies are even more rare in children (0.9%).[6] Symptoms may be nonspecific and indolent for months or even years, leading to delay in diagnosis and consequent advanced stage of disease at presentation. Epidemiological studies based on the Surveillance, Epidemiology, and End Results (SEER) database program of the National Cancer Institute (NCI) suggest that rhabdomyosarcoma (RMS) is the most common paranasal sinus malignancy in children, followed by sarcoma, lymphoma, and olfactory neuroblastoma (ONB).[6] Other histologic tumor types rarely seen in pediatric age include neuroendocrine carcinoma, yolk sac tumors, spindle cell tumors, adenoid cystic carcinoma, and mucoepidermoid carcinoma. For this reason, of the pediatric skull base are generally divided into RMS and non-RMS malignancies.[1]

RMS is the third most common extracranial solid tumor seen in children and over one-third of RMS in children occur in the head and neck region.[6] It is a highly aggressive neoplasm originating from embryonal mesenchyma with potential to differentiate to striated muscle. Incidence of this tumor is most commonly seen in the first decade, with a second peak in adolescence. Histologic subtypes include embryonal (seen more commonly in younger children), alveolar (seen more commonly in adolescence), pleomorphic, and mixed type. The embryonal subtype is associated with the highest 5-year survival rate compared to other subtypes. The therapy of RMS is guided by the extent of the disease. Surgery is generally used for diagnostic issues, since definitive radiochemotherapy usually represents the best treatment option. However, in selected cases of nonresponding tumors and when dealing with persistence of disease, surgical resection with the goal of complete tumor removal is recommended (▶ Fig. 25.1).[2]

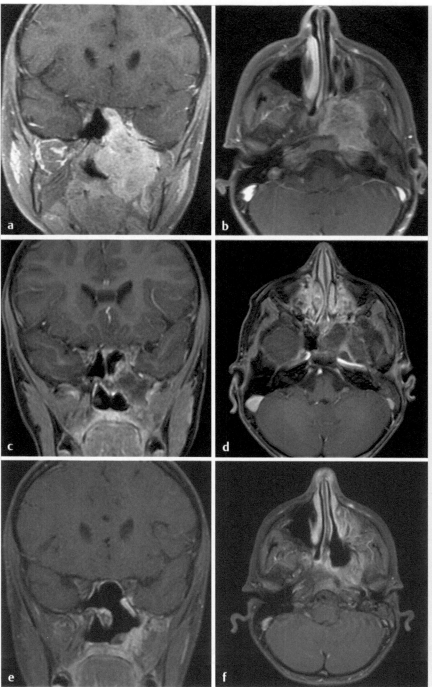

Fig. 25.1 MRI scan of a 9-year-old boy affected by anaplastic embryonal rhabdomyosarcoma of the left pterygopalatine fossa in the coronal (a) and axial (b) planes. The patient underwent induction chemotherapy and subsequent chemoradiation. The MRI performed 3 months after the initial treatment showed a persistent lesion at the level of the pterygoid recess of the left sphenoid sinus in the coronal (c) and axial (d) planes. An endoscopic endonasal transethmoid-pterygoid-sphenoid-antral procedure was performed with removal of the suspected area. The final histologic report revealed necrotic tissue with only some viable malignant cells at the level of the sphenoid sinus. The postoperative MRI after 1 year showed no evidence of disease in the coronal (e) and axial (f) planes.

Sarcomas are malignant mesenchymal tumors of unclear etiology, and are usually low grade and slow growing. Less than 10% are seen in the head and neck, and only 7 to 9% of patients are children.[6] Chondrosarcoma represents the most frequent histotype observed in childhood. For high-grade tumors, exclusive radiochemotherapy may be indicated. Surgery is used for biopsy or for persistent lesions. Nonresponding and low-grade lesions may be suitable for surgical resection.[2]

Hematolymphoid tumors including B-cell and NK/T-cell lymphomas are rare in the pediatric populations with symptoms that may be nonspecific and indolent for months or even years, leading to delay in diagnosis and consequent advanced stage disease at presentation.[1] Once the diagnosis is established through a biopsy of the nasal mass under endoscopic assistance, the treatment strategy includes different regimens of chemotherapy, eventually associated with or followed by radiotherapy.[2]

ONB, also termed esthesioneuroblastoma, is very rare in children, with an estimated incidence of less than 0.1 per 100,000 children younger than 15 years.[6] It is a malignant neoplasm that arises from the olfactory epithelium, most frequently located at the cribriform plate, the upper surface of the superior turbinates, and the upper third of the nasal septum. Because of its rarity and indolence in children, it has been difficult to develop standard treatment protocols. However, multimodal

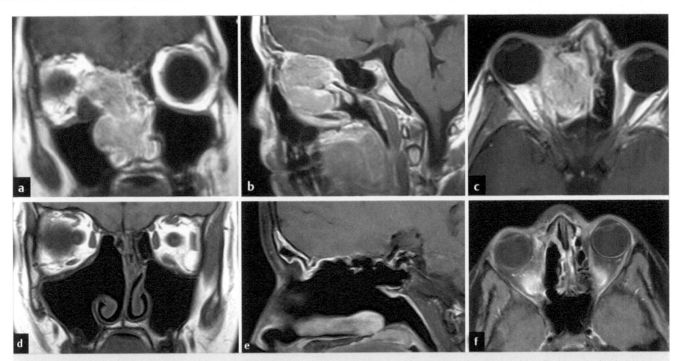

Fig. 25.2 Preoperative MRI scan with gadolinium of a 14-year-old girl with olfactory neuroblastoma of the right nasal fossa with intraorbital extension in the coronal **(a)**, sagittal **(b)**, and axial **(c)** planes. The patient underwent endoscopic transnasal resection followed by adjuvant radiotherapy. The postoperative enhanced MRI after 5 years of follow-up showed no evidence of disease in the coronal **(d)**, sagittal **(e)**, and axial **(f)** planes.

therapy including surgery followed by radiation therapy has been indicated, especially in patients with advanced disease (▶ Fig. 25.2). In patients with Hyams grade IV disease (poorly differentiated ONB), combined therapy including induction chemotherapy, surgery, and radiation therapy had better outcomes.[2]

Primitive neuroectodermal tumors (PNETs) of the sinuses are rare in children, but must be considered in the differential diagnosis of a paranasal sinus mass. Histologic features of undifferentiated small round cells elicit a differential diagnosis including Ewing's sarcoma, ONB, and RMS. Treatment may include surgery and chemoradiation.[2] Prognosis for PNET is extremely poor, with a high incidence of both local recurrences and distant metastases.

25.3 Pretreatment Workup

The role of the endoscopic skull base surgeons in these cases is variable and tailored to the histology of the disease. Endoscopic endonasal surgery can be used as a diagnostic tool for biopsy to guide chemotherapy and radiation; for resection or debulking of the tumor in order to downstage the lesion in preparation for chemotherapy or radiation therapy or both; surgery may be performed in several cases to relieve symptoms; and rarely, total resection can be planned for some non-rhabdosarcoma cases of appropriate size and location. However, it is mandatory to define the goals of treatment before surgery in every case.[2]

Imaging workup includes CT scan and contrast-enhanced MRI for all patients. Total body staging can be performed with contrast-enhanced CT scan, while PET was reserved for patients with aggressive histotypes.[7]

Remarkably, before surgery, the parents of the patient must be fully informed about the surgical proposal and of the possibility of shifting to a conventional external approach (if deemed necessary), and they must give their written consent to the treatment plan. In this respect, the patients are prepared in the operating theater for both the endoscopic and a possible external approach. Dedicated instrumentations are used. A magnetic navigation system is advisable intraoperatively and an ultrasound Doppler probe can be helpful in selected cases to identify major vessels.

25.4 Surgical Technique

Endoscopic endonasal approaches to the skull base can be used safely to manage sinonasal and skull base lesions in pediatric patients. Understanding the age-dependent pneumatization patterns of the paranasal sinuses, particularly the sphenoid and frontal sinuses, is critical for planning a safe endonasal approach in such patients. According to the site of origin, extent, and tumor histology, the endoscopic resection can be performed unilaterally (resection extended anteroposteriorly from the posterior wall of the frontal sinus to the planum sphenoidale and laterolaterally from the nasal septum to the lamina papyracea) or bilaterally (extending the resection from one lamina papyracea to the opposite one).[7] The traditional concept of oncologic surgery on en bloc resection to avoid the risk of tumor spilling is now debated, gradually being replaced by the concept of disassembling the lesion, having under view the limits between normal and diseased mucosa. The step-by-step technique of the endoscopic endonasal resection (EER) is summarized as follows (▶ Fig. 25.3):

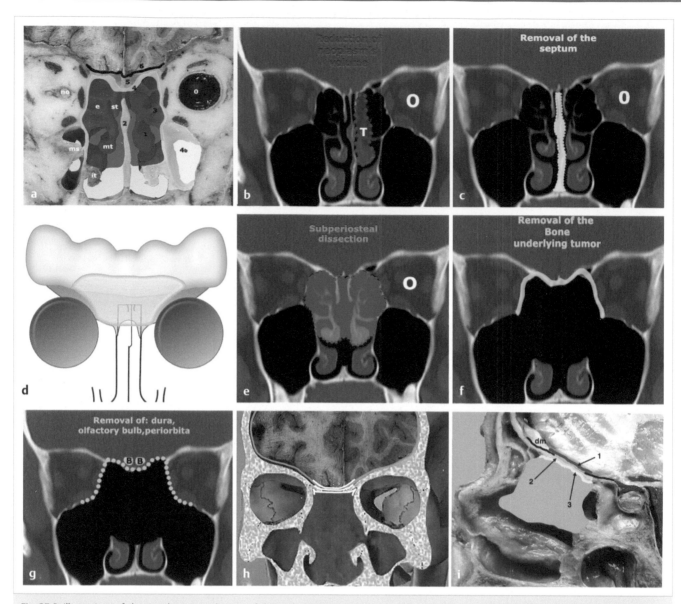

Fig. 25.3 Illustrations of the step-by-step technique of the endoscopic endonasal resection. **(a)** Schematic representation of the surgical steps: 1, debulking of the tumor; 2, removal of the septum; 3, centripetal subperiosteal resection; 4, removal of the bone in contact with the tumor; 4b, medial maxillectomy; 5, removal of the dura, the olfactory bulb, and periorbita; 6, skull base reconstruction; e, ethmoid; it, inferior turbinate; ms, maxillary sinus, mt, middle turbinate; no, optic nerve; o, orbit. **(b)** The first step consists in debulking the tumor until identification of its pedicle. O, orbit; T, tumor. **(c)** The second step requires exposure of the surgical cavity with removal of the posterior two-thirds of the nasal septum. O, orbit. **(d)** A Draf type III frontal sinusotomy is performed in order to define the anterosuperior limit of the resection. **(e)** The centripetal resection of the ethmoidal box is performed in the subperiosteal plane. O, orbit. **(f)** the bone of the skull base in contact with the tumor is removed exposing the dura. **(g)** If required, the dura as well as the olfactory bulbs and the periorbita can be removed to achieve clear margins. B, olfactory bulb. **(h)** The duraplasty is performed with a three-layer grafting technique using fascia lata intracranial intradural (1), intracranial extradural (2), and extracranial (3). In coronal view and **(I)** in sagittal view. dm, dura matter.

- *Tumor origin identification.* The lesion is gradually debulked starting from the core, in order to identify its site of origin. In this phase, it is crucial to preserve the surrounding anatomic structures, because these are useful landmarks for orientating the subsequent surgical steps.
- *Exposure of the surgical field.* In the case of bilateral resection, removal of the posterior two-thirds of the nasal septum is performed to gain better exposure of the surgical field and to optimize the endonasal maneuverability of dedicated instruments, using the two-

nostril, four-hand technique. In this step, a wide sphenoidotomy (with removal of intersinus septum and sphenoid rostrum in bilateral cases) is crucial to expose the posteroinferior margin of the dissection. The frontal sinus is approached by Draf type IIb sinusotomy in the case of unilateral EER, whereas Draf type III sinusotomy is performed if the EER involves both sides. The frontal sinusotomy represents the anterosuperior margin of the dissection, allowing precise identification of the beginning of the anterior cranial fossa.

- *Centripetal removal.* Once the posteroinferior and anterosuperior margins of the resection are exposed, a subperiosteal dissection of the nasoethmoidal–sphenoidal complex is performed unilaterally or bilaterally (according to the extension of disease), to expose the lateral margins. The lamina papyracea is included in the dissection when the tumor is in close proximity to or frankly involved in it. Sphenopalatine arteries must be cauterized and divided in this phase. Techniques to minimize and control intraoperative blood loss are critical in pediatric patients owing to their overall lower blood volume compared with adult patients. When required by the extension of the disease, an endoscopic medial maxillectomy can be performed, to achieve good control of the whole maxillary sinus. This surgical step has to be associated with nasolacrimal duct exposure and resection, just below the lacrimal sac.[8] Superiorly, the dissection is continued in the anteroposterior direction, by resecting the olfactory fibers and the basal lamella of the ethmoidal turbinates. The entire nasoethmoidal–sphenoidal complex is then isolated and pushed toward the central part of the nasal fossa (centripetal technique) to extract it transorally or through the nasal vestibule. The surgical margins are checked by frozen section and, if necessary, the dissection is continued until free margins are obtained.
- *Skull base removal.* According to the extension of the disease, the EER can be extended to include the anterior skull base (ASB) as well (endoscopic resection with transnasal craniectomy). The ethmoidal roof is exposed using a drill with a diamond burr. The anterior and posterior ethmoidal arteries are identified, cauterized, and divided. The crista galli is carefully detached from the dura and removed with blunt instruments, preserving the integrity of the dural layer.
- *Intracranial work.* The key point for subsequently performing an optimal skull base reconstruction is to properly dissect the epidural space over the orbital roofs laterally, the planum sphenoidale posteriorly, and the posterior wall of the frontal sinus anteriorly before starting the resection of the dura. The dura is then incised and circumferentially cut with scissors, far away from the suspected area of tumor spread. The falx cerebri is clipped in the anterior portion before its resection to avoid sagittal sinus bleeding, then its posterior portion at the level of the sphenoethmoidal planum is resected. The arachnoidal plane over the intracranial portion of the tumor is then dissected and separated from the brain parenchyma. The specimen, including the residual tumor, the ASB, and the overlying dura, together with one or both of the olfactory bulbs, is removed transnasally. The dural margins are sent for frozen sections.
- *Skull base reconstruction.* The resulting skull base defect is reconstructed by the endoscopic endonasal multilayer technique, performed preferably using autologous materials. Advances in skull base reconstruction after endoscopic surgery have allowed surgeons to perform more extensive resections while maintaining acceptable rates of post-reconstruction cerebrospinal fluid (CSF) leak or other potential complications. Regarding the materials used, the fascia lata and/or the iliotibial tract possess the best characteristics in terms of thickness, pliability, and strength.[7]

For the first intradural layer of duraplasty, the graft has to be at least 30% larger than the dural defect and split anteriorly on the midline to adjust to the falx cerebri in case of bilateral resection. The second layer, intracranial and extradural, needs to be precisely sized and tacked between the previously undermined dura and the residual ASB bone. Pieces of fatty tissue are placed to eliminate the dead space between the second and third layers and to flatten the residual denuded ASB. The third extracranial layer has to cover all the exposed ASB but must not overlap the frontal sinusotomies in order to avoid a postoperative mucocele. The borders of the second and third layers are properly fixed with fibrin glue. In case of a tumor not involving nasal tissues (e.g. septum, contralateral turbinates) and without multifocal localizations, the third layer of the skull base reconstruction can be performed using local flaps. Sinonasal flaps include the nasoseptal flap, the septal flip-flap, the inferior turbinate, and the middle turbinate flaps.[9,10] Their use facilitates rapid healing of the surgical cavity, especially in patients who require adjuvant irradiation. The potential size of every kind of flap is smaller in pediatric patients, and careful preoperative and intraoperative planning helps ensure the appropriateness of their use for skull base reconstruction. Reconstructions are then covered with hemostatic materials such as Surgicel (Johnson & Johnson Medical, Arlington, TX) and fibrin glues such as Tisseel (Baxter, Deerfield, IL) or DuraSeal (Covidien, Dublin, Ireland). Nasal packing with absorbable or nonabsorbable materials is kept for about 48 hours. Lumbar drains are not routinely used postoperatively. but early revision surgery is preferred in case of skull base reconstruction failure (▶ Fig. 25.4).

For lesions filling the frontal sinus or encroaching on the ASB with intradural extension over the orbital roof or with brain parenchyma infiltration, the EER has to be combined with an external transcranial approach.[11] The procedure is performed by two surgical teams (neurosurgeons and otorhinolaryngologists) working simultaneously through a transnasal and transcranial corridor, respectively.

25.5 Outcomes

Owing to the infrequency of sinonasal cancers in childhood, sufficient and significant data focusing on the different surgical approaches are difficult to obtain. Almost all the available literature regarding the surgical management of sinonasal malignancies in children is focused on the conventional approaches. The endoscopic endonasal surgery has been recently introduced in the management of such disease, and therefore case series currently available are small with short follow-up periods. One of the earlier experiences applying EER in pediatric patients has been reported by Kassam et al, which included not only malignant lesions but also different sinonasal pathologies.[12] In this series, six cases were malignant tumors, and most of them underwent either diagnostic biopsy or subtotal resection with subsequent adjuvant therapy.

The M.D. Anderson Cancer Center presented 44 pediatric cases of malignant sinonasal lesions, eight of which were resected through an endoscopic approach. Unfortunately, no specific data about the histology, extent of the disease, type of

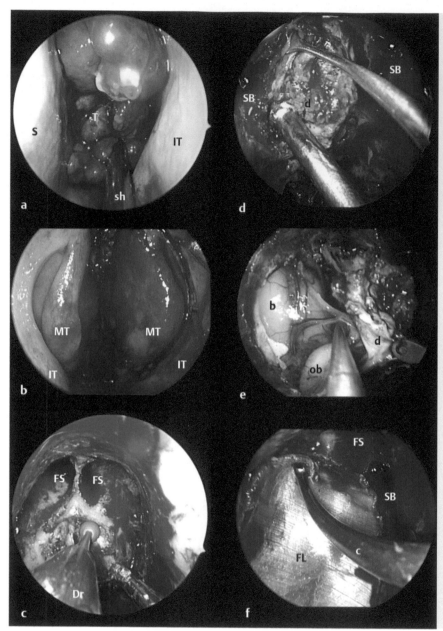

Fig. 25.4 Intraoperative images illustrating the steps of the bilateral endoscopic transnasal craniectomy. The tumor is debulked in the right nasal fossa with a microdebrider in order to identify its attachment and infiltrated areas (a). Once the posterior two-thirds of the septum is removed, the ethmoidal box is delimited and will be removed in a subperiosteal centripetal fashion (b). The skull base is removed with a diamond drill from the anterior limit, which is the posterior wall of the frontal sinus, to the planum sphenoidale posteriorly and from one orbit to the contralateral one (c). The dura is detached from the residual skull base bone over the orbits in the epidural space before its opening. In this step, it is necessary to coagulate and cut the anterior and posterior ethmoidal arteries to release the dura (d). The dura is opened and progressively removed as much as is required, together with the olfactory bulbs if needed (e). The dural reconstruction is performed in a multilayer fashion with three layers of fascia lata harvested from the thigh. The first layer is intracranial intradural, the second is intracranial extradural, and the third is extracranial (f). b, brain; c, curette; d, dura matter; Dr, drill; FL, fascia lata; FS, frontal sinus; IT, inferior turbinate; MT, middle turbinate; OB, olfactory bulb; S, septum; SB, skull base; sh, shaver; T, tumor.

resection, and status of the margins were given for these endoscopically treated patients.[13]

The Italian experience has been described by AlQahtani et al; it focused on seven patients affected by sinonasal and skull base malignancies who were treated through endoscopic endonasal approaches without complications or recurrence of disease after a mean follow-up of 65 months.[14]

Yi et al reported a case series of 20 pediatric patients affected by sinonasal cancers, four of whom were treated by means of EER. Two of them had RMS and are currently alive without evidence of the disease, and the other two had ONB and succumbed to the disease within 18 and 21 months, respectively.[15] Other smaller case series describing pediatric patients affected by malignancies arising from the cranial base in whom EER was part of the management have been summarized in ► Table 25.1.[12,13,14,15,16,17,18,19] Data currently available are encouraging: overall survival rates are comparable to those of

traditional external surgery, while morbidity and complication rates are reduced.

In the pediatric population, it is particularly important to consider the morbidity of treatment in addition to survival. Therefore, the risks of surgical resection in the sinonasal region and skull base, as well as the long-term effects of radiation therapy in this region, should be always taken into account when treating children with sinonasal malignancies. The absence of facial incisions or need for osteotomies, less postoperative pain, decreased hospitalization time, and reduced morbidity and mortality rates are the major advantages of endoscopic endonasal surgery compared to the external approach.[20] Moreover, at present, no significant complications following endoscopic endonasal surgery for skull base cancers have been described in pediatric patients, with postoperative CSF leak rates comparable to those reported in adult patients.[14] Furthermore, avoidance of surgical impairment in the growing craniofacial

Table 25.1 Summary of the case series reporting endoscopic surgery for sinonasal and skull base malignancies in pediatric patients

Author	Year	No. of cases	Histology	Aim of surgery	Complications	Status	Follow-up (mo)
Herrmann et al[16]	2003	3	3, RMS	2, biopsy 1, CR	none	3, NED	n.a.
Kassam et al[12]	2007	6	2, germinoma 1, lymphoma 1, glioma 1, NET 1, chordoma	5, biopsy 1, PR	none	4, NED 2, AWD	n.a.
Lee et al[17]	2008	1	1, lymphoma	1, biopsy	none	1, NED	n.a.
Wilson et al[18]	2010	1	1, SNUC	1, PR	none	1, NED	12
Zevallos et al[13]	2011	8	8, sarcoma	n.a.	n.a.	n.a.	n.a.
AlQahtani et al[14]	2012	7	2, ADC 1, osteosarcoma 1, ONB 1, ACC 1, RMS 1, MuEpCa	7, CR	1, diplopia 1, septic fever	6, NED 1, DOC	27–109 (mean 65)
Yi et al[15]	2012	4	2, RMS 2, ONB	4, CR	none	2, NED 2, DOD	27–40 18–21
Thompson et al[19]	2013	4	4, RMS	3, CR 1, PR	none	2, NED 1, AWD 1, DOD	13–105 16 41

Abbreviations: ACC, adenoid cystic carcinoma; ADC, adenocarcinoma; AWD, alive with disease; CR, complete resection; DOC, dead of other causes; DOD, dead of disease; MuEpCa, mucoepidermoid carcinoma; n.a., not available; NED, no evidence of disease; ONB, olfactory neuroblastoma; PR, partial resection; RMS, rhabdomyosarcoma; SNUC, sinonasal undifferentiated carcinoma.

skeleton should be considered in pediatric patients. Remarkably, the results emerging from recent literature show that no facial growth disorders were evident in any of the cases treated using an endoscopic endonasal approach during the follow-up.[12,13,14,15,16,17,18,19]

25.6 Conclusion

Although open surgical approaches are generally used in most cases, evolving endoscopic approaches to the sinonasal region and skull base are promising in limiting surgical morbidity. Moreover, several studies have demonstrated that oncologically sound resections are possible and safe using an endoscopic approach even in the pediatric population.

Therefore, in well-selected cases, endoscopic endonasal surgery can be proposed as an alternative to the traditional external approaches for either therapeutic or palliative purposes. Obviously, such an approach must be included in a multimodal treatment plan and tailored to the tumor histology and the specific needs of the case. For this reason, a multidisciplinary team approach is paramount, which should include head and neck surgeons, neurosurgeons, medical and radiation oncologists, and pediatricians.

25.7 Conflict of Interest

All the authors certify that they have no conflict of interest or financial relationship with any entity mentioned in the chapter.

References

[1] Rastatter JC, Snyderman CH, Gardner PA, Alden TD, Tyler-Kabara E. Endoscopic endonasal surgery for sinonasal and skull base lesions in the pediatric population. Otolaryngol Clin North Am. 2015; 48(1):79–99

[2] Castelnuovo P, Turri-Zanoni M, Battaglia P, Antognoni P, Bossi P, Locatelli D. Sinonasal malignancies of anterior skull base: histology-driven treatment strategies. Otolaryngol Clin North Am. 2016; 49(1):183–200

[3] Tsai EC, Santoreneos S, Rutka JT. Tumors of the skull base in children: review of tumor types and management strategies. Neurosurg Focus. 2002; 12(5):e1

[4] Hanbali F, Tabrizi P, Lang FF, DeMonte F. Tumors of the skull base in children and adolescents. J Neurosurg. 2004; 100(2) Suppl pediatrics:169–178

[5] Gil Z, Patel SG, Cantu G, et al. International Collaborative Study Group. Outcome of craniofacial surgery in children and adolescents with malignant tumors involving the skull base: an international collaborative study. Head Neck. 2009; 31(3):308–317

[6] Gerth DJ, Tashiro J, Thaller SR. Pediatric sinonasal tumors in the United States: incidence and outcomes. J Surg Res. 2014; 190(1):214–220

[7] Castelnuovo P, Battaglia P, Turri-Zanoni M, et al. Endoscopic endonasal surgery for malignancies of the anterior cranial base. World Neurosurg. 2014; 82 (6) Suppl:S22–S31

[8] Turri-Zanoni M, Battaglia P, Karligkiotis A, et al. Transnasal endoscopic partial maxillectomy: operative nuances and proposal for a comprehensive classification system based on 1378 cases. Head Neck. 2017; 39(4):754–766

[9] Battaglia P, Turri-Zanoni M, De Bernardi F, et al. Septal flip flap for anterior skull base reconstruction after endoscopic resection of sinonasal cancers: preliminary outcomes. Acta Otorhinolaryngol Ital. 2016; 36(3):194–198

[10] Shah RN, Surowitz JB, Patel MR, et al. Endoscopic pedicled nasoseptal flap reconstruction for pediatric skull base defects. Laryngoscope. 2009; 119(6):1067–1075

[11] Castelnuovo PG, Belli E, Bignami M, Battaglia P, Sberze F, Tomei G. Endoscopic nasal and anterior craniotomy resection for malignant nasoethmoid tumors involving the anterior skull base. Skull Base. 2006; 16(1):15–18

[12] Kassam A, Thomas AJ, Snyderman C, et al. Fully endoscopic expanded endonasal approach treating skull base lesions in pediatric patients. J Neurosurg. 2007; 106(2) Suppl:75–86

[13] Zevallos JP, Jain KS, Roberts D, El-Naggar A, Hanna EY, Kupferman ME. Sinonasal malignancies in children: a 10-year, single-institutional review. Laryngoscope. 2011; 121(9):2001–2003

[14] AlQahtani A, Turri-Zanoni M, Dallan I, Battaglia P, Castelnuovo P. Endoscopic endonasal resection of sinonasal and skull base malignancies in children: feasibility and outcomes. Childs Nerv Syst. 2012; 28(11):1905–1910

[15] Yi JS, Cho GS, Shim MJ, Min JY, Chung YS, Lee BJ. Malignant tumors of the sinonasal tract in the pediatric population. Acta Otolaryngol. 2012; 132 Suppl 1:S21–S26

[16] Herrmann BW, Sotelo-Avila C, Eisenbeis JF. Pediatric sinonasal rhabdomyosarcoma: three cases and a review of the literature. Am J Otolaryngol. 2003; 24(3):174–180

[17] Lee JY, Jang YD, Kim HK. The primary role of the otolaryngologist in managing pediatric sinonasal malignancies: an extranodal NK/T-cell lymphoma originating from the inferior turbinate mucosa of the nasal cavity. J Pediatr Hematol Oncol. 2008; 30(5):401–404

[18] Wilson JR, Vachhrajani S, Li J, Sun M, Hawkins C, Rutka JT. Pediatric sinonasal undifferentiated carcinoma: case report and literature review. Can J Neurol Sci. 2010; 37(6):873–877

[19] Thompson CF, Kim BJ, Lai C, et al. Sinonasal rhabdomyosarcoma: prognostic factors and treatment outcomes. Int Forum Allergy Rhinol. 2013; 3(8):678–683

[20] Castelnuovo P, Lepera D, Turri-Zanoni M, et al. Quality of life following endoscopic endonasal resection of anterior skull base cancers. J Neurosurg. 2013; 119(6):1401–1409

26 Subperiosteal Orbital Abscess

Ernesto Pasquini, Paolo Farneti, and Vittorio Sciarretta

Abstract

Pediatric periorbital cellulitis represents a common disease complicating a nasal infection warranting prompt antibiotic therapy due to catastrophic complications, such as visual loss, intracranial infection, and sepsis. Indeed, medical management is the main treatment for both preseptal and postseptal orbital cellulitis. A subperiosteal abscess, on the other hand, represents a complicated postseptal infection, developing between the bone and the periorbita. Nevertheless, there is no universally accepted guideline for the treatment of subperiosteal abscesses, and each case should be treated accordingly. Urgent surgical drainage should be considered in cases not responding to adequate medical management or those cases presenting visual deterioration.

Keywords: periorbital cellulitis, subperiosteal abscess, preseptal cellulitis, postseptal cellulitis, pediatric, orbital complication, rhinosinusitis, proptosis, ophthalmoplegia

26.1 Introduction

Periorbital cellulitis is defined as an infection of the soft tissue surrounding the eye. Although it can occur at all ages, it is prevalent in the pediatric population. In fact, orbital complications are more commonly seen in the pediatric age group, with the overall incidence of 3 to 4% in children affected by acute rhinosinusitis.[1]

Periorbital cellulitis can be subdivided into two major entities, preseptal cellulitis or postseptal cellulitis, the latter also known as orbital cellulitis. In preseptal cellulitis, the infection does not extend beyond the orbital septum and is usually due to an eyelid infection or acute rhinosinusitis, while postseptal cellulitis is generally a consequence of acute rhinosinusitis. The spreading of pathogens from the sinuses (particularly the ethmoid cells) to the nearby tissues is thought to occur directly through the lamina papyracea or through the communicating blood vessels. The lamina papyracea is a thin bony structure that contains several natural perforations. It is believed that the infection can easily spread from the ethmoid sinus to the orbit through these perforations.

Therefore, acute rhinosinusitis is the predominant cause of orbital infection in children. In general, paranasal rhinosinusitis is responsible for 66 to 75% of cases of orbital infection, and acute ethmoiditis represents the most common rhinosinusitis linked to orbital cellulitis in children. The spread of infection from the ethmoid sinus is generally very rapid, and orbital complications can develop even under antibiotic therapy. Orbital involvement can easily be suspected in the case of ophthalmoplegia and proptosis.

A diagnosis is usually reached using a combination of clinical examination and radiological findings. The Chandler classification (▶ Table 26.1) still represents the most complete and popular classification for indicating the severity of the infection.[2]

26.2 Subperiosteal Abscess

The periorbita represents the periosteum separating the orbital content from the skeleton and the neighboring structures. Anteriorly, the periorbita merges with the periosteum of the external skeleton to form the orbital septum. Infections ensuing anteriorly to the septum are defined as preseptal and rarely include preseptal abscesses. On the other hand, infections developing posteriorly to the septum are defined as postseptal and are usually considered more serious. A subperiosteal abscess represents a postseptal infection developing between the bone and the periorbita. Although these abscesses derive from a direct spread of infection from acute ethmoiditis, in rare cases they can develop from acute rhinosinusitis of the frontal or maxillary sinuses. The diagnosis of subperiosteal abscess is generally radiological via an enhanced CT scan (▶ Fig. 26.1). On CT imaging, an abscess appears as a rim-enhancing collection of fluid between the periorbita and the bone. The displacement of the orbital content can also be observed with larger purulent collections, and they are more visible in the axial and coronal planes of the CT images. MRI is generally reserved for those cases where there is suspicion of an intracranial extension of the infection.

26.3 Microbiology of Orbital Cellulitis

The most common pathogens of orbital cellulitis are the *Staphylococcus* and *Streptococcus* species. Less common causative organisms include the *Haemophilus influenzae*, *Pseudomonas*, *Klebsiella*, *Enterococcus*, *Peptostreptococcus*, *Fusobacterium*, and *Bacteroides* species.[3,4,5] Since the introduction of the *H. influenzae* (Hib) vaccine in 1985, *H. influenzae* has become an infrequent causative organism for pediatric periorbital cellulitis.[6] More recently, an increase in the incidence of methicillin-resistant *Staphylococcus aureus* (MRSA) as a causative agent has been observed.

Bacterial growth in purulent cultures may be difficult to obtain. At our institution, only 2 out of 10 patients affected by subperiosteal abscess had positive cultures for *S. pneumoniae*.[7]

26.4 Physical Examination

The ear, nose, and throat (ENT) specialist should evaluate the nasal cavity for any sign of acute rhinosinusitis (edema of the

Table 26.1 Chandler's classification of orbital complications

I	Preseptal cellulitis
II	Orbital cellulitis
III	Subperiosteal abscess
IV	Orbital abscess
V	Cavernous sinus thrombosis

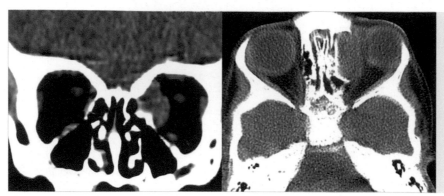

Fig. 26.1 Subperiosteal abscess on CT scan (coronal and axial views).

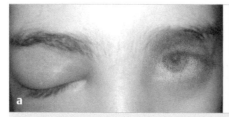
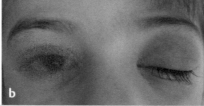
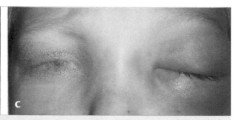

Fig. 26.2 Three different similar clinical aspects. We found a subperiosteal abscess on CT scan only in (c).

nasal mucosa and purulent secretions). If possible, nasal decongestion under endoscopic view should be performed.

An ophthalmologist should evaluate the affected eye. The lid involved is generally swollen, with loss of skin crease, and is erythematous (▶ Fig. 26.2). Visual acuity and pupil reactivity should also be evaluated. The presence of proptosis and ophthalmoplegia generally indicates postseptal orbital involvement and, therefore, the presence of a purulent collection.

Radiological assessment with a CT scan is usually obtained for every patient in whom an abscess is suspected.

A neurosurgical consultation should be requested in the presence or suspicion of any intracranial complication.

26.5 Management Options

Orbital cellulitis represents a serious infection, warranting prompt antibiotic therapy due to catastrophic complications, such as visual loss, intracranial infection, and sepsis.

Before the antibiotic era, patients affected by orbital cellulitis died from meningitis in 17% of cases or suffered from permanent visual loss in 20% of cases.

The treatment of orbital complications seems to depend on the Chandler classification stage. In fact, stages I and II of the Chandler classification are usually managed with medical therapy, while the other stages usually require a surgical approach to clear the pus collection. Stage V of this classification represents an intracranial extension of the infection rather than a mere orbital complication.

Medical therapy is usually empiric and based on a parenteral broad-spectrum antibiotic, such as combined penicillin (ampicillin-sulbactam; amoxicillin/clavulanic acid) or second- or, less frequently, third-generation cephalosporin. In cases where an association between gram-positive and anaerobes is suspected, clindamycin may be added to the combined penicillin or cephalosporin. In cases of an infection due to MRSA, vancomycin may be considered as a possible treatment.

Moreover, nasal decongestant and steroid nasal sprays may be used to reduce nasal inflammation. At our institution, we also prefer to administer IV steroids (methylprednisolone) to reduce the inflammatory component of the infection more rapidly. The use of oral or IV steroids for orbital cellulitis seems to have no particular adverse effect on children.[8,9]

Children affected by periorbital cellulitis (erythema and edema of the eyelid skin) without any proptosis or impairment of eye movements can generally be managed solely by medical therapy (▶ Fig. 26.3). Even cases of young children (younger than 9 years) presenting small periorbital abscesses without any visual impairment may be treated medically.

Children presenting with small purulent collections (≤ 5 mm) without any visual impairment and with no ophthalmoplegia or proptosis may be treated with medical treatment alone.[10] Interestingly, Arjmand et al outlined the necessity of performing surgical drainage in cases of subperiosteal orbital abscess, since visual acuity may be unchanged even in cases of rapid progression of the infection toward a serious intracranial complication.[11]

On the other hand, in older children, in the presence of large purulent collections and visual impairment, medical therapy is usually not sufficient and must be associated with surgical treatment.

When a surgical approach is required to achieve the removal of the purulent collection, the decision is mainly focused on a transnasal endoscopic approach. However, in the cases in which the transnasal approach is not able to completely clear the collection, an external approach must be added to the endoscopic one. For instance, in cases of superior and superolateral collections or eyelid abscess, an external approach must be considered. Tanna et al indicated the necessity of performing an

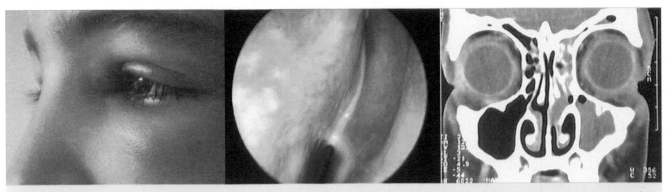

Fig. 26.3 A 9-year-old girl with mild erythema and edema without proptosis. No evident subperiosteal orbital abscess was visible at CT. Medical treatment was started with complete clinical resolution after 48 hours.

external approach when the purulent collection is located superolaterally with several orbital muscles involved.[12]

In conclusion, urgent surgical drainage should be considered in the cases that do not improve or even worsen with adequate medical management, or in those cases presenting visual deterioration (decreased vision or color vision, or afferent pupillary defect). Nevertheless, there is no universally accepted guideline for the treatment of subperiosteal abscesses, and each case should be treated independently. Cooperation among specialists, such as the ENT surgeon, the ophthalmologist, and the pediatrician, is of paramount importance in order to decide on and tailor the best treatment.

If the patient has improved sufficiently to be discharged, the antibiotic therapy can be changed to oral therapy and usually continued for 2 or 3 weeks.

26.6 The Role of Endoscopic Endonasal Surgery

A pediatric subperiosteal abscess is considered an abscess pocket localized between the lamina papyracea and the periorbita. The transnasal endoscopic approach seems to have a major role in clearing this purulent collection, mainly due to the relative ease with which this anatomic area endonasally can be reached. Although several authors have pointed out the effectiveness of antibiotic therapy for subperiosteal abscess in children younger than 9 years, our philosophy is to drain the abscess as soon as possible.[13,14,15] All the patients in our series who received surgical treatment had already been treated for several days by oral and IV antibiotics without any significant improvement.

The procedure always requires general anesthesia. Topical vasoconstriction is usually obtained through vasoconstrictor-soaked cottonoids. To perform the entire procedure, 4- or 2.7-mm 0- or 30-degree endoscopes are generally used. In rare cases, angled scopes such as 45 degrees, can become useful in visualizing the maxillary sinus.

A dedicated set of instruments for pediatric functional endoscopic sinus surgery must always be available to carry out the surgery. A microdebrider with a pediatric 2.9-mm blade is also generally useful in facilitating the dissection.

The procedure starts with medialization of the middle turbinate, and uncinate process removal. Middle turbinate resection (partial or total) is generally avoided. Uncinate resection

exposes the natural ostium of the maxillary sinus and the anterior ethmoid. The bulla is then entered, and the anterior ethmoidotomy is completed. The ground lamella is then breached to enter the posterior ethmoid. All the partitions are removed to complete the ethmoidotomy. The mucosa covering the lamina papyracea is also removed to expose the bone. At this stage, an opening of the lamina papyracea at the level of the abscess pocket is carried out in order to safely clear the purulence collected between the periorbita and the bone. Gentle orbital pressure should be applied to facilitate purulent drainage through the defect. The periorbita should not be breached, and the resection of the lamina papyracea should only be partial and performed over the pus collection. The opening of the periorbita should be reserved for those cases also having an orbital abscess.

Nasal packing can be accomplished with absorbable or nonabsorbable material. If nonabsorbable material is used, it must be removed the day after in order to guarantee maximum ventilation of the surgical cavity.

26.7 Case Example

A 14-year-old patient was referred to the ENT department of the University of Bologna for a definitive surgical treatment of a persistent subperiosteal orbital abscess of the left eye.

This patient had been operated on transnasally elsewhere 3 days earlier with partial left ethmoidotomy to resolve acute ethmoiditis associated with orbital cellulitis and possible subperiosteal abscess. This surgical treatment was pursued without any opening of the lamina papyracea and drainage of the purulent collection. Unfortunately, the eyelid erythema and edema worsened dramatically the day after this first surgery (▶ Fig. 26.4). When ophthalmoplegia ensued, a new CT scan of the orbit and paranasal sinuses was obtained (▶ Fig. 26.5). This radiological assessment showed a large purulent collection at the level of the left orbit, with pressure on the periorbita and displacement of the globe. Although ophthalmoplegia was in fact present, the ophthalmologic examination did not show any visual loss.

The patient was referred to our institution, where it was decided to immediately drain the purulent collection. The transnasal endoscopic route was chosen to resolve the infection; a revision of the middle meatotomy, complete sphenoethmoidectomy, and partial lamina papyracea removal were sufficient to completely drain the purulent collection. The

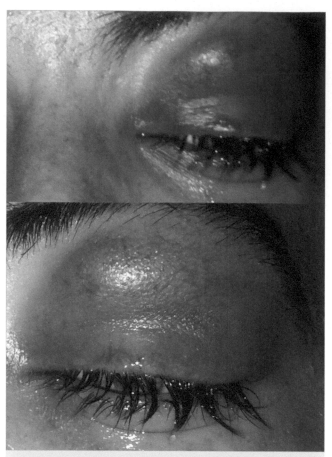

Fig. 26.4 A 14-year-old boy referred to our institution for the transnasal endoscopic drainage of a subperiosteal abscess of the left orbit.

microbiologic result did not show any growth on pus sampling. The symptoms of this patient, such as ophthalmoplegia and eyelid appearance, improved in just few hours after the definitive surgery (▶ Fig. 26.6). After 5 years of follow-up, the patient is still free from any recurrent periorbital infection.

26.8 Operative Pearls

An anteroposterior ethmoidotomy is usually performed to completely expose the lamina papyracea. The opening of the lamina papyracea is essential for obtaining complete drainage of the purulent collection. The removal of the lamina papyracea is generally not complete, and the opening should be carried out on the area of the purulent collection. Curved suction tubes (possibly with a blunt tip) should be used to apply pressure on the periorbita and facilitate drainage of the pus. Opening of the periorbita is not recommended, but is usually required when the suppurative process is extended within the orbital content.

26.9 Operative Pitfalls

The otolaryngologist should be familiar with the endoscopic approach in general and orbital decompression. Incomplete surgeries, such as partial ethmoidectomies, are not sufficient for approaching subperiosteal abscesses. A pediatric set of instruments for endoscopic sinus surgery along with pediatric telescopes must be available. Timely ophthalmologic and ENT examinations are essential for deciding whether surgical drainage is required in order to prevent disastrous complications.

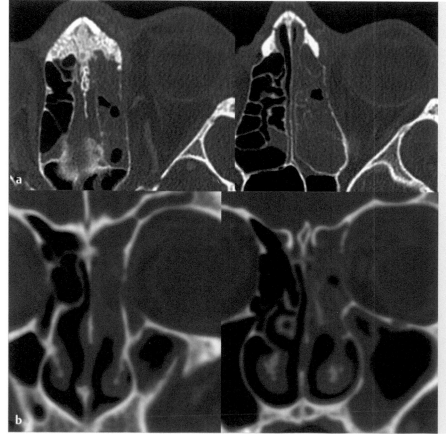

Fig. 26.5 Axial (a) and coronal (b) views of the left orbital cellulitis and subperiosteal abscess.

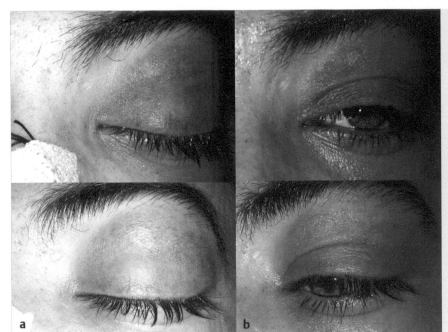

Fig. 26.6 The same patient immediately and 48 hours after the surgical procedure.

26.10 Conclusion

Medical treatment seems to remain the mainstay of management for subperiosteal abscess, although it should be associated with surgical drainage in some cases. Surgical drainage of a subperiosteal abscess is dependent on the presence of visual impairment, ophthalmoplegia, and proptosis. Decision-making is also dependent on the progression of the disease and failure to improve with antibiotic therapy. Coordinated specialist evaluations of patients are essential for avoiding the serious complications of orbital cellulitis.

If surgical drainage is needed, the transnasal endoscopic approach is usually sufficient for clearing the purulent collection. However, in cases of subperiosteal abscesses extending superiorly and superolaterally or in cases of eyelid abscesses, an external approach must be considered.

References

[1] Giusan AO, Kubanova AA, Uzdenova RKh. Rhinosinusogenic orbital complications: the prevalence and principles of treatment. Vestn Otorinolaringol. 2010(4):64–67

[2] Chandler JR, Langenbrunner DJ, Stevens ER. The pathogenesis of orbital complications in acute rhinosinusitis. Laryngoscope. 1970; 80(9):1414–1428

[3] Brook I. Microbiology and antimicrobial treatment of orbital and intracranial complications of rhinosinusitis in children and their management. Int J Pediatr Otorhinolaryngol. 2009; 73(9):1183–1186

[4] Liao S, Durand ML, Cunningham MJ. Sinogenic orbital and subperiosteal abscesses: microbiology and methicillin-resistant Staphylococcus aureus incidence. Otolaryngol Head Neck Surg. 2010; 143(3):392–396

[5] McKinley SH, Yen MT, Miller AM, Yen KG. Microbiology of pediatric orbital cellulitis. Am J Ophthalmol. 2007; 144(4):497–501

[6] Barone SR, Aiuto LT. Periorbital and orbital cellulitis in the Haemophilus influenzae vaccine era. J Pediatr Ophthalmol Strabismus. 1997; 34(5):293–296

[7] Sciarretta V, Macrì G, Farneti P, Tenti G, Bordonaro C, Pasquini E. Endoscopic surgery for the treatment of pediatric subperiosteal orbital abscess: a report of 10 cases. Int J Pediatr Otorhinolaryngol. 2009; 73(12):1669–1672

[8] Yen MT, Yen KG. Effect of corticosteroids in the acute management of pediatric orbital cellulitis with subperiosteal abscess. Ophthal Plast Reconstr Surg. 2005; 21(5):363–366, discussion 366–367

[9] Hongguang P, Lan L, Zebin W, Guowei C. Pediatric nasal orbital cellulitis in Shenzhen (South China): etiology, management, and outcomes. Int J Pediatr Otorhinolaryngol. 2016; 87:98–104

[10] Oxford LE, McClay J. Complications of acute rhinosinusitis in children. Otolaryngol Head Neck Surg. 2005; 133(1):32–37

[11] Arjmand EM, Lusk RP, Muntz HR. Pediatric rhinosinusitis and subperiosteal orbital abscess formation: diagnosis and treatment. Otolaryngol Head Neck Surg. 1993; 109(5):886–894

[12] Tanna N, Preciado DA, Clary MS, Choi SS. Surgical treatment of subperiosteal orbital abscess. Arch Otolaryngol Head Neck Surg. 2008; 134(7):764–767

[13] Harris GJ. Subperiosteal abscess of the orbit. Age as a factor in the bacteriology and response to treatment. Ophthalmology. 1994; 101(3):585–595

[14] Garcia GH, Harris GJ. Criteria for nonsurgical management of subperiosteal abscess of the orbit: analysis of outcomes 1988–1998. Ophthalmology. 2000; 107(8):1454–1456, discussion 1457–1458

[15] Brown CL, Graham SM, Griffin MC, et al. Pediatric medial subperiosteal orbital abscess: medical management where possible. Am J Rhinol. 2004; 18(5):321–327

Part III

Skull Base Closure, Complication Management, and Postoperative Care

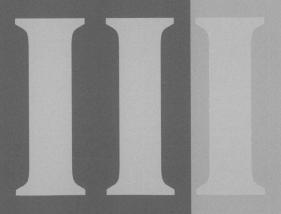

27 Closure Techniques for the Pediatric Skull Base: Vascularized Flaps

Cristine N. Klatt-Cromwell, Brian D. Thorp, Charles S. Ebert, Deanna M. Sasaki-Adams, Matthew G. Ewend, and Adam M. Zanation

Abstract

Endoscopic endonasal surgery has significantly evolved to provide various options for the resection of skull base lesions. These options pioneered in the adult population, have expanded to address the needs of the pediatric population. Anatomical differences and the constant changing of the pediatric skull make pediatric endonasal work more challenging. Meticulous pre-surgical planning and realistic goals are imperative. This paper discusses the multiple reconstructive options and how they were developed in and studied in the adult population and how the same techniques can serve the pediatric population.

Keywords: skull base reconstruction, nasoseptal flap, pericranial flap, temporoparietal fascia flap, CSF leak, endoscopic skull base surgery, pediatric

27.1 Introduction to Vascularized Flaps

Over recent years, endoscopic endonasal surgery has dramatically evolved and expanded to provide diverse options for the resection of skull base lesions. Extensive understanding of anatomy, combined with advances in instrumentation and technique, have allowed for significant evolution in these procedures. These expanded endonasal approaches (EEA) are being used to treat a multitude of complex intradural and extradural processes; although EEA were pioneered in the adult population, they have been progressively expanded to address the pediatric population.

A thorough understanding of anatomy has allowed surgery to encompass not only the paramedian skull base but also the orbit and upper cervical spine. With the use of more extensive approaches, evolution of reconstructive techniques has comparably followed. Initially, the bulk of skull base reconstruction was performed with cellular or acellular grafts. In a meta-analysis by Hegazy et al,[1] cerebrospinal fluid (CSF) leaks resulting from trauma were repaired with cellular and acellular grafts. The study included 289 patients, with an overall success rate of 90%. As techniques expanded, reconstructive efforts began to encompass techniques using vascularized tissue. In a study by Thorp et al,[2] 152 patients underwent skull base reconstruction with vascularized tissue, including primarily the nasoseptal flap (NSF) and the pericranial flap (PCF), but also several other vascularized tissue reconstructions. Overall, the study found a CSF leak rate of 3.3%, demonstrating success of these reconstructions. Further discussion of these reconstructive techniques will take place later in this chapter.

As with adult surgical procedures, approaches to the pediatric skull base through an endoscopic endonasal route have significantly evolved over the recent years. Advantages include the absence of external skin incisions and the need for craniotomy. While endonasal surgery overall has multiple advantages, careful attention to the differences between the pediatric and adult skull base anatomy is vital to success, as the developing cranium undergoes progressive pneumatization, further emphasizing thorough understanding of the relationship of critical structures. The literature includes several studies describing successful approaches to the midline skull base through EEA in the pediatric population.[3,4,5] This chapter will describe the differences between adult and pediatric endonasal surgeries and will discuss available surgical reconstructive techniques.

27.2 The Pediatric Skull Base

In the pediatric patient, the cranium and endonasal skull base are constantly changing. Pneumatization of the sinuses generally begins around the age of 2 years and continues into puberty, with different sinuses pneumatizing at different times and rates. In a study by Waitzman et al,[6] CT scans were used to demonstrate that cranial growth increased rapidly in the first few years of life, leveling off at about the age of 10 years. In comparison, this same group found that upper midface structures did not increase dramatically early in life, instead increasing when children were older. In a retrospective radioanatomical study by Shah et al, CT scans were used to assess the anatomic limitations for transsphenoidal EEA in pediatric patients.[5] All the patients included in the study were divided by age and compared to adult controls. CT scans were assessed, and measurements for expected skull base defects including those for transsellar, transcribriform, and transclival approaches were made by both a neuroradiologist and an otolaryngologist. For each of the defects, calculations compared the NSF area for skull base reconstruction. Patients included in the study were divided by age. The study concluded that before the age of 10 years, the NSF should be used with caution, as its size may not permit its use in skull base reconstruction, depending on the defect size. The group emphasized that careful assessment of the predicted defect for each patient should be performed prior to surgery for optimal reconstructive considerations.[5]

Relative anatomic differences in the pediatric skull base compared to adults may make pediatric endonasal work more challenging. In a separate study, Tatreau et al assessed the role of developmental immaturity of the skull base and its relationship to the surrounding neurovasculature.[7] In this study, three separate bony anatomic limitations were discussed. The first anatomic limitation is the piriform aperture, which is the first superficial bony structure encountered during skull base surgery. In the developing pediatric population, soft tissues may be displaced; however, it is important to avoid damage to this area to avoid problems with normal development. Moreover, the size of this area is important in the passage of instruments during skull base surgery. Tatreau et al found that this area was prohibitively small for expanded EEA in patients younger than 24 months. From this age to approximately age 6 or 7 years, the space is narrow but not prohibitive, and after that age, it resembles the size of an adult nose. Because of this, sublabial approaches may be required to approach cases in the youngest of patients.[7]

The second anatomic limitation in pediatric skull base surgery is incomplete pneumatization of the sphenoid sinus. The patterns of pneumatization of the sphenoid sinus have previously been described in the literature.[8,9,10] Studies have found that the pneumatization patterns can be classified into three categoriespresellar/conchal, sellar, and postsellarand follow a pattern of aeration from anterior to posterior. Tatreau et al found that by the age of 6 or 7 years, the anterior wall of the sphenoid sinus was fully pneumatized. They also found that by this same age, 77% of patients had anterior sellar wall pneumatization and 32% had sellar floor pneumatization; additionally, 88 ± 17% of the planum was pneumatized as well. Other findings included the pneumatization of the dorsum sellae, which was not evident in 84% of patients younger than 16 years. Spread of pneumatization to the clival recess was not seen before the age of 10 years, but was present in 89% of patients older than 15 years.[7] While incomplete sphenoid sinus pneumatization does correlate with the need for more drilling during surgery, this is not prohibitive to endonasal approaches. In a study by Cavallo et al, several anatomical conditions that limit the use of endoscopic surgery were also discussed. This includes thicker bone overlying the planum and tuberculum, making approaches more complex.[11] However, careful surgical planning and adequate imaging can overcome these challenges, allowing EEA in the pediatric population.

With the advantages of pediatric endonasal skull base surgery clearly evident, it is important to reflect on the risks and morbidity associated with injuries to neurovascular structures in this area. There is an inherent relationship between the internal carotid arteries (ICAs) and ongoing sphenoid sinus pneumatization that occurs in a developing skull base. Tatreau et al assessed the pediatric patients included in their study, measuring minimum distances between the carotid arteries at the level of the cavernous sinus and at the level of the superior clivus, immediately below the sellar floor. Around age 12 years, 89% of patients were found to have some degree of prominence in the vertical portion of the ICA.[7] Based on CT measurements, the study found that intercarotid distances at the superior clivus were relatively fixed after 24 months. At the cavernous sinus, the intercarotid distance was significantly smaller in patients younger than 24 months and up to 6 to 7 years, compared to 9- to 10-year-old patients. There was no statistically significant difference in patients after age 9 to 10 years compared to adults. Overall, the average distance at the level of the cavernous sinus in adults is approximately 12 to 18 mm, which decreases only to about 10 mm in 3- and 4-year-old patients. Because of this, endoscopic transsellar surgery could be performed in all except the youngest of patients. Yilmazlar et al discussed how a narrow intercarotid distance at the level of the cavernous sinus could be considered a relative contraindication to transsphenoidal surgery.[12] Several studies emphasize that this largely depends on the experience and confidence of the surgeon.

27.3 Approaches to Skull Base Reconstruction

With the anatomical considerations outlined earlier, skull base surgery in the pediatric population has the same goals and

objectives as it does in the adult population. These goals include safe resection of pathology followed by watertight closure of the defect separating the nasal cavity from the intracranial space/structures. These goals prevent potential complications that result in postoperative morbidity including pneumocephalus, CSF leak, meningitis, or death. Preoperative planning and careful patient selection are critical for safe surgical outcomes. Meticulous surgical planning for skull base surgery in the pediatric population is especially important, and while pediatric patients have a decreased incidence of comorbid conditions, including smoking and obesity, prior radiation remains an important factor to be considered. Kassam et al also emphasize the importance of considering the size of pediatric patients, as younger children may have smaller blood volumes. Because of this, procedures may require staging to keep the patient safe.[3] In addition, because children are still growing, surgical effects on craniofacial growth should also be considered. While endonasal work typically does not disrupt growth centers, combined open procedures may disrupt growth plates and dentition in pediatric patients. Even with special considerations, care for pediatric patients should be as standardized as possible for optimization of outcomes.

Historically, skull base surgery has involved the use of lumbar drains. As described by Stokken et al, lumbar drains were frequently used in skull base surgery for CSF diversion postoperatively.[13] As the field has evolved and changed, the literature now reflects a preference to not use drains in skull base surgery unless patient-specific factors require its use. As described by Ransom et al,[14] lumbar drains were independently assessed and found to have a complication rate of 12.3%. A combination of improved reconstructive techniques and associated lumbar drain complications have driven the field to use drains more judiciously, specifically in patients with recurrent leaks requiring multiple reconstruction or those with confounders that elevate intracranial pressure. Zanation et al identified that patients with defects along both the clivus and anterior skull base were more likely to have leaks after surgery.[15] In the pediatric population, lumbar drains are further complicated due to patient discomfort, associated complications, and difficulty in placement. While no true consensus exists for which patients require lumbar drain use, the surgical team should carefully assess the patient and expected procedures prior to surgery to determine the need for lumbar drainage concurrently.

27.3.1 Reconstructive Options

Acellular Grafts

In the skull base reconstructive ladder, there is extensive literature describing multiple reconstructive options. As they were traditionally developed and studied in the adult population, many of the techniques that will be described here have limited data in the pediatric skull base surgery literature. However, these techniques serve as the workhorse for pediatric skull base reconstruction and will be carefully delineated.

Acellular grafts have always played a vital role in skull base reconstruction. Several products, including acellular dermal matrix (AlloDerm LifeCell, Branchburg, NJ) and collagen matrix (Duragen, Integra Life Sciences, Plainsboro, NJ), have been used as adjuncts to skull base reconstruction. For inlay techniques,

Alloderm has been used in the subdural or epidural plane. If used as an onlay over the bony skull base, all underlying mucosa must be removed to prevent mucocele formation, and it must be fully hydrated prior to use. For surgical procedures that require the removal of dura, collagen matrix Duragen may be used as either an inlay, between the brain and dura in a subdural plane, or in the epidural plane, between the dura and bony skull base. This graft has been used to seal the defect and eliminate CSF leakage from dural resection. With surgical resection in which bony margins are limited, this may also be used as an onlay graft. All acellular grafting techniques must be bolstered into place using a combination of packing tissues that will be delineated further in the text.

Cellular Grafts

In addition to acellular options, cellular grafts were among the first techniques used for skull base reconstruction. As with all reconstruction, it is important to emphasize the importance placed on multilayer closure. In a study by Harvey et al, free tissue was used to repair smaller defects (< 1 cm) in conjunction with multilayer closure and was found to have a success rate of greater than 90%.[16] Several options can be used, which are described here.

Free Mucosal Graft

Mucosal grafts are available from tissue throughout the nasal cavity and can be used for reconstruction of skull base defects. Grafts can be taken from the septum, nasal floor, and/or middle turbinate. This reconstructive technique does not require a second surgical site. However, nasal malignancies may preclude the use of mucosa from within the nose for reconstruction due to concerns for underlying disease. During surgery, surgeons may elect to remove the middle turbinate and/or the septum as part of the approach or resection. With these resections, harvest of the mucosa from these structures may serve as free mucosal grafts. In addition, surgical approach and resection provides wide access to the nasal floor, which may also be used for reconstruction. To harvest nasal floor mucosa, needle-tip bovie electrocautery is bent to 45 degrees, and used to make circumferential incisions. Variations in size of the mucosal graft can be made with extension onto the septum and under the inferior turbinate. The graft is then carefully elevated with a Cottle elevator, and the graft is kept in saline until it is required for reconstruction. Meticulous hemostasis is confirmed along the donor site prior to use of the graft for reconstruction. As previously described, it is vital to remove all underlying mucosa from the reconstruction site in order to prevent mucocele formation. Multilayer bolstering for closure is used following graft placement as described below.

Abdominal Fat

Abdominal fat grafts are frequently used as a component of skull base reconstruction. These grafts are traditionally used to obliterate space within a defect in order to create a more laminar reconstructive site. This graft may be used in conjunction with other reconstruction tools, including acellular grafts and/or vascularized reconstructions. The incision must be made at a second surgical site, either the periumbilical region, lower abdominal area, or lateral hip and must be prepped and draped

separately. The incision is made, and circumferential dissection is performed in order to obtain the adequate volume required for reconstruction. Once complete, the wound is irrigated, hemostasis is confirmed, and it is closed in multiple layers. A drain may be used if the size of the defect requires it; however, this is rarely required in children. Caution must be undertaken in this harvest, as many children are thin and have only small amounts of fat. Also, with extensive harvest, cosmetic deformity may result, thereby precluding large periumbilical grafts. Recently, dermal fat grafts have been used in skull base reconstruction. To harvest, an ellipse incision is made. Leaving the dermis attached to the fat, the epidermis is removed to obtain the composite graft. Fat can still be circumferentially dissected around the dermal component, but it remains attached for use. The dermis allows for a stronger reconstruction that is easier to manipulate during insertion and further graft placement. Just like traditional fat grafts, the dermal fat graft can be used with further acellular and cellular reconstructions as part of the multilayer closure.

It should be noted that in a study by Hadad et al, resections that were reconstructed with free tissue grafts, which resulted in a greater than 3-cm defect, were found to have a CSF leak rate of 20 to 30%, a rate that was unacceptable. Because of this, they recommended vascularized reconstruction techniques.[17] These will be further described in the next section.

Vascularized Flaps

Vascularized skull base reconstruction has become a technique widely used in adjunct to the acellular and cellular techniques described earlier. Initially described in 2006 by Hadad et al, the NSF has become the chosen technique for skull base reconstruction.[17] Comprised of mucoperiosteum and mucoperichondrium from the septum, this vascularized flap obtains its vascular supply from the posterior septal artery, a branch of the sphenopalatine artery. In adults, one of the greatest advantages is the strong pedicle and the expansile nature of the flap, able to reach from orbit to orbit and from sella to frontal sinus.[15] The flap also eliminates the need for a second surgical site and is associated with minimal morbidity. Its primary disadvantage is that in all patients, adult and pediatric, its harvest must occur prior to surgical resection. In addition, tumor involvement or vascular compromise eliminates this as a surgical reconstructive option. Previous nasal surgery is not an absolute contraindication to the use of this flap; however, great care must be taken to elevate the flap, and an alternative reconstructive option must be planned if warranted. This flap has specific potential disadvantages in the pediatric population that must be considered prior to surgery. In a study by Shah et al, radioanatomical measurements were taken to hypothesize the size of the skull base resection and NSF.[5] Measurements required for reconstruction of transcribriform, transsellar, and transclival defects were measured in patients of all age groups. Pediatric patients were assessed for adequacy of the NSF size and CSF leak rate. Based on CT measurements, transcribriform defects reconstructed with an NSF would not be sufficient until after age of 9 to 10 years. Prior to this, the length of the NSF would not cover the length of the defect. For transsellar procedures, the NSF reconstruction would be adequate in 6- to 7-year-old patients. At this point, it would be long enough to span the defect. The width of the flap is sufficient except for the youngest of patients. For transclival procedures, the study found that only three adults had adequate length to reconstruct the area sufficiently; therefore, all pediatric patients did not have enough septal length to make this a viable reconstructive option. Overall, the study noted that the NSF may not provide a viable reconstructive option for patients undergoing skull base surgery prior to the age of 10 years.[5] However, the study does not take into account patient-specific variations, which may further include or exclude the NSF as a reconstructive option. Because of this, presurgical planning is vital to success.

27.3.2 Nasoseptal Flap Technique

Once the independent patient data have been extensively reviewed and physical examination performed, the NSF may be selected for skull base reconstruction. The patient is positioned and prepped, and image guidance is in place. The procedure begins with gentle outfracturing of bilateral inferior turbinates, and the middle turbinate on the side of the NSF is removed or lateralized based on surgeon preference. Control of bleeding from the middle turbinate basal lamella remnant must be done with care to prevent damage to the underlying pedicle. The remaining superior turbinate is then outfractured gently, allowing identification of the sphenoid ostium in the sphenoethmoidal recess. Once the position is confirmed, attention is turned to incisions. The extended-length needle-tip monopolar cautery bent at 45 degrees is then used to make parallel incisions in the septum. The first incision is made inferiorly, beginning at the posterior choanal margin and then transitioning to the nasal septum at its junction with the nasal floor. The second incision is placed vertically anteriorly within the nasal vestibule, extending as far forward as possible to the mucocutaneous junction. The third superior incision begins at the natural os of the sphenoid sinus, and comes forward and superiorly. This is done approximately 1 to 2 cm from the roof of the cavity to prevent damage to the olfactory epithelium. The Cottle elevator is used to begin flap elevation, typically starting at each of the incision lines to prevent tearing. Once the front of the flap is elevated, more posterior elevation can be performed with less risk to flap continuity. Once the flap is completely elevated and the pedicle isolated, the flap is tucked into the nasopharynx or ipsilateral maxillary sinus. It can remain in either location until the extirpative portion of the surgery is complete and the defect is ready to be reconstructed. The flap must be removed with care from either location to ensure that the flap pedicle is not inadvertently twisted. It is then used as part of a multilayer reconstruction, and can be used with the previously described acellular and cellular techniques. Once the flap is ready to be placed into position, it is important that it be in direct contact with the surrounding bone margin with no mucosal overlap. The flap is then bolstered in the fashion described below. If during resection the defect required is larger than expected and cannot be adequately covered with the NSF, it is important to consider alternative reconstructive options to prevent postoperative complications.

27.3.3 Endoscopic-Assisted Pericranial Flap

In the pediatric patient population, open craniofacial resections were traditionally reconstructed with locoregional flaps. Including the PCF or the temporalis muscle flap. [18] While these reconstructions require both a second surgical site and external incisions, one of their benefits is that the tissue is unaffected by underlying pathology. In addition, cranial growth is typically faster than facial growth in the young population, allowing for abundant tissue for reconstruction.[19] It is for this same reason that the limitations of the NSF were discussed earlier. Should the surgical resection be extensive, or should intranasal tissues be inadequate for skull base reconstruction, the endoscopic-assisted PCF is a good reconstructive option. Described by Zanation et al, this robust flap is based on the supraorbital and supratrochlear arteries.[20] Its expansive size allows for extensive reconstruction of challenging defects, and it can be used in children in whom the NSF is inadequate. The flap must be harvested from a second incision using a multitude of techniques, including endoscopic-assisted, hemicoronal, or coronal approaches. The flap is then inserted into the nose through a small glabellar incision with an underlying bony defect through the nasion. When the endoscopic-assisted PCF is planned for reconstruction, the hair and face must be prepped and draped in the standard sterile fashion. The hair is stapled away from the marked incision line, not shaved. In order to protect the pedicle, the supraorbital notch is identified, and 1.5-cm markings are made on each side, allowing maintenance of a 3-cm flap pedicle. In addition, the midline is marked to avoid violation of the contralateral PCF, which can be preserved for further reconstructive efforts if warranted. Once the surgical resection is complete, attention is turned to elevation of the PCF for reconstruction. The incision is made and carried down to the subgaleal plane. The endoscope may be used during this process. Once elevation of the pocket is complete, the extended-length needle-tip bovie is used to harvest the pericranium. Lateral incisions are placed and connected posteriorly, ensuring that a large flap can be harvested without violation of the pedicle or contralateral PCF. The flap is then elevated carefully with or without the use of the endoscope, depending on the approach utilized. Once the flap has been elevated, attention is turned to the glabella, where an incision is made down to the level of the periosteum. The high-speed drill is then used to drill through the bone of the nasion to enter the nasal cavity. It is important that this bony opening is not restrictive, or it will compromise the pedicle of the flap when it is placed into the nose. With the nasionectomy complete, the flap is moved into the nasal cavity and placed into position as part of the skull base reconstruction. As with other flaps, it is important that the flap be in contact with surrounding bone margin. As with the NSF, this flap may be used with other acellular and cellular reconstructive techniques and is bolstered as described below. The external wounds are then copiously irrigated and closed in a multilayer fashion. A drain is typically used to close the dead space in the scalp and prevent seroma or hematoma formation.

27.3.4 Turbinate Flaps

While the NSF and the endoscopic-assisted PCF comprise the bulk of skull base reconstructions in the pediatric population, inferior turbinate and middle turbinate flaps may be used, but are done so less commonly. Zanation et al describe these two flaps, pedicled on their respective arteries, which are branches of the posterior lateral nasal artery, a terminal branch of the sphenopalatine artery.[15] The inferior turbinate flap has a role in smaller skull base defects, specifically those in the parasellar and midclival regions. When used, bilateral inferior turbinate flaps can provide better coverage. The middle turbinate flap is less commonly used due to thin mucosa and difficulty of harvest.

27.3.5 Bolstering Technique

After any reconstructive technique, it is vital to have a standardized approach to bolstering to produce reliable and consistent results. Once skull base reconstruction has been completed, Surgicel (Ethicon US, LLC) is used circumferentially around the margins of the reconstruction. Following its placement, firm Nasopore (Polyganics, Groningen, the Netherlands) is used to further support key portions of the repair. Once this is in adequate position, a biologic glue-like Duraseal (Confluent Surgical Inc., Waltham, MA) is placed over the entire reconstruction, providing a 3D bolster. Nasopore is then used in multiple layers to further support the entire reconstruction to prevent any movement during the initial period of healing and to ensure adequate support for adherence to the skull base. Finally, nondissolvable packs or a Foley balloon are placed under direct visualization to support the repair, which are typically removed prior to discharge from the hospital. The Foley catheter or nonabsorbable packs are typically kept in place anywhere from 3 to 7 days following surgery, and are removed prior to discharge. Nasal saline irrigations are typically started a week after surgery.

27.4 Conclusion

As previously described, presurgical planning and adequate preparation are vital to success in the pediatric patient population. Careful planning of reconstructive options reduces complications intraoperatively and allows consideration of secondary options when surgical resections are larger than expected and/or primary reconstructive options are inadequate. While medical comorbidities are less common in this patient population, patient age, size, and estimated blood volume should be assessed prior to surgery. Large tumors or those with expected large volume blood loss may require staged procedures in order to keep the patient safe. Embolization should be used selectively in certain tumor pathologies to reduce intraoperative blood loss. Consideration of prior radiation therapy and other healing complications are also vital to intraoperative safety and postoperative success. With all factors in mind, standardization should be attempted for pediatric patients much as it is for adults.

As previously discussed, anatomy is a vital component in pediatric skull base surgery. Therefore, an image guidance system loaded with fine-cut CT and MRI data are used throughout all pediatric surgeries. Careful induction to anesthesia is vital, especially in cases with intracranial extension. In addition, careful blood pressure control, avoiding hypotension and hypertension, is important to limit intraoperative blood loss and prevent intracranial complications. Fluid balance is carefully monitored with a foley catheter. Attention to proper positioning is also vital to success. The bed is typically turned 90 degrees away from the care of anesthesia, with the head of the bed just slightly elevated. Careful attention is placed on adequate positioning to ensure all pressure points are padded prior to the commencement of procedures. The patient is also adequately prepped and draped in the standard sterile fashion for any reconstructive procedures that require different surgical sites, including the abdomen, scalp, or thigh. Once the patient is positioned and prepped, the image guidance system is brought onto the field and registration is completed.

27.4.1 Postoperative Care and Complications

Standardization of care for pediatric patients undergoing skull base resections and reconstructions is vital to reduce complications. While the varying ages of pediatric patients make this more challenging than in adults, adherence to a routine helps identify problems that present in the postoperative period. As discussed, multilayer closure is emphasized in all reconstructions, including the use of a Foley catheter or nondissolvable packs as a final bolster for the repair. Patients are monitored closely following surgery to identify complications as soon as possible. Patel et al found that intraoperative high-flow CSF leak was the most reliable predictor of postoperative CSF leak.[21] Because of this, children are monitored closely after surgery. Bed rest and foley catheters may be employed to help reduce movement following surgery, thus decreasing the risk of CSF leak during the acute healing period. Fluid balance in children is delicate; therefore, large intraoperative blood loss can require staging of procedures to keep the child safe.

Complications exist in endoscopic skull base surgery as with all surgeries. As described by Kassam et al, complications including CSF leak, pneumocephalus, meningitis, and graft failure exist following skull base surgery.[22] These are the same in pediatric patients. In a meta-analysis by Harvey et al, 38 separate studies were assessed for postoperative complications. In assessing all techniques for skull base reconstruction, the overall postoperative CSF leak rate was 11.5% (70/609).[16] The study further assessed that free tissue grafts had a leak rate of 15.6% (51/326), and vascularized flaps had a leak rate of 6.7%. While most outcome data are typically done for adult patients, the results can be interpreted for pediatric cases as well.

With expanding skull base surgical options for the pediatric population, we have discussed potential skull base reconstructive options. Overall, emphasis must be placed on meticulous presurgical planning, with realistic discussion of the planned resection and reconstruction. Pediatric patients and their families should be counseled about the potential for multiple reconstructive options prior to surgery, especially if a second surgical site may be required. In patients requiring large resections, the possibility of staged procedures should also be discussed. Additionally, facial growth defects pose a hypothetical risk. We do not know if facial growth defects are going to be a true risk for endoscopic skull base surgery. A discussion with the parents and long-term follow-up and future research regarding facial growth is important. While children present a complex challenge in skull base surgery and reconstruction, current techniques are well suited for optimal outcomes in these patients and continue to evolve over time.

References

[1] Hegazy HM, Carrau RL, Snyderman CH, Kassam A, Zweig J. Transnasal endoscopic repair of cerebrospinal fluid rhinorrhea: a meta-analysis. Laryngoscope. 2000; 110(7):1166–1172

[2] Thorp BD, Sreenath SB, Ebert CS, Zanation AM. Endoscopic skull base reconstruction: a review and clinical case series of 152 vascularized flaps used for surgical skull base defects in the setting of intraoperative cerebrospinal fluid leak. Neurosurg Focus. 2014; 37(4):E4

[3] Kassam A, Thomas AJ, Snyderman C, et al. Fully endoscopic expanded endonasal approach treating skull base lesions in pediatric patients. J Neurosurg. 2007; 106(2) Suppl:75–86

[4] Pirris SM, Pollack IF, Snyderman CH, et al. Corridor surgery: the current paradigm for skull base surgery. Childs Nerv Syst. 2007; 23(4):377–384

[5] Shah RN, Surowitz JB, Patel MR, et al. Endoscopic pedicled nasoseptal flap reconstruction for pediatric skull base defects. Laryngoscope. 2009; 119(6):1067–1075

[6] Waitzman AA, Posnick JC, Armstrong DC, Pron GE. Craniofacial skeletal measurements based on computed tomography: part II. Normal values and growth trends. Cleft Palate Craniofac J. 1992; 29(2):118–128

[7] Tatreau JR, Patel MR, Shah RN, et al. Anatomical considerations for endoscopic endonasal skull base surgery in pediatric patients. Laryngoscope. 2010; 120 (9):1730–1737

[8] Gruber DP, Brockmeyer D. Pediatric skull base surgery. 1. Embryology and developmental anatomy. Pediatr Neurosurg. 2003; 38(1):2–8

[9] Spaeth J, Krügelstein U, Schlöndorff G. The paranasal sinuses in CT-imaging: development from birth to age 25. Int J Pediatr Otorhinolaryngol. 1997; 39 (1):25–40

[10] Hamid O, El Fiky L, Hassan O, Kotb A, El Fiky S. Anatomic variations of the sphenoid sinus and their impact on trans-sphenoid pituitary surgery. Skull Base. 2008; 18(1):9–15

[11] Cavallo LM, de Divitiis O, Aydin S, et al. Extended endoscopic endonasal transsphenoidal approach to the suprasellar area: anatomic considerations: part 1. Neurosurgery. 2007; 61(3) Suppl:24–33, discussion 33–34

[12] Yilmazlar S, Kocaeli H, Eyigor O, Hakyemez B, Korfali E. Clinical importance of the basal cavernous sinuses and cavernous carotid arteries relative to the pituitary gland and macroadenomas: quantitative analysis of the complete anatomy. Surg Neurol. 2008; 70(2):165–174, discussion 174–175

[13] Stokken J, Recinos PF, Woodard T, Sindwani R. The utility of lumbar drains in modern endoscopic skull base surgery. Curr Opin Otolaryngol Head Neck Surg. 2015; 23(1):78–82

[14] Ransom ER, Palmer JN, Kennedy DW, Chiu AG. Assessing risk/benefit of lumbar drain use for endoscopic skull-base surgery. Int Forum Allergy Rhinol. 2011; 1(3):173–177

[15] Zanation AM, Thorp BD, Parmar P, Harvey RJ. Reconstructive options for endoscopic skull base surgery. Otolaryngol Clin North Am. 2011; 44(5): 1201–1222

[16] Harvey RJ, Parmar P, Sacks R, et al. Endoscopic skull base defects: a systematic review of published evidence. Laryngoscope. 2012; 122:452–459

[17] Hadad G, Bassagasteguy L, Carrau RL, et al. A novel reconstructive technique after endoscopic expanded endonasal approaches: vascular pedicle nasoseptal flap. Laryngoscope. 2006; 116(10):1882–1886

[18] Demonte F, Moore BA, Chang DW. Skull base reconstruction in the pediatric patient. Skull Base. 2007; 17(1):39–51

[19] Scott JH. The growth of the human face. Proc R Soc Med. 1954; 47(2):91–100

[20] Zanation AM, Snyderman CH, Carrau RL, Kassam AB, Gardner PA, Prevedello DM. Minimally invasive endoscopic pericranial flap: a new method for endonasal skull base reconstruction. Laryngoscope. 2009; 119(1):13–18

[21] Patel MR, Stadler ME, Snyderman CH, et al. How to choose? Endoscopic skull base reconstructive options and limitations. Skull Base. 2010; 20(6):397–404

[22] Kassam AB, Thomas A, Carrau RL, et al. Endoscopic reconstruction of the cranial base using a pedicled nasoseptal flap. Neurosurgery. 2008; 63(1) Suppl 1:ONS44–ONS52, discussion ONS52–ONS53

28 Closure Techniques for the Pediatric Skull Base: Multilayer Closure

João Mangussi-Gomes, Felipe Marconato, Leonardo Balsalobre, Eduardo Vellutini, and Aldo C. Stamm

Abstract

Endoscopic skull base reconstruction (ESBR) in children is not a trivial task. This is especially true for those large defects usually associated with high-flow cerebrospinal fluid leaks. Certainly, the best option is trying to repair them in a multilayer fashion. The mnemonic "**triple-F**" technique reminds the surgeon of the most commonly used materials for multilayer ESBR: **F**at, **F**ascia lata, and **F**lap. Fat grafts harvested from the thigh or the abdomen are quite useful to fill large cavities. Placement of large pieces of fascia lata and/or synthetic dural substitutes inlay and/or onlay is also an excellent option. Although using septal bone and cartilage as free grafts is quite interesting, there are some concerns that surgical manipulation of the nasal septum in children might interfere with further craniofacial growth. The order and position in which all these materials are placed might vary, but whatever the technique used, closure should be as watertight as possible. The use of nasoseptal flap (NSF) has become a mainstay in ESBR and should be placed on top of the reconstruction plane whenever viable. In spite of that, NSF is not always available or long enough, especially in very young infants. Other mucosal flaps and free mucosal grafts are very good alternatives to the classical NSF. Correct nasal packing prevents displacement of the materials used to reconstruct the skull base and is key at the end of the procedure.

Keywords: skull base reconstruction, multilayer, pediatric population, children, skull base defects, free grafts, mucosal flaps

28.1 Introduction

Endoscopic endonasal approaches (EEA) to skull base lesions in the pediatric population is a new and emerging field. The first clinical studies on this issue began to be published just around a decade ago.[1] Because of that, there are no guidelines or solid consensuses in this area, and the principles and techniques of EEA and endoscopic skull base reconstruction (ESBR) in children have been largely imported from the experience already gained with adults.[2]

Techniques used for ESBR in children may vary largely, depending mainly on the experience and preferences of the surgical team and on the case itself. Whatever the strategy used, it is essential to completely separate the intracranial content from the nasal cavity and consequently prevent postoperative complications. This is usually achieved after a watertight multilayer closure of the skull base defect, especially for those large openings associated with high-flow cerebrospinal fluid (CSF) leaks.[3,4]

28.2 Multilayer ESBR in Children: Principles, Materials, and Peculiarities

Multilayer ESBR, rather than a technique itself, should be considered a surgical reasoning or principle—as more layers are correctly selected and placed, the greater are the chances of success. The mnemonic "triple-F" technique reminds surgeons of the most commonly used materials for multilayer ESBR: **F**at, **F**ascia lata, and **F**lap.[4]

Fat serves as an autologous graft, which is useful to fill large surgical cavities. Fat grafts can be most commonly harvested from the following sites:

- Abdominal wall, via an infraumbilical or suprapubic incision: it provides large volumes of fat and resulting scars are minimal and discrete.
- Thigh, via a lateral longitudinal incision: it gives good amounts of fat, except in patients with very low body mass indexes. It is the site of choice when fascia lata is also needed, although it may result in unwanted scars.

Fascia lata can also be readily acquired from the lateral aspect of the thigh. It is an excellent autologous graft that is most commonly used as inlay and/or onlay graft to nicely close dural openings. Synthetic dural substitutes (e.g., DuraGen) might be used as alternatives or complements to fascia lata. They are quite useful when fascia lata is not sufficiently available (e.g., in young infants with very large skull base defects) or when skin incisions are undesired.

Harder grafts might also be used to reinforce the skull base closure. Pieces of **bone** and **cartilage** harvested from the nasal septum are useful in this context. There is some concern, however, regarding the effects that removal of these grafts might exert on children's nasal and craniofacial growth. Most recent studies indicate that septoplasty can be safely performed in children ≥ 6 years of age (and possibly in younger infants), without adverse consequences to their nasal and craniofacial development.[5] Therefore, such grafts are best used when septoplasty is required prior to ESBR (e.g., when a nasal septum deviation precludes EEA) or when reinforcement of the skull base closure is extremely desirable.[6]

Since the **nasoseptal flap** (NSF) was described, it has become the workhorse for ESBR, including the pediatric population.[7] It is a versatile flap and should be used whenever possible.[8] It is known, however, that septal growth occurs more rapidly between 10 and 13 years of age and nasal septum reaches adult measures only in patients ≥ 14 years of age. Because of that, NSF may not cover the more anterior skull base or even sellar defects in very young infants.[9] In such situations, harvesting other mucosal flaps, like the lateral nasal wall flap, and using free mucosal grafts, taken from nasal floor or from middle turbinates, are very well-accepted alternatives to the classical NSF.

28.3 Decision-Making and Operative Technique

Some factors should guide the decision on how to perform a multilayer ESBR in children. Besides the patient's age and diagnosis, the following variables must be considered[8]:

- History of prior radiotherapy and/or nasal surgeries.
- Location, width, and depth of the skull base defect.
- Occurrence of intraoperative dural violation and high-flow CSF leak.
- Presence and thickness of bony and dural ledges around the skull base defect.
- Availability of grafts, synthetic materials, and regional mucosal flaps.

For small skull base defects (diameter < 1 cm) with low-flow CSF leaks, the use of various layers of grafts and flaps is not usually necessary. However, medium to large defects (diameter ≥ 1–3 cm) located in the anterior cranial fossa or sellar region deserve a bilayer or multilayer reconstruction technique. Examples of how such defects might be reconstructed are depicted in ► Fig. 28.1.[6,10]

The best indication for the multilayer "triple-F" technique is for very large skull base defects, like those resulting from extirpation of clival chordomas, which are usually associated with high-flow CSF leak. ESBR of defects like these are challenging, especially in the pediatric population. For such cases, performing a watertight closure that necessarily includes a vascularized mucosal flap is key.[4,11]

Reconstruction should begin with the obliteration of any large surgical cavity with fat. Besides preventing the formation of dead spaces, fat grafts also avoid seeping of CSF through the borders of the defect, because of its hydrophobic properties. When large intradural tumors have been removed, fat can also be carefully placed intradurally, without putting neurovascular structures at risk. After that, fascia lata and/or dural substitutes are layered in an inlay or onlay fashion. In some cases, more fat might be layered or used to obliterate normal cavities, which increases the reach of pedicled mucosal flaps. Finally, the NSF is placed on top of the other layers.

There are various other ways in which the multiple layers can be placed. Some examples can be appreciated in ► Fig. 28.2 and ► Fig. 28.3.

28.4 Nasal Packing and Postoperative Considerations

After the multiple layers are nicely positioned, nasal packing is performed (see ► Fig. 28.4)[4]:

- Surgicel patties might be used to picture frame the mucosal flap(s) and to control minor bleedings.
- Spongostan Powder followed by Gelfoam are layered directly over the mucosal flap and help secure all the layers in place; Fibrin glue is not typically necessary.
- Nasal cavity is packed with synthetic gauze soaked in antibiotic ointment.
- Packing is supported by nasal tampons, such as Rapid Rhino.

Nasal tampons are left in place for 3 to 5 days and synthetic gauze is removed only after 5 to 7 days from surgery. Lumbar drainage is not routinely used. Nevertheless, it must always be considered when high-flow CSF leak is identified intraoperatively; if used, lumbar drain is kept in place for 3 to 5 days. Broad-spectrum antibiotics are used for 10 days or as long as necessary.

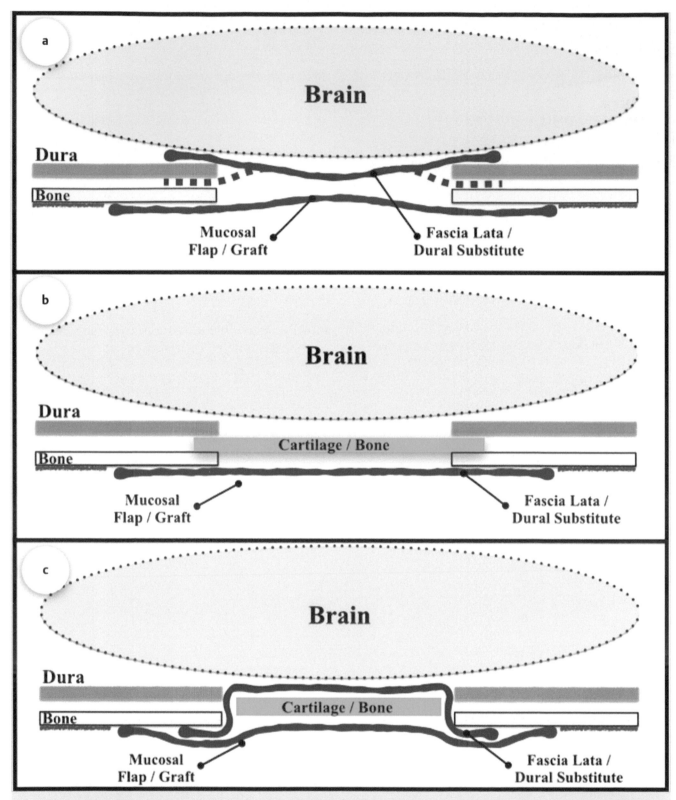

Fig. 28.1 Correction of medium to large skull base defects located in the anterior cranial fossa or sellar region demands a bilayer or multilayer technique. (a) Large pieces of fascia lata or dural substitutes are placed inlay or onlay. (b) When bony ledges are clearly identified, it is a good option to carefully position grafts of septal bone or cartilage in the epidural space (onlay). (c) A combination of fascia lata and cartilage might also be employed (similarly to the "gasket-seal" technique.[6] A mucosal graft or flap is then used to secure the grafts in place and to promote adequate healing.

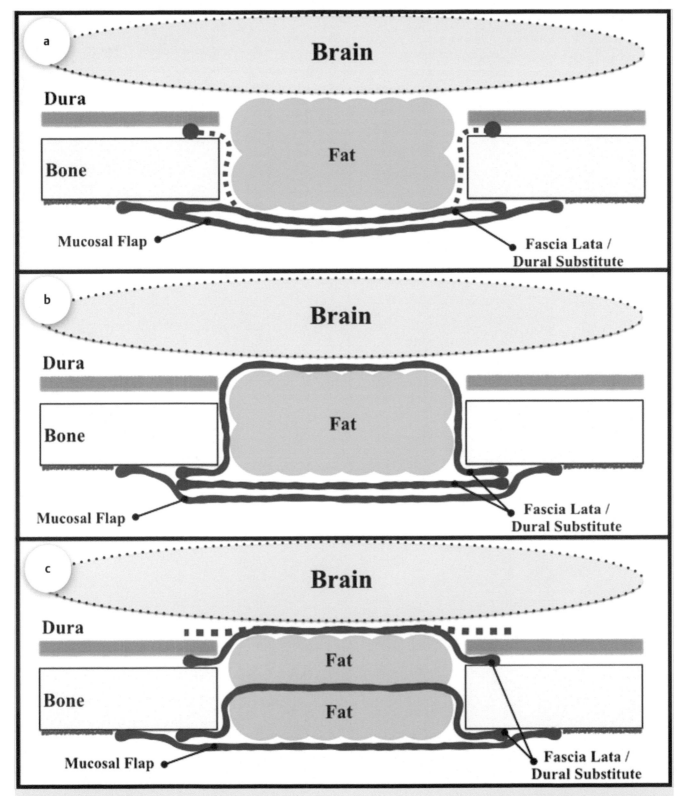

Fig. 28.2 Examples of how large skull base defects in children, like those located in the clival region, can be nicely reconstructed with the classical multilayer "triple-F" technique (a). Fat grafts and fascia lata can be positioned inlay or onlay. The same type of material can be layered more than once (b,c). In all situations, the closing layer should be a vascularized mucosal flap. Care must be taken to correctly place the flap—its mucoperichondrial/osteal surface must cover the defect completely and its borders must be in close contact to the previously denuded bone.[4,7]

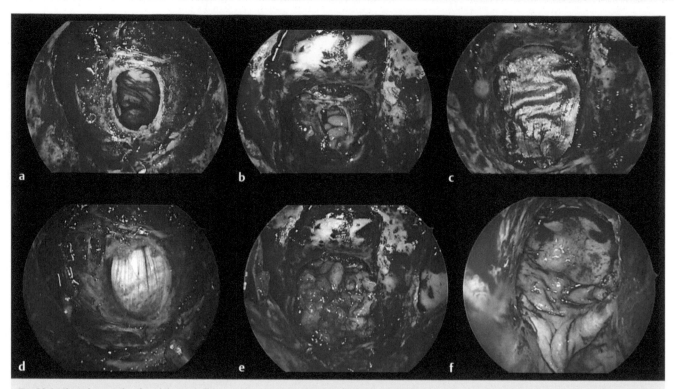

Fig. 28.3 Clinical example of multilayer skull base closure in a 14-year-old female patient who had undergone resection of a clival chordoma. The resulting dural defect is shown in (a). Fat (b) and fascia lata (c,d) grafts harvested from her thigh were positioned inlay. Another layer of fat was placed onlay (e). Finally, the nasoseptal flap was used to cover the other grafts (f).

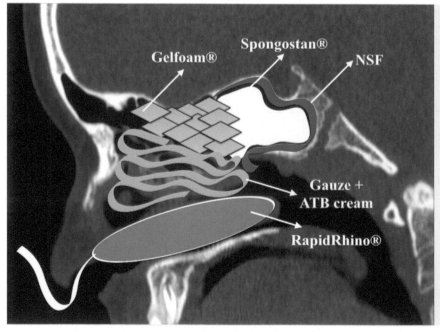

Fig. 28.4 Didactic example of how nasal packing is performed at the end of the procedure.[4] ATB, antibiotics; NSF, nasoseptal flap. (Refer to text for more information.)

References

[1] Kassam A, Thomas AJ, Snyderman C, et al. Fully endoscopic expanded endonasal approach treating skull base lesions in pediatric patients. J Neurosurg. 2007; 106(2) Suppl:75–86

[2] Khalili S, Palmer JN, Adappa ND. The expanded endonasal approach for the treatment of intracranial skull base disease in the pediatric population. Curr Opin Otolaryngol Head Neck Surg. 2015; 23(1):65–70

[3] Hachem RA, Elkhatib A, Beer-Furlan A, Prevedello D, Carrau R. Reconstructive techniques in skull base surgery after resection of malignant lesions: a wide array of choices. Curr Opin Otolaryngol Head Neck Surg. 2016; 24(2):91–97

[4] Mangussi-Gomes J, Beer-Furlan A, Balsalobre L, Vellutini EAS, Stamm AC. Endoscopic endonasal management of skull base chordomas: surgical technique, nuances, and pitfalls. Otolaryngol Clin North Am. 2016; 49(1):167–182

[5] Lawrence R. Pediatric septoplasty: a review of the literature. Int J Pediatr Otorhinolaryngol. 2012; 76(8):1078–1081

[6] Leng LZ, Brown S, Anand VK, Schwartz TH. "Gasket-seal" watertight closure in minimal-access endoscopic cranial base surgery. Neurosurgery. 2008; 62 (5) Suppl 2:E342–E343, discussion E343

[7] Hadad G, Bassagasteguy L, Carrau RL, et al. A novel reconstructive technique after endoscopic expanded endonasal approaches: vascular pedicle nasoseptal flap. Laryngoscope. 2006; 116(10):1882–1886

[8] Zanation AM, Carrau RL, Snyderman CH, et al. Nasoseptal flap reconstruction of high flow intraoperative cerebral spinal fluid leaks during endoscopic skull base surgery. Am J Rhinol Allergy. 2009; 23(5):518–521

[9] Shah RN, Surowitz JB, Patel MR, et al. Endoscopic pedicled nasoseptal flap reconstruction for pediatric skull base defects. Laryngoscope. 2009; 119(6): 1067–1075

[10] Patel MR, Stadler ME, Snyderman CH, et al. How to choose? Endoscopic skull base reconstructive options and limitations. Skull Base. 2010; 20(6):397–404

[11] Harvey RJ, Parmar P, Sacks R, Zanation AM. Endoscopic skull base reconstruction of large dural defects: a systematic review of published evidence. Laryngoscope. 2012; 122(2):452–459

29 Closure Techniques for the Pediatric Skull Base: Gasket Seal

Harminder Singh, Vijay K. Anand, and Theodore H. Schwartz

Abstract

The gasket seal is based on the concept of creating a "gasket" that forms a watertight seal, isolating the intracranial contents from the sinonasal space. The indications, technique, and limitations of this closure will be discussed in this chapter.

Keywords: gasket seal, facia lata, rigid buttress, watertight seal, nasoseptal flap

29.1 Introduction to Gasket Seal

As endoscopic endonasal surgery extended across the skull base, the difficulty of achieving a watertight closure through the endoscope became a central preoccupation for skull base surgeons. Most effective closure techniques are based on a few simple principals. These include (1) multilayer closure (redundancy is effective in case any one layer by itself is inadequate); (2) buttressing (fluctuations in intracranial pressure during the early postoperative period can dislodge closure material); and (3) vascularized tissue (allows for long-term security in closure).

The first principle was initially addressed with inlay and only graft materials such as fat, fascia lata, alloderm. and matrix materials. Although fat has historically been the mainstay in transsphenoidal closures, it has been used mostly for adenomas, where the sella holds the fat and the opening requiring closure is a small arachnoidal opening. For extended transsphenoidal approaches, placement of intracranial fat can have certain drawbacks. First, intradural fat can impair the interpretation of postoperative imaging and the ability to discern residual or recurrent tumors. Second, fat grafts are not initially vascularized and can become infected, particularly when dragged through the nostrils. Fat grafts in the sphenoid can also have drawbacks, as they are bulky and can impair mucous drainage and necrose, creating a foul smell.

Fascia lata is an attractive material, since it is an autograft and has the appropriate thickness and malleability for skull base repair. Buttressing is also important to prevent graft dislodgement and can be addressed in several ways. Initial use of a foley balloon was effective, but it was difficult to know exactly how much to inflate the balloon, and the round contour never perfectly fitted the sphenoid sinus, so it was difficult to control the amount of pressure exerted in each region. Moreover, the patient had a catheter emerging from their nostril that may need to be left in place for several days, which is uncomfortable and can impair nasal drainage and slow down patient discharge.

Grafts that wedge into the bone around the opening can be useful to reconstruct the defect and hold softer grafts in place, as is done when reconstructing the floor of the sella after pituitary surgery. Autologous vomer is often used for this purpose, but with extended skull base approaches, the defects are often large and irregularly shaped, and one cannot rely on having the

perfect vomer graft in every case. MEDPORE (Porex) provides a nice alternative that can be cut to custom sizes based on need and has some flexibility to wedge into exiting bone defects more easily. Bone cement is also an option, but the initial soft consistency makes it difficult to control and the speed of hardening is also difficult to manage.

The advent of the pedicled nasoseptal flap (NSF) was a giant step forward in managing high-flow cerebrospinal fluid (CSF) leaks. To address several of the issues and limitations described, the "gasket seal" was developed at Cornell as a workhorse closure for extended skull base approaches.[1,2] The combination of the NSF with the *gasket seal* produces the lowest rate of CSF leak of any closure technique published to date.[3,4,5,6] The indications, technique, and limitations of this closure will be discussed in this chapter.

29.2 Procedure

The gasket seal technique is based on the concept of creating a "gasket" that forms a watertight seal, isolating the intracranial contents from the sinonasal space. For conceptual understanding, this technique can be broken down into four steps.

29.2.1 Step 1: Harvesting of Fascia Lata

A piece of autologous fascia lata is harvested from the contralateral thigh from which the primary surgeon is standing, so as to not disrupt the endonasal procedure while the harvest is being performed. The fascia lata graft is fashioned such that it circumferentially extends 1 cm beyond the margins of the bony defect. The vertical and horizontal diameters of this defect are measured either with a ruler or with a cottonoid. If fascia lata is unavailable for any reason, bovine pericardium or alloderm may be used as a substitute. The harvested graft is placed over the bony opening (▶ Fig. 29.1a, b).

29.2.2 Step 2: Fashioning of Rigid Buttress

A piece of rigid material, such as vomer (harvested during the exposure) or MEDPOR graft (Stryker, Kalamazoo, MI) is cut to be the same size as the bony defect. Nasal cartilage or bioabsorbable plates are not used, because they may not last long enough or be rigid enough to ensure a stable closure.

29.2.3 Step 3: Creating a "Gasket"

A MEDPOR graft is wedged into the defect over the fascia lata graft. The MEDPOR pushes down on the center of the fascia lata and holds it in place. The built-in handle of the MEDPOR graft helps in manipulating it inside the nose using pituitary forceps. The fascia lata graft is drawn circumferentially into the defect around the rigid MEDPOR buttress, forming a watertight gasket

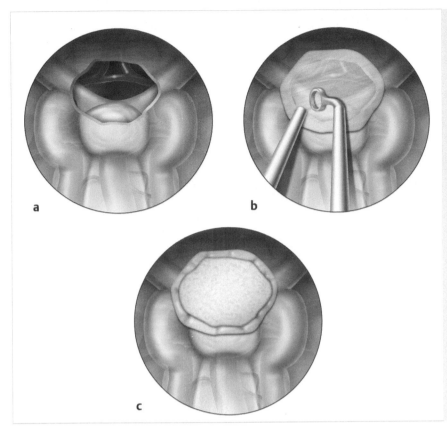

Fig. 29.1 Creation of a "gasket" seal. (a) The skull base opening after resection of tumor. The bony edges of the defect are defined. (b) The fascia lata graft is fashioned such that it circumferentially extends 1 cm beyond the margins of the bony defect. (c) A MEDPOR graft is wedged into the defect over the fascia lata graft. The MEDPOR pushes down on the center of the fascia lata and holds it in place. The fascia lata graft is drawn circumferentially into the defect around the rigid MEDPOR buttress, forming a watertight gasket seal.

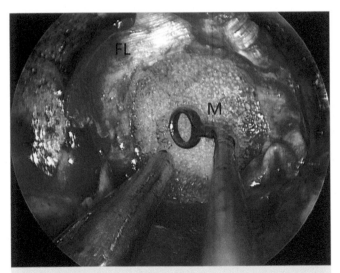

Fig. 29.2 Gasket seal used for skull base reconstruction, using fascia lata (FL) and MEDPOR (M) graft wedged into the bony opening. The previously harvested vascularized nasoseptal flap is layered over this closure.

seal (▶ Fig. 29.1c). The ideal gasket is formed when the MEDPOR graft is wedged into the bone without countersinking. However, in some cases a perfect wedge cannot be created, and slight countersinking is acceptable. For the gasket seal to be effective, the defect in the skull base must be surrounded by a rim of bone, into which the MEDPOR can be wedged (▶ Fig. 29.2).

29.2.4 Step 4: Deploying the Vascularized Nasoseptal Flap

The gasket seal is then covered by the NSF. It is crucial that the margins of the NSF extend beyond the margins of the fascia lata graft; otherwise, the flap is not in direct opposition with the bone of the skull base. The NSF is then sprayed with polymerized hydrogel (Duraseal, Integra) to hold it in place. Alternately, fibrin glue (Tisseel, Baxter) may also be used. Bioabsorbable Nasopore (Stryker) dressing is left in the sinonasal cavity to reduce adhesions, and minimize sinonasal bloody exudate.

29.3 Advantages

The rigid buttress obviates the need for an inflated intranasal balloon, with its inherent risks of overinflation, local infection, sinusitis, and postoperative distress to the patient. The skull base defect is reconstructed in a rigid fashion, and graft migration is rarely seen. The gasket seal technique for closing the cranial base after extended endonasal endoscopic approaches has lowered our CSF leak rates to approximately 3% for high-flow leaks, even approaching 0% in the latter half of our series.[2,5,6]

29.4 Disadvantages

Factors that may limit the utility of this technique include the absence of a solid bone surrounding the cranial defect, into which the rigid buttress has to be wedged. Likewise, if the defect traverses two separate geometric planes, the gasket may fail because the buttress is not curved and exists in only one plane in space. In these cases, the use of a *bilayer button* graft (refer to Bilayer Button, Chapter 30) may be advantageous. There is also some morbidity associated with the lateral thigh incision used for harvesting the fascia lata graft, such as wound infection, wound dehiscence, and persistent pain.

29.5 Conclusion

The gasket seal closure is an effective method for achieving watertight closure of the anterior cranial base after endoscopic intradural surgery. Combining this technique with a vascularized NSF and/or brief postoperative lumbar drainage may further reduce the risk of CSF leak after endoscopic anterior skull base surgery.

References

[1] Leng LZ, Brown S, Anand VK, Schwartz TH. "Gasket-seal" watertight closure in minimal-access endoscopic cranial base surgery. Neurosurgery. 2008; 62 (5) Suppl 2:E342–E343, discussion E343

[2] Garcia-Navarro V, Anand VK, Schwartz TH. Gasket seal closure for extended endonasal endoscopic skull base surgery: efficacy in a large case series. World Neurosurg. 2013; 80(5):563–568

[3] McCoul ED, Anand VK, Singh A, Nyquist GG, Schaberg MR, Schwartz TH. Long-term effectiveness of a reconstructive protocol using the nasoseptal flap after endoscopic skull base surgery. World Neurosurg. 2014; 81(1):136–143

[4] Hu F, Gu Y, Zhang X, et al. Combined use of a gasket seal closure and a vascularized pedicle nasoseptal flap multilayered reconstruction technique for high-flow cerebrospinal fluid leaks after endonasal endoscopic skull base surgery. World Neurosurg. 2015; 83(2):181–187

[5] Mascarenhas L, Moshel YA, Bayad F, et al. The transplanum transtuberculum approaches for suprasellar and sellar-suprasellar lesions: avoidance of cerebrospinal fluid leak and lessons learned. World Neurosurg. 2014; 82(1–2): 186–195

[6] Patel KS, Komotar RJ, Szentirmai O, et al. Case-specific protocol to reduce cerebrospinal fluid leakage after endonasal endoscopic surgery. J Neurosurg. 2013; 119(3):661–668

30 Closure Techniques for the Pediatric Skull Base: Bilayer Button

Douglas R. Johnston, Alan Siu, Mindy R. Rabinowitz, Sanjeet V. Rangarajan, Marc R. Rosen, and James J. Evans

Abstract

The bilayer fascia lata button graft is a useful multilayer skull base reconstruction technique. The graft's versatility allows it to conform to irregular defects with multiple planes, such as the planum sphenoidale-tuberculum sella interface.

At our institution, it has lowered post-operative CSF leak rates in high-flow CSF leak cases to less than 3%, when used in conjunction with the nasoseptal flap.

Keywords: bilayer button, transnasal, multilayer closure, graft, cranial base defect, facia lata autograft

30.1 Introduction to Bilayer Button

Extended endoscopic transnasal approaches have benefited greatly from the development of multilayered closures to dramatically decrease the incidence of postoperative cerebrospinal fluid (CSF) leaks. In 2010, we described our initial experience with a technique developed at Thomas Jefferson University for the primary closure of skull base defects using a "bilayer button graft" of fascia lata to repair high-flow CSF leaks.[1] Since 2010, we have utilized this closure technique to primarily repair the dural defect in cases with high-flow CSF leaks, along with the nasoseptal flap as an adjunct,[2] which has yielded a CSF leak rate of ≤ 3%.

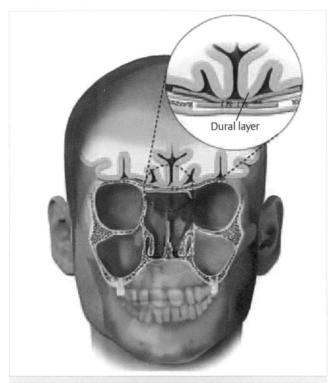

Fig. 30.1 Coronal schematic of the bilayer button in relation to the dural defect. The dural edge is sandwiched circumferentially between the two leaflets of the bilayer button.

30.2 Procedure

The "bilayer button graft" consists of two layers of fascia lata sutured together to form an inlay and an onlay component. The inlay portion sits within the subdural space, while the onlay portion covers the epidural space to create a tight primary dural closure (▶ Fig. 30.1). A vascularized mucosal second layer, often a nasoseptal flap, can then lay over the button graft and cranial base defect for a multilayered closure.

A pituitary rongeur or cottonoid is first used to measure the size of the dural defect. A template is created from a piece of sterile paper the exact size of the dural defect. A 4- to 6-cm linear incision is made along the lateral thigh halfway between the greater trochanter and the knee. The incision is carried through the subcutaneous tissue, fat is removed, and the fascia lata is identified (▶ Fig. 30.2). A piece of fascia lata is harvested with blunt and sharp dissection. The graft harvest size is individualized to the defect size and allows two pieces of fascia: one 10% larger than the defect for the onlay portion, and the other approximately 25 to 30% larger for the inlay portion. The rationale for the smaller onlay is to allow the nasoseptal flap direct contact with the dural edge circumferentially, since, in our experience, nasoseptal flap heals to exposed dura more robustly than exposed bone. The inlay and onlay fascial layers are then sutured together with four 4–0 Nurolon sutures (Ethicon, Bridgewater, NJ), with all sutures placed just inside the size of the actual dural defect (▶ Fig. 30.3a, b). One side of the graft is colored with a surgical marker to aid with orientation when placing the graft (▶ Fig. 30.3c). The bilayer button graft is placed into the defect with a pituitary rongeur. It is then maneuvered into position with ring curettes such that the inlay portion is inserted through the defect and made flush with the surrounding inner dural surface, while the onlay portion only sits over the defect flush with the outer dural surface (▶ Fig. 30.1). Since the two layers are sutured together, the inlay portion can

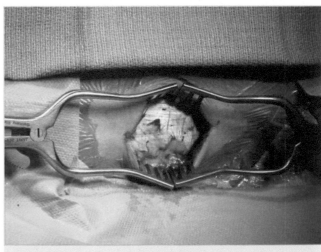

Fig. 30.2 Intraoperative view of fascia lata harvest.

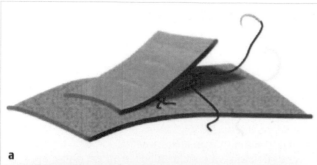

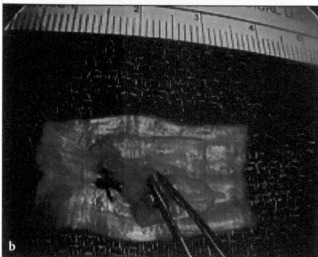

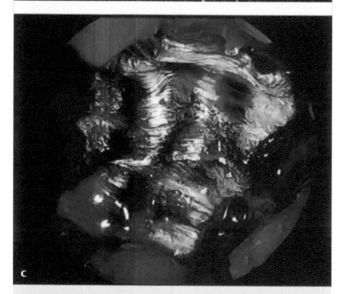

Fig. 30.3 (a) Bilayer button illustration. (b) intraoperative photo with Nurolon suture placement. (c) graft placement with inked onlay portion to aid in orientation.

be manipulated and positioned by grasping and moving the onlay portion. The onlay portion is sequentially lifted to confirm the inlay graft is completely approximated to the dura. The nasoseptal flap is then reflected over the button graft, biological glue is applied along its edges, and a single piece of absorbable packing is placed centrally along the flap for stability.

30.3 Advantages

The primary reason for failure of large cranial base defects is graft migration, which is not likely with the malleable button design in that a watertight seal is created and that the two allograft surfaces can heal to the surrounding intracranial and intranasal surfaces. The graft's versatility allows it to conform to defects with multiple planes, such as the planum sphenoidale–tuberculum sella interface. The bilayer button graft has significantly decreased our postoperative CSF leak rate from 45 to 3% for high-flow leaks. With the use of an adjunct vascularized graft, such as the nasoseptal flap, the button graft obviates the need for a perioperative lumbar drain, placement of a foley balloon catheter, or fat packing of the sphenoid sinus, potentially decreasing morbidity. The fascia lata autograft can often be simultaneously harvested while the primary surgery is taking place, thus saving operative time.

30.4 Disadvantages

The morbidity associated with the lateral thigh incision and postoperative wound care is the major disadvantage. However, we have not encountered wound complications or lasting postoperative complaints. We have never seen aseptic meningitis as has been described with some synthetic grafts.

30.5 Conclusion

The bilayer fascia lata button graft is a versatile skull base repair technique that is associated with low morbidity and dramatic reductions in postoperative CSF leaks. Its adoption as a crucial component to our multilayered skull base reconstruction for extended endonasal approaches has yielded a robust closure technique with improved outcomes.

References

[1] Luginbuhl AJ, Campbell PG, Evans J, Rosen M. Endoscopic repair of high-flow cranial base defects using a bilayer button. Laryngoscope. 2010; 120(5):876–880

[2] Kassam AB, Thomas A, Carrau RL, et al. Endoscopic reconstruction of the cranial base using a pedicled nasoseptal flap. Neurosurgery. 2008; 63(1) Suppl 1:44–52, discussion 52–53

31 Closure Techniques for the Pediatric Skull Base: Lumbar Drains

Nathan T. Zwagerman, Paul A. Gardner, and Elizabeth C. Tyler-Kabara

Abstract

The endoscopic endonasal approach has presented new opportunities to safely remove tumors of the skull base; however, one of the most difficult hurdles to overcome has been closure of dural defects. This is particularly true in children as the anatomy and size are different than adults and present unique challenges. This chapter discusses the adjunctive use of a lumbar drain in the pediatric population to help prevent postoperative cerebral spinal fluid leaks, and it reviews the current literature regarding this practice. Much of the known literature on lumbar drains is from adult series but can be applied to pediatric patients. The authors present their experience and useful information regarding the proper use of lumbar drains in the pediatric population after endoscopic endonasal skull base surgery.

Keywords: pediatric, endoscopic endonasal approach, lumbar drain, CSF leak

31.1 Introduction to Lumbar Drains

The pediatric population presents many challenges to the surgeon applying the endoscopic endonasal approach (EEA) for skull base tumor resection. One of the most difficult of these challenges is the repair of skull base defects, as many of these patients are in various phases of skull base and sinonasal development. Many times, defects created by surgery result in high-flow cerebrospinal fluid (CSF) leaks, and repair of these may be limited by pediatric anatomy. Failure of a successful closure may result in pneumocephalus, postoperative CSF leak, meningitis, and other morbidities. To this end, postoperative CSF diversion in the form of lumbar drains may be used in the postoperative period to provide CSF diversion and prevent postoperative CSF leaks.[1,2] Lumbar drains have been used in the adult population with success; however, this is rarely addressed in the pediatric literature. In addition, CSF-leak risk appears to be higher in pediatric patients compared to adult patients with similar tumors. In our series (unpublished data), we found that the postoperative CSF leak for chordoma was 40% for pediatrics compared with 22% for adults.

The pediatric population, in addition to the challenges presented from the surgical anatomy, presents challenges associated with the use of lumbar drains. The adult produces approximately 500 mL of CSF daily, whereas children (ages 4–13 years) produce only 65 to 150 mL,[3] making small children particularly at risk for overdrainage complications. A smaller body habitus may increase risk of overpenetration of the stylet and needle, causing bleeding from the ventral venous plexus or even penetration of the retroperitoneal cavity. A useful recommendation for needle depth in the pediatric population may be estimated by the following formula: *depth of LP* = 0.77 cm + (2.56 × body surface area [BSA; m²]).[4] Postimplantation challenges exist as well. The pediatric

population may be at greater risk of drain dislodgement and noncompliance resulting in over- or underdrainage. To counter this, a well-educated nursing staff is critical for successful postoperative drain care. These are in addition to the known risks of lumbar drain placement, which include postural headaches, nausea, meningitis, tonsillar herniation, intracranial hypotension, and retained catheters.[1,5,6,7]

Despite these challenges, several studies have documented successful use of lumbar drains in the pediatric population for a variety of reasons, including fulminant idiopathic intracranial hypertension and traumatic and postoperative CSF leaks.[8] Levy et al describe the successful use of lumbar drains for the diversion of CSF in 16 pediatric severe traumatic brain injury patients without complications associated with lumbar drain placement or care.[9] Lumbar drainage after surgical intervention is less well documented. Lumbar drainage has been used after operative repair of a traumatic CSF leak.[10] Zhan published a series of 11 patients who underwent EEA for sellar region pathology and noted the use of a lumbar drain in one patient who developed a postoperative CSF leak. No complications were listed.[11]

Di Rocco et al published a series of 28 pediatric patients with anterior skull defects repaired through an endoscopic approach. In patients with a significant preoperative CSF leak, lumbar drains were placed (*n* = 5). Also, a lumbar drain was placed in one patient who developed a postoperative CSF leak. The drains were in place for 3 to 8 days. They found that lumbar drainage increased hospital stay, constrained the patients, and increased risk of drain-related complications. They recommend drains be placed in cases of abundant CSF leak or in early recurrence of CSF leakage, but they could not draw any definitive conclusions.[12] The largest series of EEA for pediatric patients included 133 patients and noted that a perioperative lumbar drain was placed in 25 patients, but no complications of drain management was mentioned.[13] This series was later revisited and evaluated for risk factors for CSF leak in this population. Drains were not associated with postoperative CSF leak or lack thereof in the series; however, this is likely a reflection of the fact that lumbar drains were only placed in cases with high-flow intraoperative leaks.[14] This lends support to the usage of drains in this setting, as it seems to lower the risk of lower-flow leaks without drains.

Our clinical practice is to use a lumbar drain in cases of high-flow CSF leak created during EEA (▶ Fig. 31.1). These drains are then kept in place for 72 hours and removed to avoid increased risk of drain-associated meningitis, which can increase with prolonged drainage. Typically, 5 to 10 mL of CSF is removed per hour depending on patient size (similar in adults). Although no association between CSF leak and lumbar drain was discovered during the aforementioned analysis (suggesting appropriate usage of lumbar drains), a recent randomized trial was concluded, demonstrating clear lumbar drain utility in adults.[17] Lumbar drains in this adult population significantly decreased CSF leaks after endoscopic endonasal surgery for pathology in

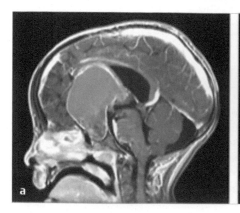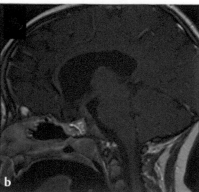

Fig. 31.1 Sagittal MRI T1 with contrast indicating a large craniopharyngioma before (**a**) and after (**b**) resection. Lesions such as this require a large skull base defect for resection, and lumbar drains are used to prevent postoperative cerebrospinal fluid leaks.

the anterior or posterior cranial fossa. This is likely a result of defect size and was independent of patient BMI or surgical history.

The use of a lumbar drain when a patient develops a postoperative leak is much more controversial. In general, our philosophy has been to NOT use lumbar drainage as the primary modality in this setting. Rather, if postoperative CSF leak is suspected or proven, early re-exploration is recommended. Several studies have shown a success rate of lumbar drainage of 50% as the primary treatment of postoperative leak.[15,16] While this may avoid re-exploration in a few patients, leak is never confirmed, and the patients in whom it fails end up with significantly prolonged courses and increased risk of meningitis and subsequent complications that are entirely avoidable.

Contraindications to placement of lumbar drains also exist and are important to recognize. Patients with large residual posterior fossa lesions or small posterior fossa cavities are at particular risk for downward herniation after lumbar drain placement. Patients with pneumocephalus may also suffer from overdrainage/herniation with lumbar drain placement. For these reasons, it is important to get postoperative imaging prior to opening of a lumbar drain. Patients with myelomeningocele/meningoceles may not have a lumbar cistern, and a lumbar drain would be contraindicated.

The decision to place a lumbar drain after endoscopic endonasal surgery is largely up to the individual surgeon and defect created after tumor removal. There is some class 1 evidence for the usage of drains in large anterior or posterior fossa defects in adults, but this can only be extrapolated to children. However, given that CSF leaks appear to be more prevalent in the pediatric population, lumbar drain usage in the setting of large or high-flow defects seems prudent.

References

[1] Ackerman PD, Spencer DA, Prabhu VC. The efficacy and safety of preoperative lumbar drain placement in anterior skull base surgery. J Neurol Surg Rep. 2013; 74(1):1–9

[2] Rastatter JC, Snyderman CH, Gardner PA, Alden TD, Tyler-Kabara E. Endoscopic endonasal surgery for sinonasal and skull base lesions in the pediatric population. Otolaryngol Clin North Am. 2015; 48(1):79–99

[3] Bonadio WA. The cerebrospinal fluid: physiologic aspects and alterations associated with bacterial meningitis. Pediatr Infect Dis J. 1992; 11(6):423–431

[4] Bonadio WA, Smith DS, Metrou M, Dewitz B. Estimating lumbar-puncture depth in children. N Engl J Med. 1988; 319(14):952–953

[5] Kim YS, Kim SH, Jung SH, Kim TS, Joo SP. Brain stem herniation secondary to cerebrospinal fluid drainage in ruptured aneurysm surgery: a case report. Springerplus. 2016; 5:247

[6] Kitchel SH, Eismont FJ, Green BA. Closed subarachnoid drainage for management of cerebrospinal fluid leakage after an operation on the spine. J Bone Joint Surg Am. 1989; 71(7):984–987

[7] Samadani U, Huang JH, Baranov D, Zager EL, Grady MS. Intracranial hypotension after intraoperative lumbar cerebrospinal fluid drainage. Neurosurgery. 2003; 52(1):148–151, discussion 151–152

[8] Jiramongkolchai K, Buckley EG, Bhatti MT, et al. Temporary lumbar drain as treatment for pediatric fulminant idiopathic intracranial hypertension. J Neuroophthalmol. 2017; 37(2):126–132

[9] Levy DI, Rekate HL, Cherny WB, Manwaring K, Moss SD, Baldwin HZ. Controlled lumbar drainage in pediatric head injury. J Neurosurg. 1995; 83(3):453–460

[10] Kumar R, Deleyiannis FW, Wilkinson C, O'Neill BR. Neurosurgical sequelae of domestic dog attacks in children. J Neurosurg Pediatr. 2017; 19(1):24–31

[11] Zhan R, Xin T, Li X, Li W, Li X. Endonasal endoscopic transsphenoidal approach to lesions of the sellar region in pediatric patients. J Craniofac Surg. 2015; 26(6):1818–1822

[12] Di Rocco F, Couloigner V, Dastoli P, Sainte-Rose C, Zerah M, Roger G. Treatment of anterior skull base defects by a transnasal endoscopic approach in children. J Neurosurg Pediatr. 2010; 6(5):459–463

[13] Chivukula S, Koutourousiou M, Snyderman CH, Fernandez-Miranda JC, Gardner PA, Tyler-Kabara EC. Endoscopic endonasal skull base surgery in the pediatric population. J Neurosurg Pediatr. 2013; 11(3):227–241

[14] Stapleton AL, Tyler-Kabara EC, Gardner PA, Snyderman CH, Wang EW. Risk factors for cerebrospinal fluid leak in pediatric patients undergoing endoscopic endonasal skull base surgery. Int J Pediatr Otorhinolaryngol. 2017; 93:163–166

[15] Dehdashti AR, Ganna A, Witterick I, Gentili F. Expanded endoscopic endonasal approach for anterior cranial base and suprasellar lesions: indications and limitations. Neurosurgery. 2009; 64(4):677–687, discussion 687–689

[16] Dehdashti AR, Karabatsou K, Ganna A, Witterick I, Gentili F. Expanded endoscopic endonasal approach for treatment of clival chordomas: early results in 12 patients. Neurosurgery. 2008; 63(2):299–307, discussion 307–309

[17] Zwagerman NT, Wang EW, Shin SS, Chang YF, Fernandez-Miranda JC, Snyderman CH, Gardner PA. Does lumbar drainage reduce postoperative cerebrospinal fluid leak after endoscopic endonasal skull base surgery? A prospective, randomized controlled trial. J Neurosurg. 2018 Oct 1:1–7

32 Complication Management in Pediatric Endonasal Skull Base Surgery

Paul A. Gardner, Elizabeth C. Tyler-Kabara, Juan C. Fernandez-Miranda, Eric W. Wang, and Carl H. Snyderman

Abstract

Endoscopic endonasal skull base surgery (EESBS) has gained significant popularity for the management of ventral skull base pathologies, from the frontal sinus to the odontoid process. The application of EESBS to pediatric patients presents its own challenges, from size limitations to lack of sinus pneumatization to limited reconstructive options. These challenges, combined with the significant learning curve of EESBS and rarity of pediatric cases, create an environment ripe for complications. Understanding the source and management of these complications can minimize their occurrence and impact.

Keywords: complications, endonasal, pediatric, cerebrospinal fluid leak, injury

32.1 Introduction

Endoscopic endonasal skull base surgery (EESBS) has revolutionized the care of ventral, midline cranial base tumors.[1,2] Although it has reduced morbidity by minimizing neurovascular manipulation and avoidance of brain retraction, EESBS introduces its own set of new and unique complications. While some of these may be unavoidably related to the tumor, many are a result of the approach. In either case, they can be magnified in the pediatric population, given the long-term impact of tumor-related morbidity and the diminutive sinonasal cavities.

Proper approach selection undertaken by a combined pediatric/cranial base surgical team helps mitigate the risks. In addition, an understanding of the potential complications, methods of avoidance, and management is critical to the success of these complex approaches.

Complications can be divided into those that occur intraoperatively, such as nerve or vascular injury, and those that will occur during the postoperative period as sequelae of intraoperative decisions or technique, such as pituitary dysfunction or cerebrospinal fluid (CSF) leak. Complications can occur from the moment the patient enters the operating theater. It is a useful exercise to discuss all complications that may occur at the start of each surgery. Prevention and management of such complications is discussed in detail in this chapter.

32.2 Intraoperative Complications

For EESBS, patients are normally placed in head-pin fixation (using pediatric pins and dual support with a horseshoe in small patients) to ensure proper positioning (slight extension and head tilted toward the surgeon), facilitate image-based navigation, and avoid movement during critical periods of dissection. Ergonomic positioning improves access while minimizing surgeon fatigue, especially for long cases. In pediatric patients, improper placement of head pins over the thin squamosal bone can result in a skull fracture with risk of injury to the middle meningeal artery. Neurophysiological monitoring with unexplained intraoperative changes in somatosensory evoked potentials (SSEPs) can alert the surgeon to an unidentified epidural hematoma in this setting.

Blood loss is extremely difficult to monitor during EESBS. It is difficult to assess the volume of bleeding in an endoscopic field, and the suctioned blood is mixed with saline irrigation. As a result, careful and regular irrigation counts must be maintained in order to subtract this from the suction counts for a reasonable estimate of blood loss and to avoid both the hypoperfusion and coagulopathy associated with excessive blood loss. Given the lower overall blood volume of pediatric patients, careful monitoring of blood loss is more critical. For cases that may require staging, such as juvenile nasal angiofibroma (JNA), a target for maximal blood loss should be established preoperatively for staging of the surgery.

32.2.1 Vision Loss

Many suprasellar tumors, such as macroadenomas or craniopharyngiomas or even large chordomas, may present with occult but significant vision loss. Children are often not cooperative for reliable formal visual field testing. Simple threat testing or visual stimulus in all fields of vision can be used to detect significant deficits. Any patient with clinical or radiographic evidence of significant visual apparatus compromise should be closely monitored to avoid perioperative hypotension, which can result in hypoperfusion and can be devastating, even if transient. Weight-based corticosteroids can be used liberally in these cases as well.

One advantage of endonasal surgery, especially using an endoscope, is the ability to identify and preserve the subchiasmatic perforators from the superior hypophyseal arteries. Their anatomy should be closely studied by any surgeon operating in this region and branches identified and preserved intraoperatively.[3] This can be especially challenging for tumors such as craniopharyngiomas, which may receive partial supply from an occasional branch.

32.2.2 Cranial Nerve Injury

Avoidance of cranial nerve (CN) injury is a primary goal of any skull base surgery. Endonasal approaches were developed in large part to provide a corridor within the confines of the CNs, thus avoiding manipulation and injury. This advantage has been demonstrated in case series for many different tumor types.[4,5,6,7] The abducens nerve, however, remains at high risk given its ventral origin (at the vertebrobasilar junction), long course, fragility, and frequent involvement with tumors that are ideal for EESBS (e.g., chordomas). It is particularly susceptible to injury at Dorello's canal, where the nerve is interdural. Monitoring of CNs with electromyography can help localize them at the margin of the tumor and prevent injury.[8,9,10] Establishing a threshold for stimulation also provides prognostic information for recovery when there has been manipulation of the nerve.

32.2.3 Vascular Injury

Vascular injury is the most potentially devastating complication of any skull base surgery, but concern over vascular control adds a degree of fear to this complication with EESBS. However, the options for vascular control are the same as with "open" surgery, with the exception of suturing. The two-surgeon, four-hand technique becomes most critical during management of any vascular injury. This is especially critical for maintenance of view, troubleshooting/problem solving, and applying technical maneuvers such as holding pressure while increasing exposure. Skull base tumors can contact or encase vessels, and management strategies are different for petrous or cavernous segments of the internal carotid artery (ICA) and intracranial contributions to the circle of Willis (▶ Fig. 32.1).

In the event of an ICA injury, control of hemorrhage with suction and tamponade with a cottonoid are the first steps. Rapid notification of the rest of the surgical team and anesthesia providers is critical for optimal patient management. Evaluation of the injury and potential for wider exposure, proximal and distal control, and repair options are all part of the dialogue between co-surgeons. Options for repair are somewhat limited due to the inability to reliably suture.[11] Very small holes, such as perforator avulsions, can often be sealed with careful bipolar coagulation of the side wall with little or no stenosis of the artery. Well-visualized injuries can often be pinched off with an aneurysm clip, applied via a single-shaft clip applier, with potential preservation of flow. For larger injuries, or for any poorly controlled injury, packing with muscle tissue is a proven, reliable option. Muscle tissue can be obtained from the rectus abdominis, temporalis, sternocleidomastoid, quadriceps (fascia lata exposure), or even nasopharynx/rectus capitis muscles. Muscle should be crushed to flatten it and release calcium to augment hemostasis. Any time there is significant, repetitive compression or manipulation of the ICA, consideration should be given to anticoagulation. This can be counterintuitive in the setting of ICA injury, but would be standard for any planned arteriotomy.

ICA preservation should always be the goal of any repair, with sacrifice as a last resort. However, sacrifice is tolerated in most patients and, as a result, is preferable to uncontrolled hemorrhage.

Intracranial arterial injury can be equally devastating and difficult to control. Packing is not a good option in this setting, as it can lead to devastating intracranial hemorrhage, and controlled suction alone is frequently used to localize and control bleeding. Sidewall bipolar coagulation on a low setting can be used as a vessel preserving technique. Microaneurysm clips are another option. Bleeding from very small perforator injuries often stops with warm saline irrigation, which optimizes conditions for activation of the coagulation cascade. Occlusion of any intracranial artery should be avoided whenever possible, but communicating arteries may be sacrificed if necessary, often without consequence. Control of hemorrhage is always the primary goal, however, and other techniques, such as those mentioned above, or simple compression with cotton or other similar material should be attempted prior to coagulation or clip sacrifice. For example, posterior cerebral artery (PCA) injury during craniopharyngioma resection can be managed with sacrifice of the P1 segment if the patient has an adequate posterior communicating artery, but loss of thalamic perforators can be devastating.

Any time there is a risk of vascular injury, neurophysiologic monitoring should be employed. Simple SSEPs can provide critical information about the consequence of maneuvers, such as sacrifice, and help guide intraoperative decision-making, especially in the absence of preexisting balloon test occlusion (BTO).

Immediate angiographic follow-up is essential after any significant vascular injury. Unless the artery is easily and convincingly controlled during surgery, continued tumor dissection should generally be aborted in favor of angiographic evaluation. Stenosis, thrombus (which can embolize), and pseudoaneurysm can all require urgent treatment that is delayed by prolonged tumor resection. Most of these conditions have reasonable endovascular salvage, and urgent bypass is rarely a practical consideration. High-risk tumors, such as chordomas with significant ICA involvement, especially if recurrent or radiated, should be evaluated with preoperative BTO, often relying on neurophysiologic testing (SSEPs or TCD [transcranial Doppler]) combined with evaluation of filling time or venous transit times under anesthesia in younger, less cooperative children.

32.3 Postoperative Complications

32.3.1 Cerebrospinal Fluid Leak

CSF leak is the most common complication following intradural EESBS. Vascularized reconstruction, primarily with the nasoseptal flap based on the posterior nasal branch of the sphenopalatine artery, is the definitive component of a multilayer reconstruction. CSF leak rates have declined dramatically and approach those of many open approaches with the use of this and other local intranasal flaps.[12,13,14,15] CSF leak rates are higher in children than in adults for several reasons, including delayed nasal development, resulting in smaller flaps, poor compliance with packing and postoperative restrictions, and difficulties with postoperative assessment.[16] All of these are amplified in tumors such as clival or craniocervical junction chordomas, where large defects are at the limits of the flap, and CSF leak may present only as retropharyngeal drainage.

CSF leak should be evaluated and treated urgently. If available, beta-2 transferrin testing can be used to confirm the nature of clear drainage. CT scan can be used to assess for an increase in pneumocephalus. Any increase with serial postoperative scans is clear evidence of a fistula. Persistent drainage (nasal sprays should be stopped) should be assumed to be CSF and treated accordingly. Lumbar drainage is not recommended as the primary treatment, since it is not effective in the majority of cases and will delay definitive treatment and increase risk of meningitis. Rather, a CSF leak is treated with re-exploration at the soonest reasonable time (▶ Fig. 32.2).

Nasoseptal flap necrosis is a rare event but can have devastating consequences if not correctly diagnosed.[17] It presents approximately 2 weeks postoperatively with signs of meningitis and frequently a foul smell from the surgical site. Diagnosis is confirmed with MRI that shows lack of flap enhancement. Treatment includes lumbar puncture and/or drain, re-exploration, flap debridement, and coverage with additional vascularized tissue when possible. Intravenous antibiotics complete the treatment, and prognosis is good, with low risk of developing a delayed CSF leak.

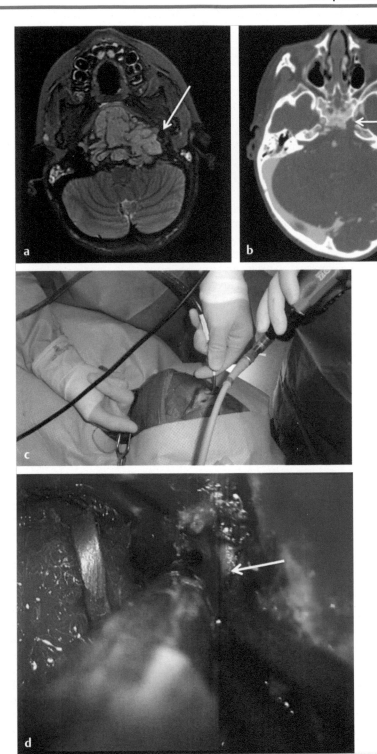

Fig. 32.1 (a) T2-weighted axial MRI image showing an extensive chordoma in contact with the left parapharyngeal internal carotid artery (ICA; *arrow*). (b) Preoperative CT angiography (CTA) showing further involvement of the left petrous ICA, with resultant stenosis. (c) Proximal left ICA control was obtained at the beginning of the surgery via a small cervical incision in preparation for potential ICA injury. (d) Intraoperative endoscopic endonasal view showing the cut end of the left petrous ICA (*arrow*). The patient had no change in neuromonitoring with proximal ICA occlusions via the cervical incision, so the ICA was sacrificed with bipolar coagulation.

32.3.2 Hematoma

Postoperative tumor bed hematoma can have significant short- and long-term impacts. Meticulous intraoperative hemostasis, confirmed with prolonged, copious warm water irrigation, combined with control of postoperative hypertension is a good recipe to avoid this frustrating complication. Residual tumor, especially pituitary adenoma, can undergo apoplexy, a factor that should be considered when contemplating staging or subtotal resection.

Hematoma can present variably depending on the location. Delayed vision loss is common in the suprasellar space, whereas decreased responsiveness or quadriparesis can occur in the clival region. Lesser hematomas can also interrupt reconstructive layers, interposing between bone, dura, and vascularized flaps. Finally, any intracranial blood can increase the risk of vasospasm, which often occurs in a delayed fashion and, as such, can prove relatively untreatable and is often diagnosed in retrospect.

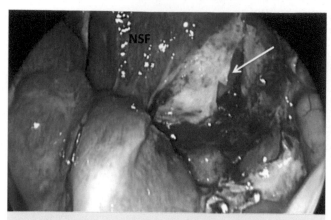

Fig. 32.2 Intraoperative endoscopic endonasal view during re-exploration in a patient with postoperative cerebrospinal fluid leak following endoscopic endonasal approach. The allograft has pulled away from the native dura, exposing the underlying collagen graft (Duragen, *arrow*). This type of defect will never seal with lumbar drainage alone and requires early reoperation. NSF, nasoseptal flap.

32.3.3 Pituitary Dysfunction

Loss of hormone function early in life can have significant long-term consequences and even lead to a shorter lifespan. As a result, every attempt at preservation of function should be made during resection of tumors involving the pituitary axis. Pituitary adenomas have a low risk of dysfunction, and so should their treatment. Surgery for upper clival tumors, such as chordomas, may require pituitary transposition; this is best done via the interdural method, which generally preserves anterior gland function but carries some risk to the posterior gland.[18] Craniopharyngiomas, which often involve the stalk, have an extremely high risk of dysfunction.[6,19,20] Loss of pituitary function may prove inevitable for many pediatric craniopharyngiomas, as incomplete resection in favor of preservation of function leads to frequent recurrence, the treatment of which usually results in hypopituitarism and poorer tumor control. In general, all attempts should be made to preserve the stalk and gland, but if this is the only obstacle to complete resection, then sacrifice is reasonable and recommended. The main exception would be approaching puberty, when anterior gland function is difficult to properly mimic. In addition to stalk preservation, preservation of the superior hypophyseal arteries is important, given their dual importance for both optic apparatus and pituitary stalk function.

32.3.4 Sinonasal Complications

All surgery is traumatic, and the trade-off for direct access to the entire ventral skull base is the impact on sinonasal function. Studies in adults show that quality of life following EESBS is excellent, with the exception of sinonasal symptoms, which do not return to baseline for 3 to 6 months, especially if a nasoseptal flap is used.[21] Debridement is a regular part of postoperative care following EESBS, but endoscopy may not be well tolerated by young children. Indeed, initial packing removal may require sedation or general anesthesia in the operating room. Merocel tampon strings should be cut completely so that the patient cannot pull them. Despite inability to debride as often or as effectively, children heal quite well with few long-term issues. Proper identification and coagulation (when necessary) of the sphenopalatine artery or its branches avoids significant postoperative epistaxis. Saddle nose deformity due to nasal dorsum collapse occurs in approximately 5% of all patients and is related to the nasoseptal flap.[22]

32.4 Long-Term Impact

The long-term impact of any surgery is often a reflection of complications. The same is true for EESBS, with rare persistent nasal or neurological impact. Of note, there does not seem to be any impact of EESBS on midfacial growth. A recent study[23] (Pediatric endoscopic endonasal skull base surgery and long-term impact on midface growth, in preparation) at our center found no difference in cephalometric analysis compared with age-matched controls for children when operated below or above age 7 years (the age at which midfacial growth is driven by the cranial base). Future studies should assess this prospectively, especially in patients with nasoseptal flaps.

32.5 Complication Avoidance

Time and effort spent on complication avoidance is always rewarded. There are many adjuvant tools that can limit some of the more common complications. Much of the inadvertent nasal morbidity occurs from introduction of instrumentation through the nasal passages. Placement of nasal protection sleeves, which are just becoming commercially available (SPIWay, LLC, Carlsbad, CA), can make introduction easier and also avoid mucosal injury. CSF diversion (lumbar spinal drainage) is recommended for any patient with a large dural defect, especially in the anterior or posterior fossa (can be avoided in small or low-flow sellar/suprasellar defects).[24] Pre-existing obstructive hydrocephalus should be treated with an external ventricular drain with a low threshold for shunting.

When complications occur, post hoc analysis in the form of a root cause analysis can help identify contributory system, technical, surgeon, equipment, or patient factors. This exercise always increases attention to these factors and can help prevent a repeat of similar complications.

Endonasal approaches were designed to access midline tumors that displace critical neurovascular structures laterally, thereby limiting or completely avoiding manipulation of these structures. Proper case selection following this basic principle of not "crossing" CNs limits their damage. Some tumors are best managed with an alternative extranasal/transcranial approach or a combination of approaches.

32.6 Learning Curve

Endoscopic endonasal approaches have a significant learning curve associated with them. This is due to unfamiliar anatomy, the 2D endoscopic view, new technical skills, reconstruction challenges, and the two-surgeon team learning to work together. All of these factors require that any surgical team or surgeon slowly progress from simpler cases (such as pituitary

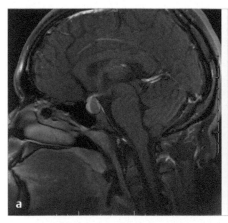
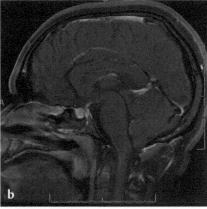

Fig. 32.3 Preoperative (a) and postoperative (b) sagittal MRI showing a level II (of V) case, a Rathke cleft cyst, treated via endoscopic endonasal approach.

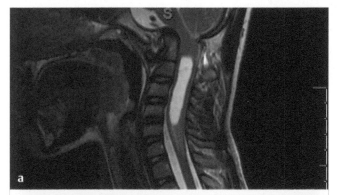
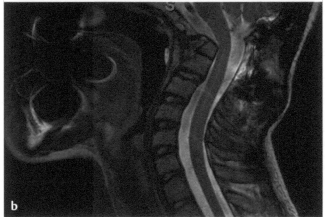

Fig. 32.4 Preoperative (a) and postoperative (b) sagittal T2-weighted MRI of the cervical spine showing significant basilar invagination with associated syringomyelia, successfully treated with endoscopic endonasal approach and occipitocervical fixation. Extradural surgery such as this represents a level III case.

Table 32.1 Training program for endoscopic endonasal surgery

Level I
- Sinus surgery

Level II
- Advanced sinus surgery
- Cerebrospinal fluid leaks
- Sella/pituitary (intrasellar)

Level III
- Sella/pituitary (extrasellar)
- Optic nerve decompression
- Orbital surgery
- Extradural skull base surgery

Level IV
- Intradural skull base surgery

Level V
- Coronal plane (carotid dissection)
- Vascular surgery

adenomas and CSF leaks) to more complicated ones (like intradural, suprasellar craniopharyngiomas) and, ultimately, large intra- and extradural pathologies at the extremes of access with vascular involvement (e.g., extensive chordomas; Table 32-1; ► Fig. 32.3, ► Fig. 32.4, ► Fig. 32.5, ► Fig. 32.6). Respecting this learning curve is critical for avoiding major complications and preserving or surpassing the results provided by established skull base approaches.

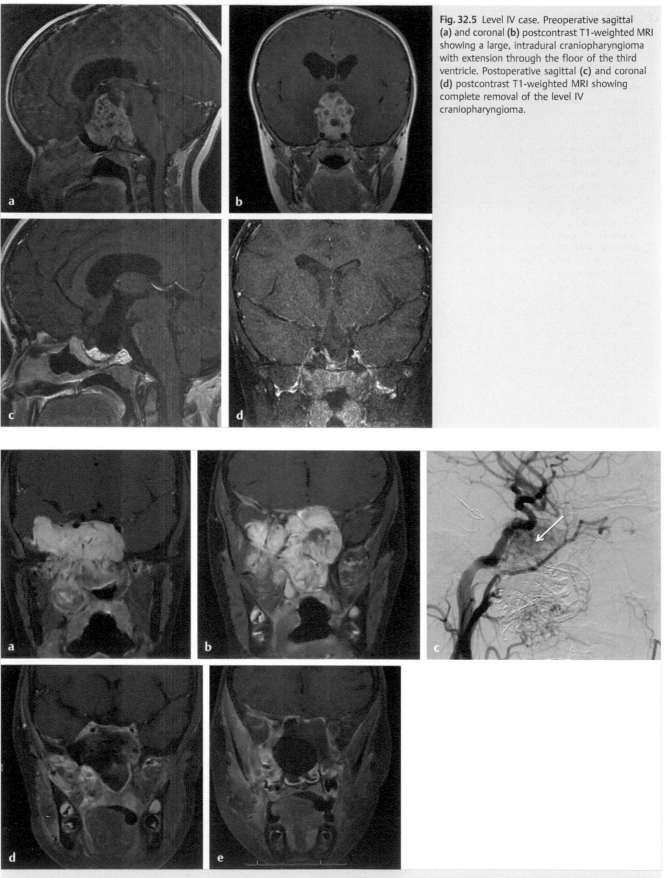

Fig. 32.5 Level IV case. Preoperative sagittal (a) and coronal (b) postcontrast T1-weighted MRI showing a large, intradural craniopharyngioma with extension through the floor of the third ventricle. Postoperative sagittal (c) and coronal (d) postcontrast T1-weighted MRI showing complete removal of the level IV craniopharyngioma.

Fig. 32.6 Level V case. Preoperative postcontrast T1-weighted coronal MRI images (a,b) showing an extensive juvenile nasal angiofibroma with middle and infratemporal fossa cextension as well as right intracranial artery (ICA) encasement. (c) Common carotid artery injection after extensive tumor embolization showing residual blush (arrow) from the ICA. Postcontrast T1-weighted coronal MRI images (d,e) showing complete removal of this level V tumor via two stages, including an endoscopic endonasal approach and endoscopic anterior transmaxillary approach.

References

[1] Kassam A, Snyderman CH, Mintz A, Gardner P, Carrau RL. Expanded endonasal approach: the rostrocaudal axis. Part I. Crista galli to the sella turcica. Neurosurg Focus. 2005; 19(1):E3

[2] Kassam A, Snyderman CH, Mintz A, Gardner P, Carrau RL. Expanded endonasal approach: the rostrocaudal axis. Part II. Posterior clinoids to the foramen magnum. Neurosurg Focus. 2005; 19(1):E4

[3] Patel CR, Fernandez-Miranda JC, Wang WH, Wang EW. Skull base anatomy. Otolaryngol Clin North Am. 2016; 49(1):9–20

[4] Koutourousiou M, Gardner PA, Tormenti MJ, et al. Endoscopic endonasal approach for resection of cranial base chordomas: outcomes and learning curve. Neurosurgery. 2012; 71(3):614–624, discussion 624–625

[5] Koutourousiou M, Fernandez-Miranda JC, Stefko ST, Wang EW, Snyderman CH, Gardner PA. Endoscopic endonasal surgery for suprasellar meningiomas: experience with 75 patients. J Neurosurg. 2014; 120(6):1326–1339

[6] Koutourousiou M, Gardner PA, Fernandez-Miranda JC, Tyler-Kabara EC, Wang EW, Snyderman CH. Endoscopic endonasal surgery for craniopharyngiomas: surgical outcome in 64 patients. J Neurosurg. 2013; 119(5):1194–1207

[7] Khattar N, Koutourousiou M, Chabot JD, et al. Endoscopic endonasal and transcranial surgery for microsurgical resection of ventral foramen magnum meningiomas. Oper Neurosurg (Hagerstown). 2018; 14(5):503–514

[8] Thirumala PD, Mohanraj SK, Habeych M, et al. Value of free-run electromyographic monitoring of lower cranial nerves in endoscopic endonasal approach to skull base surgeries. J Neurol Surg B Skull Base. 2012; 73(4):236–244

[9] Thirumala PD, Potter M, Habeych ME, et al. Value of electromyographic monitoring of cranial nerve V during endoscopic endonasal surgery. Neurosurg Q. 2013; 23:264–267

[10] Elangovan C, Singh SP, Gardner P, et al. Intraoperative neurophysiological monitoring during endoscopic endonasal surgery for pediatric skull base tumors. J Neurosurg Pediatr. 2016; 17(2):147–155

[11] Gardner PA, Tormenti MJ, Koutourousiou M, Fernandez-Miranda JC, Wang EW, Snyderman CH. Carotid injury during endoscopic endonasal surgery: incidence and outcomes in 2015 cases. J Neurol Surg B Skull Base. 2012; 73 Suppl 2:127–128

[12] Harvey RJ, Parmar P, Sacks R, Zanation AM. Endoscopic skull base reconstruction of large dural defects: a systematic review of published evidence. Laryngoscope. 2012; 122(2):452–459

[13] Zanation AM, Carrau RL, Snyderman CH, et al. Nasoseptal flap reconstruction of high flow intraoperative cerebral spinal fluid leaks during endoscopic skull base surgery. Am J Rhinol Allergy. 2009; 23(5):518–521

[14] Prevedello DM, Barges-Coll J, Fernandez-Miranda JC, et al. Middle turbinate flap for skull base reconstruction: cadaveric feasibility study. Laryngoscope. 2009; 119(11):2094–2098

[15] Choby GW, Pinheiro-Neto CD, de Almeida JR, et al. Extended inferior turbinate flap for endoscopic reconstruction of skull base defects. J Neurol Surg B Skull Base. 2014; 75(4):225–230

[16] Stapleton AL, Tyler-Kabara EC, Gardner PA, Snyderman CH, Wang EW. Risk factors for cerebrospinal fluid leak in pediatric patients undergoing endoscopic endonasal skull base surgery. Int J Pediatr Otorhinolaryngol. 2017; 93: 163–166

[17] Chabot JD, Patel CR, Hughes MA, et al. Nasoseptal flap necrosis: a rare complication of endoscopic endonasal surgery. J Neurosurg. 2018; 128(5):1463–1472

[18] Fernandez-Miranda JC, Gardner PA, Rastelli MM, Jr, et al. Endoscopic endonasal transcavernous posterior clinoidectomy with interdural pituitary transposition. J Neurosurg. 2014; 121(1):91–99

[19] Patel VS, Thamboo A, Quon J, et al. Outcomes following endoscopic endonasal resection of craniopharyngiomas in the pediatric population. World Neurosurg. 2017

[20] Chivukula S, Koutourousiou M, Snyderman CH, Gardner PA, Tyler-Kabara EC. Endoscopic endonasal skull base surgery in the pediatric population. Skull Base. 2012; 22 Suppl 1:28

[21] Pant H, Bhatki AM, Snyderman CH, et al. Quality of life following endonasal skull base surgery. Skull Base. 2010; 20(1):35–40

[22] Rowan NR, Wang EW, Gardner PA, Fernandez-Miranda JC, Snyderman CH. Nasal deformities following nasoseptal flap reconstruction of skull base defects. J Neurol Surg B Skull Base. 2016; 77(1):14–18

[23] Chen W, Gardner PA, Branstetter IV BF, Liu SD, Chang YF, Snyderman CH, Goldstein JA, Tyler-Kabara EC, Schuster LA. Long-term impact of pediatric endoscopic endonasal skull base surgery on midface growth. J Neurosurg Pediatr, accepted for publication, August 2018.

[24] Zwagerman NT, Wang EW, Shin S, Chang YF, Fernandez-Miranda J, Snyderman CH, Gardner PA. Does lumbar drainage reduce postoperative cerebrospinal fluid leak after endoscopic endonasal skull base surgery? A prospective, randomized controlled trial. J Neurosurg, accepted for publication, April 2018.

33 Postoperative Care for Pediatric Skull Base Patients: The Neurosurgery Perspective

Jonathan A. Forbes, Georgiana Dobri, Theodore H. Schwartz, and Jeffrey P. Greenfield

Abstract

Endonasal surgery in pediatric patients is associated with a unique set of complications, the individual likelihood of which varies with the underlying pathologic abnormality as well as the specifications of the treatment chosen. Despite the heterogeneity that exists among all lesions treated via the endonasal approach in children, a handful of postoperative complications are commonly encountered. These include postoperative cerebrospinal fluid fistula, new anterior pituitary endocrinopathy, transient/permanent diabetes insipidus, panhypopituitarism, syndrome of inappropriate antidiuretic hormone, postoperative hydrocephalus, and emergent postoperative complications which include hematoma and epistaxis. Appropriate postoperative care requires vigilance in timely detection and treatment of these complications, which are discussed in the chapter.

Keywords: pediatric, endonasal, postoperative complications, endocrinopathy, CSF fistula, diabetes insipidus, SIADH, Hematoma, epistaxis

33.1 Introduction

Endonasal surgery in pediatric patients is associated with a unique set of complications, the individual likelihood of which varies based upon the underlying abnormality/tumor as well as the specifications of the treatment chosen. Despite the considerable heterogeneity that exists among all lesions treated via the endonasal approach in children, a handful of postoperative complications are commonly encountered. In one study of 133 pediatric patients who underwent endonasal approaches, postoperative cerebrospinal fluid (CSF) leaks were detected in 14 patients (10.5%), new anterior pituitary endocrinopathy in 14 (10.5%), panhypopituitarism in 2 (1.8%), permanent diabetes insipidus (DI) in 12 (9.0%), transient DI in 8 (6.0%), syndrome of inappropriate antidiuretic hormone (SIADH) in 3 (2.3%), and development of hydrocephalus in 6 (4.5%).[1] Additionally, postoperative hematoma and epistaxis were noted in 3 (2.3%) and 8 patients (6.0%), respectively. This is a significant complication burden for a delicate patient population.

Postoperative DI and SIADH can be categorized as disorders of fluid and electrolyte balance associated with dysfunction of the posterior pituitary. Anterior pituitary endocrinopathy and hypopituitarism are postoperative disorders of anterior pituitary function. CSF leaks and hydrocephalus involve postoperative disturbances of CSF homeostasis. Postoperative hematoma and epistaxis fall under emergent postoperative complications. Appropriate postoperative care requires vigilance in timely detection and treatment of these complications, which are discussed in the ensuing sections.

33.2 Detection and Management of Postoperative Posterior Pituitary Dysfunction

A proper understanding of normal physiology is beneficial in the diagnosis and management of postoperative disorders of fluid and electrolyte balance. Thorough knowledge of osmolality homeostasis, in particular, is essential. Elevations in plasma osmolality stimulate osmostat receptors in the anterolateral hypothalamus, which respond by signaling for the release of antidiuretic hormone (ADH). ADH, also known as L-arginine vasopressin, is produced in the bodies of magnocellular neurons in the paired supraoptic and paraventricular nuclei of the hypothalamus and transported down the pituitary stalk for storage in the posterior pituitary. Following release into the bloodstream, circulating ADH binds to V_2 receptors in the kidneys, which leads to synthesis of aquaporin-2 water channels and subsequent increased reabsorption of free water. This feedback loop tightly maintains plasma osmolality at 280 to 290 mOsm/kg.[2]

Increases in serum osmolality result in high levels of circulating ADH, which serves to promote the retention of free water in the kidneys and normalize serum tonicity. On occasion, disruption of this feedback loop is encountered in pediatric patients following endonasal surgery. This is especially common in patients whose pituitary stalk has been manipulated or transected. Trauma to the stalk can result in a temporary or permanent inability to synthesize and/or release stores of ADH termed central DI. In assessing the risk that central DI poses to the patient, perhaps the most important variable is the integrity of the patient's thirst mechanism. In the context of a compromised thirst mechanism (e.g., a patient who is obtunded or comatose or a very young patient unable to communicate thirst or gain access to water), the inability to concentrate urine can rapidly lead to life-threatening levels of hypernatremia. In these patients, vigilance in ensuring timely diagnosis and treatment of central DI is imperative.

In pediatric patients who undergo endonasal approaches in which the hypothalamus, pituitary stalk, pituitary gland, or superior hypophyseal arterial supply is subjected to operative manipulation, appropriate steps are taken postoperatively to optimize early diagnosis and/or treatment of DI. In this population, the foley catheter is continued following surgery for hourly measurement of urinary output. Urine samples are sent for specific gravities no less than every 6 hours. The arterial line is kept following surgery as well to allow for every 6 hour measurements of sodium (in setting of florid DI, this frequency can be increased as needed). In the immediate postoperative period, a low urine-specific gravity (≤ 1.005) combined with a high urine volume (> 4 mL/kg/h for 2–3 consecutive hours) raises suspicion for early development of DI. If the thirst mechanism is intact and the patient is permitted to have unrestricted access to water, any small associated increase in osmolality results in increased thirst, and normal osmolality is restored with the generous oral intake of free water.[3] Florid DI can sometimes result in a large free water deficit that can be uncomfortable to recover using oral intake alone; additionally, copious urinary output—especially during nighttime hours—can adversely affect patient rest and comfort. In this instance, treatment with an ADH analog such as dDAVP (desmopressin) is often advised to help improve patient comfort. When actively receiving dDAVP, the serum sodium and osmolality are periodically measured to help assess the efficacy of the treatment. In cases of postoperative DI in which the thirst mechanism is not intact, treatment with dDAVP and calculated free water supplementation with input from an endocrinology or pediatric intensive care service is imperative.

Many options exist for replacing ADH in the postoperative patient with central DI. Pitressin is a synthetic form of L-arginine vasopressin that has potent antidiuretic effects. However, because of its short half-life and effect on blood pressure, it is uncommonly utilized for management. dDAVP is an alternative medication that lacks the hypertensive effects of Pitressin and is associated with a longer half-life.[4] This medication is well suited for the management of DI and can be obtained in intranasal, oral, and parental forms. In patients who have undergone endonasal surgery, the intranasal preparation is sometimes avoided. In small children, however, use of the endonasal preparation in conjunction with the rhinal tube sometimes allows administration of lower doses of dDAVP (≤ 5 mcg) that can be titrated more readily. When this strategy is employed (often in small children or patients with high receptor sensitivity), the medication should be administered in the nostril where the nasal mucosa was not disrupted to ensure maximal absorption. Use of bilateral nasoseptal flaps is a contraindication to use of intranasal dDAVP. Initial oral dDAVP doses in pediatric patients older than 4 years often begin at 0.05 mg (half of a 0.1-mg tablet). Initial IV or subcutaneous doses in pediatric patients range from 0.1 to 0.5 mcg based on age and weight. The duration of ADH-related effects is usually 6 to 12 hours. Subsequent doses, often delivered twice a day, are titrated according to the effect of the initial dose. Following initiation of desmopressin, a graduated regimen for monitoring sodium has been recommended, with measurement of serum sodium every 6 hours for the first 24 to 48 hours, every 8 hours for the next 24 hours, and every 12 hours thereafter until stabilization. As overtreatment of transient DI remains a common and preventable source of unnecessary increased length of hospital stay, it is preferable in many cases to aim for return of increase in urinary output prior to redosing.

Treatment with dDAVP results in a state of nonsuppressible ADH activity. For this reason, perhaps the greatest risk associated with treatment is progressive hyponatremia and related sequelae (e.g., hyponatremia-related seizures). While peak onset of DI is on the second postoperative day, previous studies have noted new onset as late as 11 days following surgery.[5] Infrequently, the neurosurgeon will be faced with a scenario where DI has gone undetected until presentation at an advanced stage. In this instance, formal calculation of water deficit is useful to guide strategies for correction. The following formula is used to calculate overall water deficit: water deficit = $0.6 \times$ preoperative weight $\times (1 - 140/[Na^+])$. The hyperosmolarity should be corrected over a protracted period to avoid issues relating to cerebral edema.[6] Oral replacement with water or IV supplementation with D5W (dextrose in 5% water) is utilized. In the vast majority of cases unrelated to treatment of craniopharyngioma and/or stalk resection, DI is transient and resolves within a few days of the procedure. Permanent DI is incurred if $\geq 90\%$ of the vasopressin-secreting neurons are destroyed and involves long-term follow-up with the endocrinology service.[7]

In addition to DI, providers should remain aware of the SIADH—which complicated the postoperative course of 2.3% of patients in the pediatric endonasal series by Chivukula et al.[1] SIADH, in contrast to DI, peaks in incidence on the seventh postoperative day.[8] Comparatively speaking, SIADH is much less common following endonasal procedures than DI. However, as it is relatively common for patients to have been discharged home prior to onset of SIADH, education regarding the possibility of this occurrence is of paramount importance. In patients who have noted any form of subacute decline after discharge home following endonasal surgery, it is important to obtain a serum sodium level. The authors routinely obtain an outpatient serum sodium in all patients with sellar pathology who have been discharged from the hospital on postoperative day 6. An early diagnosis of hyponatremia in this setting helps avoid severe clinical sequelae.

Symptomatic hyponatremia requires readmission for evaluation and correction. Fluid restriction with occasional IV or oral sodium supplementation is recommended if SIADH is present. Vasopressin receptor antagonists can also be considered on an individual basis in severe cases. Hypothyroidism and adrenal insufficiency should be ruled out, as both can cause hyponatremia that is falsely attributed to SIADH. Dual etiologies sometimes exist, which can make correction and management of hyponatremia cumbersome. The occurrence of cerebral salt wasting (CSW), while sometimes encountered following craniotomies, tends to be rare following endonasal procedures. While SIADH is statistically more common in this setting, differentiation of SIADH from CSW is occasionally challenging. CSW involves renal loss of sodium following intracranial surgery and results in characteristic hypovolemic hyponatremia. This phenomenon may relate to increased release of brain natriuretic peptide (BNP) from the hypothalamus secondary to physiologic or traumatic disturbance.[2] In contrast to CSW, patients with SIADH exhibit euvolemic hyponatremia. Volume status is the most important characteristic used to differentiate the two pathologies; trends of weight gain and water balance, central venous pressure (CVP), and urine sodium help with confirmation. CSW is managed by treatment of the underlying problem if reversible (e.g., meningitis, hydrocephalus, adrenal insufficiency) followed by volume replacement. Oral or IV sodium supplementation and/or fludrocortisone can be added in an iterative manner if necessary. In treatment of all causes of hyponatremia, care is taken to avoid overexuberant correction of hyponatremia that may predispose to central pontine myelinolysis.

33.3 Detection and Management of Postoperative Anterior Pituitary Dysfunction

All pediatric patients scheduled to undergo endonasal surgery undergo routine assessment of hypothalamic and pituitary function prior to surgery. In the event this assessment demonstrates some element of insufficiency, supplementation is provided prior to surgical intervention. In patients with normal preoperative pituitary function, endonasal surgery is often associated with some degree of risk for subsequent development of anterior pituitary insufficiency. This risk is heavily dependent on the pathology at hand (craniopharyngioma, in particular, is associated with a high risk of postoperative anterior pituitary insufficiency) in addition to specific details of the procedure. In the cases in which the pathology and operative findings support a high postoperative risk to anterior pituitary dysfunction, patients are often maintained on glucocorticoids prior to clinical reevaluation in an outpatient setting 4 to 12 weeks following surgery. Patients with preexistent anterior pituitary deficiency sometimes recovery pituitary function following surgery. In these patients, the hormonal supplementation should continue until evidence of recovery at the first outpatient endocrine visit.

In pediatric patients who undergo endonasal surgery for sellar pathology, our practice has been to pretreat with a single dose of hydrocortisone prior to surgery. If the operative findings are consistent with low risk to the stalk and gland, an attempt is made to wean hormonal supplementation in the early postoperative period. Determination of the postoperative integrity of the hypothalamic–pituitary–adrenal (HPA) axis integrity is of vital importance.[9] Multiple studies conducted in the adult population have attempted to designate a cortisol-level threshold predictive of HPA axis sufficiency; levels between 10 and 17 µg/dL have been entertained.[10,11] However, others continue to favor the insulin hypoglycemia test as perhaps a more accurate assessment.[12] In patients known to have intact HPA axis integrity prior to surgery, the authors prefer to give a single dose of stress-dose hydrocortisone immediately prior to surgery. A cortisol level is subsequently obtained a minimum of 24 hours following the initial dose of hydrocortisone (in procedures that begin at 7:30 am, this level is obtained the morning of postoperative day 1; in all other cases, this level is obtained the morning of postoperative day 2). If the cortisol level is less than 15 µg/dL, the patient is placed on daily glucocorticoid supplementation with plans to electively reevaluate the HPA axis approximately 6 weeks following surgery with an adrenocorticotropic hormone (ACTH) stimulation test.

The ability to detect anterior pituitary dysfunction following endonasal surgery is of paramount importance. In pediatric patients who have undergone endonasal surgery and remain off glucocorticoid supplementation, it is good practice to routinely consider signs and symptoms of cortisol deficiency—including hypotension, nausea, malaise, hyponatremia, and

difficulties with thermoregulation. Although multiple corticosteroid preparations are available, hydrocortisone prescribed at 7 to 20 mg/m^2/d (5–15 mg/d) given orally in two or three divided doses is considered the most physiologic replacement. Hypothyroidism is usually detected 3 to 7 days after surgery and can be picked up with a free T4 serum measurement. Thyroid supplementation is usually initiated immediately after insufficiency is detected. Total replacement levothyroxine dose is 100 mcg/m^2/d. However, the authors' practice has been to initiate thyroid replacement at much lower doses and titrate higher if necessary, as pituitary–thyroid axis deficiency is often incomplete and/or transient. Growth hormone deficiency and hypogonadism are evaluated and addressed at the first endocrine evaluation after surgery 4 to 12 weeks, as diagnosis is not accurate in the immediate postoperative period, and there is no urgency in replacement either.

33.4 Detection and Management of Postoperative CSF Fistula

Another notable complication that can affect pediatric patients who have undergone endonasal surgery is postoperative CSF fistula. In the cases in which expanded endonasal approaches have been utilized, extensive preoperative planning and intraoperative modification are important components to minimize the incidence of this complication. Following simple transsphenoidal approaches, the need to reoperate for a CSF leak is relatively rare. In one study of 592 adult patients who underwent transsellar approaches, 26 (4.4%) developed evidence of CSF leakage a mean of 25 days (range from 4 to 180 days) postoperatively.[13] In another smaller study of pediatric patients who underwent limited transsellar approaches, 9.1% of patients developed postoperative CSF leakage (of note, nasoseptal flaps were not utilized in this series).[14] In the aforementioned series of 133 pediatric patients who underwent endonasal approaches for a variety of skull base pathologies, postoperative CSF leaks were detected in 14 patients (10.5%).[1] In general, expanded endonasal approaches (particularly those associated with increased arachnoid dissection) are associated with higher rates of CSF leakage than routine transsellar approaches. Use of the vascularized nasoseptal flap has been shown to decrease the rate of CSF leakage following endonasal approaches.[15] Although increased preparation appears to be necessary to ensure optimal utilization of the nasoseptal flap in pediatric patients, successful coverage has been demonstrated in patients as young as 3 years.[16]

In select pediatric patients who undergo endonasal surgery for intradural pathology, our practice has been to proceed with lumbar drain insertion for injection of intrathecal (IT) fluorescein prior to surgery. Benadryl and glucocorticoids are given prior to administration of IT fluorescein. The fluorescein allows for easy identification of intraoperative CSF leakage. This is especially important at the end of the case, where a watertight closure is desired. The lumbar drain is kept, in most instances, for 24 to 48 hours following surgery set to drain at a predetermined rate of 5 mL/h. Perioperative antibiotics are continued until the lumbar drain is removed.

Inspection for postoperative CSF fistula is an important part in the routine care of patients who have undergone endonasal surgery. When IT fluorescein has been used in the OR, the characteristic fluorescent appearance on gauze often makes the occurrence of early postoperative CSF leakage obvious to the provider. In the cases in which IT fluorescein has not been used or the leak is delayed in nature, diagnosis of postoperative CSF leakage can be more difficult. The patient is routinely asked about drainage from the nose, a salty taste in the back of the mouth, or the sensation of a continuous drip down the back of the throat. The patient is queried about headaches that may be positional in nature. A "Dandy maneuver" is performed during clinical evaluation, whereby the patient is asked to lean forward and flex his or her head; CSF that has pooled in the sphenoid sinus, if present, will often drain from the nose following this maneuver. If the volume is such that the drainage can be collected in a tube, the fluid can be sent for analysis of markers such as beta-transferrin, prostaglandin-D synthase, and transthyretin to help differentiate CSF from postoperative nasal discharge. However, in most cases the diagnosis of postoperative CSF leakage is made using clinical findings alone.

When a postoperative CSF leak is suspected, the next step is to obtain a noncontrast CT scan of the head to assess for pneumocephalus. If significant pneumocephalus is present, a return to the OR for revision of closure is favored. If pneumocephalus is absent, a trial of lumbar drainage is sometimes considered. Prolonged CSF leakage places patients at risk for subsequent development of bacterial meningitis. Because CSF rhinorrhea may not become obvious until well after discharge home, proper patient education in this regard is imperative.

In rare instances, underlying hydrocephalus can predispose to postoperative CSF leakage with subsequent failed attempts at repair of CSF fistula. Fraser et al reported preoperative hydrocephalus, as determined by the radiologic evidence of preoperative ventriculomegaly, to be a significant risk factor for postoperative CSF leak following endonasal surgery.[17] In this study, 25 of 35 patients (71.4%) found to have preoperative hydrocephalus were treated with perioperative CSF diversion with placement of a VP (ventriculoperitoneal) shunt.

33.5 Emergent Postoperative Complications

Endoscopic endonasal procedures in pediatric patients are associated with a host of potential emergent postoperative complications. Injury to the carotid artery has been roughly estimated to occur in 0.9% of routine transsphenoidal procedures.[18] However, the risk of injury appears to increase in the setting of expanded approaches and with certain pathologies. For instance, the risk of internal carotid artery injury in expanded endonasal approaches for chordoma and chondrosarcoma has been estimated to be 10 times higher than with routine transsphenoidal approaches alone.[19]

When a carotid arterial injury is encountered intraoperatively, the laceration can infrequently be addressed with endonasal bipolar cautery alone. In the majority of cases, hemostasis is urgently obtained via endonasal packing (the use of muscle for hemostatic material has been advocated), and the patient is taken urgently to the angiography suite. Depending on a variety of factors, the neurointerventionalist contemplates vessel sacrifice versus attempt at endoluminal reconstruction with either PTFE-covered stents or flow-diversion devices.[18] Following endovascular intervention, the patient is placed on antiplatelet medication and monitored accordingly.

In addition to risk of injury to the carotid artery, endonasal procedures are occasionally associated with new postoperative neurological deficit. The new development of visual loss, cranial neuropathy, or alteration in mental status is addressed with emergent CT of the head. When this deficit is felt to potentially relate to mass effect from hematoma or closure-related material (e.g., fat), urgent return to the OR for endoscopic re-exploration is indicated. Mild deficits that develop in a subacute manner should be investigated using MRI.

33.6 Conclusion

Disorders of anterior/posterior pituitary dysfunction and CSF fistula compose the majority of complications encountered following endonasal surgery in pediatric patients. Other less frequent complications include postoperative neurologic deficit secondary to postoperative hematoma or carotid laceration. Proper understanding of associated physiology of these conditions allows for timely identification and treatment. Input from endocrinology and otolaryngology services is essential in delivery of optimal care.

References

[1] Chivukula S, Koutourousiou M, Snyderman CH, Fernandez-Miranda JC, Gardner PA, Tyler-Kabara EC. Endoscopic endonasal skull base surgery in the pediatric population. J Neurosurg Pediatr. 2013; 11(3):227–241

[2] Greenfield JP, Anad VJ, Schwartz TH. Post-operative management of patients undergoing endonasal endoscopic transsphenoidal surgery. In Anand VJ, Schwartz TH, eds. Practical Endoscopic Skull Base Surgery. San Diego, CA: Plural Publishing; 2007

[3] Johnson AK, Buggy J. Periventricular preoptic-hypothalamus is vital for thirst and normal water economy. Am J Physiol. 1978; 234(3):R122–R129

[4] Seckl JR, Dunger DB, Bevan JS, et al. Vasopressin antagonist in early postoperative diabetes insipidus. Lancet. 1990; 335(8702):1353–1356

[5] Kristof RA, Rother M, Neuloh G, Klingmüller D. Incidence, clinical manifestations, and course of water and electrolyte metabolism disturbances following transsphenoidal pituitary adenoma surgery: a prospective observational study. J Neurosurg. 2009; 111(3):555–562

[6] Gullans SR, Verbalis JG. Control of brain volume during hyperosmolar and hypoosmolar conditions. Annu Rev Med. 1993; 44:289–301

[7] Mishra G, Chandrashekhar SR. Management of diabetes insipidus in children. Indian J Endocrinol Metab. 2011; 15 S uppl 3:S180–S187

[8] Ausiello JC, Bruce JN, Freda PU. Postoperative assessment of the patient after transsphenoidal pituitary surgery. Pituitary. 2008; 11(4):391–401

[9] Inder WJ, Hunt PJ. Glucocorticoid replacement in pituitary surgery: guidelines for perioperative assessment and management. J Clin Endocrinol Metab. 2002; 87(6):2745–2750

[10] Auchus RJ, Shewbridge RK, Shepherd MD. Which patients benefit from provocative adrenal testing after transsphenoidal pituitary surgery? Clin Endocrinol (Oxf). 1997; 46(1):21–27

[11] Marko NF, Gonugunta VA, Hamrahian AH, Usmani A, Mayberg MR, Weil RJ. Use of morning serum cortisol level after transsphenoidal resection of pituitary adenoma to predict the need for long-term glucocorticoid supplementation. J Neurosurg. 2009; 111(3):540–544

[12] Erturk E, Jaffe CA, Barkan AL. Evaluation of the integrity of the hypothalamic-pituitary-adrenal axis by insulin hypoglycemia test. J Clin Endocrinol Metab. 1998; 83(7):2350–2354

[13] Han ZL, He DS, Mao ZG, Wang HJ. Cerebrospinal fluid rhinorrhea following trans-sphenoidal pituitary macroadenoma surgery: experience from 592 patients. Clin Neurol Neurosurg. 2008; 110(6):570–579

[14] Zhan R, Xin T, Li X, Li W, Li X. Endonasal endoscopic transsphenoidal approach to lesions of the sellar region in pediatric patients. J Craniofac Surg. 2015; 26(6):1818–1822

[15] Soudry E, Turner JH, Nayak JV, Hwang PH. Endoscopic reconstruction of surgically created skull base defects: a systematic review. Otolaryngol Head Neck Surg. 2014; 150(5):730–738

[16] Ghosh A, Hatten K, Learned KO, et al. Pediatric nasoseptal flap reconstruction for suprasellar approaches. Laryngoscope. 2015; 125(11):2451–2456

[17] Fraser S, Gardner PA, Koutourousiou M, et al. Risk factors associated with postoperative cerebrospinal fluid leak after endoscopic endonasal skull base surgery. J Neurosurg. 2017; 9:1–6

[18] Sylvester PT, Moran CJ, Derdeyn CP, et al. Endovascular management of internal carotid artery injuries secondary to endonasal surgery: case series and review of the literature. J Neurosurg. 2016; 125(5):1256–1276

[19] Gardner PA, Tormenti MJ, Pant H, Fernandez-Miranda JC, Snyderman CH, Horowitz MB. Carotid artery injury during endoscopic endonasal skull base surgery: incidence and outcomes. Neurosurgery. 2013; 73(2) Suppl Operative:ons261–ons269, discussion ons269–ons270

34 Postoperative Care for Pediatric Skull Base Patients: The Otolaryngology Perspective

Patrick C. Walz, Daniel M. Prevedello, and Ricardo L. Carrau

Abstract

Endoscopic endonasal techniques have been adapted to the pediatric population, expanding their indications and implementation. However, the use of these techniques in the pediatric age group carries its own set of challenges, including adapting standard operative and postoperative techniques and technologies utilized in adults to address the specific needs of pediatric patients. While there are many similarities in the postoperative care of patients after endoscopic skull base surgery, this chapter will focus on the nuances that set apart the postoperative care of pediatric patients.

Keywords: pediatric skull base, postoperative care, pediatric endoscopic skull base surgery

34.1 Introduction

The development and advancement of endoscopic techniques and their application to disorders of the skull base has revolutionized the care of patients afflicted with lesions in this area. As with most technologic advancements in medicine, initial endeavors in this field centered around the care of adult patients with skull base lesions. Over time, endoscopic skull base surgical techniques were adapted and modified for use in pediatric patients, and with this transition, new challenges were encountered. While the anatomic constraints of the pediatric nose and skull base are covered elsewhere in this text, the psychological and interpersonal challenges of the pediatric patient weigh heavily in the safe and effective administration of postoperative care following skull base surgery.

34.2 General Postoperative Measures

34.2.1 Location and Duration of Hospital Stay

After endoscopic skull base surgery (ESBS), patients are routinely monitored in the pediatric intensive care unit (PICU). In the first 24 hours after surgery, ICU care is necessary for neuromonitoring and close assessment of fluid balance and blood pressure. In addition, monitoring of fluid balance (in and out) and frequent serum electrolyte balance is necessary in cases involving manipulation of the pituitary gland and/or stalk to help identify early signs of hormonal dysfunction (diabetes insipidus [DI] and syndrome of inappropriate antidiuretic hormone [SIADH]). Whenever possible, the patient should be extubated immediately following postsurgical imaging (noncontrasted CT immediately performed after surgery), facilitating his/her neurologic assessment. In patients who require mechanical ventilation, we generally stop the sedation to complete a neurologic examination every hour.

The patient should be transitioned to a general surgical floor when neurologic examination, fluid balance, and endocrine function are determined to be stable. This typically occurs on the first or second postoperative day but varies with pathology, surgical approach, and comorbidities.[1] Similarly, the overall length of stay is dependent on healing time of the surgical site and endocrine control, with lengths of stay ranging from 3 to 7 days in uncomplicated cases.[1] Complications can greatly extend length of stay.

34.2.2 Pain Control

The objective of pain management following ESBS is to obtain maximum patient comfort while maintaining appropriate responsiveness to ensure a reliable neurologic assessment. The use of oral acetaminophen as a primary analgesic supplemented with narcotics when necessary is the mainstay of treatment. Intravenous narcotic medication is reserved for refractory pain. While adequate pain control is the goal, progressive headaches that do not respond to increasing doses of narcotic analgesics must be thoroughly and closely evaluated for potential risk of cerebrospinal fluid (CSF) leak with concomitant pneumocephalus, and other possible intracranial complications as such as hemorrhage and vasospasm.[2]

Narcotics may induce nausea/vomiting and constipation, possibly causing an increase in intracranial pressure (ICP), displacement of the skull base reconstruction, and subsequent CSF leakage. Therefore, narcotic analgesia must be employed judiciously, administering the lowest dosage possible. Stool softeners and nonstimulant laxatives are routinely utilized in the postoperative setting for this purpose.

Nonsteroidal anti-inflammatory drugs are avoided in the postoperative period to minimize the risk of bleeding complications. Nonpharmacologic pain control strategies such as distraction have also shown efficacy in management of acute pain in the pediatric patient; therefore, therapeutic recreation, child life, or similar services can be utilized for this purpose.[3]

34.2.3 Diet

Following surgery, the patient's diet should be routinely advanced to the least restrictive diet as soon as possible. Following posterior fossa intervention with concern for alteration in function of lower cranial nerves, clinical assessment of the safety of swallow is performed before advancing the diet.

Fluid intake monitoring is necessary in patients with DI to prevent significant hyponatremia or dehydration while their medical management is optimized.

34.2.4 Monitoring

Continuous telemetry and pulse oximetry monitoring is utilized in the immediate postoperative period and during the length of

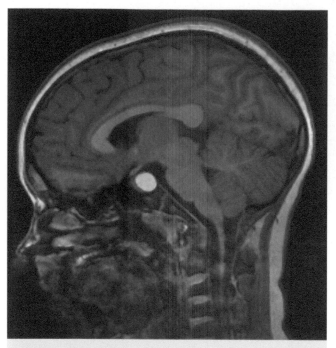

Fig. 34.1 Preoperative T1-weighted, noncontrasted spoiled gradient reconstruction (SPGR) MRI revealing a hyperintense posterior sellar lesion in a 15-year-old adolescent boy. Pathology demonstrated xanthogranuloma.

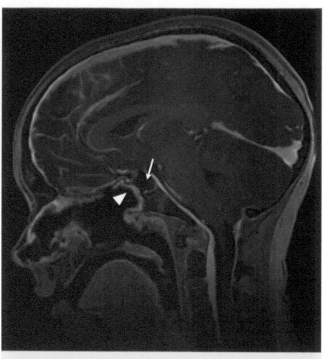

Fig. 34.2 Postoperative sagittal T1 postcontrast spoiled gradient reconstruction (SPGR) MRI of the patient seen in ▶ Fig. 34.1. Imaging demonstrates enhancing vascularized nasoseptal flap (arrowhead) and the sellar cavity with absence of sellar tumor (arrow).

stay in the ICU to ensure any changes in hemodynamic stability are quickly identified. Arterial line blood pressure monitoring is typically utilized intraoperatively and continued for the first 24 hours after surgery. After the first postoperative day, the arterial line is removed unless needed for frequent blood draws (as in the case of frequent sodium monitoring), and blood pressure monitoring is continued with cuff pressures. Upon transfer to the postsurgical floor, hemodynamic monitoring should be continued with vital sign measurements every 4 to 6 hours.

Neurologic status is typically assessed every hour in the first 24 hours after surgery and every 4 to 6 hours thereafter. Accurate assessment of neurologic status in the pediatric patient can be challenging due to stranger anxiety, fear of discomfort, and uneasiness in an unfamiliar setting. Patience during this process, establishing rapport, and utilizing examination aids to maintain the patient's interest are helpful. For example, a small toy with a flashing light can capture the patient's interest and enable complete visual field examination.

As in adults, sedating medications that could mimic a compromised neurologic condition should be avoided in most pediatric patients following ESBS. In rare instances, patients can become so agitated that they compromise their own postoperative outcome due to straining and Valsalva-like activity. Should this be the case, judicious use of short-acting sedatives is selected, and limitations of the examination are documented.

34.2.5 Imaging in the Acute Period

In the immediate postoperative period, a noncontrasted CT scan is obtained to rule out intracranial complications such as hematoma, subarachnoid bleeding, tension pneumocephalus, or dilated ventricles. This is repeated as needed to follow any finding or to rule out a possible postoperative CSF leak. Postoperative CSF leaks can present with increased pneumocephalus, illustrating the importance of obtaining a baseline scan for comparison.[4] Patients who require a staged procedure undergo a CT scan with image guidance protocol (axial fine-cut images [1-mm cuts or thinner] with cuts extending from the vertex to the maxillary incisors).

MRI is also obtained within the first 24 hours (to avoid artifact) to assess neurovascular integrity and adequacy of resection in patients with malignancies, recurrent tumors, and other select pathologies. As a secondary but significant gain, the MRI allows assessment of the multilayer reconstruction and flap placement (▶ Fig. 34.1; ▶ Fig. 34.2).

34.2.6 Nasal Precautions

After ESBS, it is imperative to avoid blind instrumentation of the nose. Clear communication to the nursing staff is necessary to prevent nasal suctioning, placement of nasal trumpets, or placement of nasogastric feeding or other nasal tubes. These interventions could potentially compromise the skull base repair and precipitate a CSF leak or even injure the brain or other neurovascular structures.[5] In addition, the patient should be instructed to avoid activities that generate positive or negative pressure in the nose, as pressure changes can lead to pneumocephalus and unnecessarily challenge a skull base repair early in the healing period. Nose blowing and sneezing with mouth closed are avoided for the first 4 to 6 weeks after surgery. Clear explanation to the pediatric patient and his/her caregivers regarding the rationale behind these restrictions and consequences of these behaviors can help improve compliance. Nasal saline should be provided as a replacement for nose blowing.

The use of straws has been debated in the postoperative period due to concern for generation of negative pressure. However, the pressure generated by straw use is similar to that generated during respiration, and the negative pressure with straw utilization is created in the oral cavity with minimal transfer to the nasopharynx. Therefore, straw use is permitted in the postoperative setting.

34.2.7 Activity

Activity level after ESBS is dependent on the extent of skull base defect and type of repair employed.

No Cerebrospinal Fluid Leak or Dural Injury

If no CSF leak or transgression of dura occurs intraoperatively, only restrictions on vigorous activity are employed. The patient is encouraged to ambulate and be up and out of bed during recovery to avoid pulmonary or thromboembolic complications.

Low-Flow Cerebrospinal Fluid Leak

If a low-flow CSF leak is present, this typically results from a small communication between the sinuses and intracranial space. Examples include a small dural tear at a fracture line or intermittent leakage or transudation of CSF through or around the diaphragma sellae. Positioning measures are employed to optimize CSF outflow; thus, the patient's bed should be elevated to 30 degrees. Light activity such as ambulation is encouraged, but activities that would elevate ICP like bending, lifting, and straining are restricted. Stool softeners are routinely employed to avoid Valsalva related to constipation.

High-Flow Cerebrospinal Fluid Leak

If a high-flow CSF leak, defined by communication of the operative defect with the ventricular system or more than one cistern, is encountered and repaired (▶ Fig. 34.3), positioning measures as in low-flow CSF leak and the use of stool softeners are employed, but activity is further limited with restriction to bed/chair rest for 3 to 5 days. After the packing/drain securing the repair is removed and the repair is noted to be intact, activity is slowly advanced to mirror that of low-flow CSF leak repair patients.

Considerations for Compliance

The youngest of patients undergoing ESBS are at considerable risk for noncompliance with nasal precautions and activity restrictions given their limited ability to understand the situation and the potential impact of their actions to their overall healing. Employing additional measures to ensure the greatest degree of compliance possible can be of assistance in the pediatric population. Enlisting the assistance of the patient's caregivers to reinforce restrictions and utilizing child life or similar enrichment activities to distract patients from these restrictions aid in this effort. In rare circumstances, compliance continues to be poor despite these efforts. In these situations, an

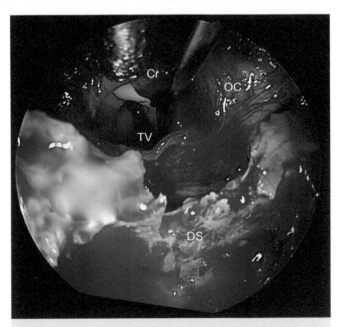

Fig. 34.3 Endoscopic endonasal view with 30-degree endoscope during resection of craniopharyngioma (Cr) in a 14-year-old adolescent. Disease extended into the third ventricle (TV), leading to high-flow cerebrospinal fluid leak requiring nasoseptal flap reconstruction. The dorsum sella (DS) is seen in the foreground and optic chiasm (OC) is displaced leftward.

honest evaluation of the potential risk the patient is posing to him/herself with these behaviors needs to be undertaken. If the risk for surgical failure and attendant morbidity is high, or if a patient has proven themselves unable to tolerate standard precautions, a period of sedation during the critical healing period is employed.

34.2.8 Nasal Saline Use

Nasal saline spray should be initiated on the day of surgery to decrease crusting buildup on splints and within the nares. Most pediatric patients will tolerate nasal saline spray. On day 5 to 7 (or after packing and splints are removed), nasal saline spray is transitioned to nasal saline irrigations. This facilitates clearance of crusts and absorbable packing.[6] If not tolerating nasal saline irrigation or if attempts at administration lead to severe irritation, risking the integrity of the skull base repair, continuation of nasal saline spray and close monitoring for excessive crusting with low threshold for surgical debridement is a reasonable alternative.

34.2.9 Surgical Site Care

Splints placed at the time of surgery to stabilize the nasoseptal flap site repair (if needed) or help prevent synechiae are removed between postoperative days 5 and 7. This is typically coordinated with removal of any nonabsorbable packing material such as finger cots or Merocel sponges (Medtronic, Minneapolis, MN). If CSF leak is encountered at the time of surgery, a challenge of the repair is undertaken at this time by having the patient hang his/her head forward for several minutes (head tilt test) and potentially adding a mild Valsalva maneuver. Following packing removal, nasal endoscopy to evaluate extent of crusting and debridement of the nasal cavity is performed. Care is taken to avoid debridement over the repair (flap or graft) or its immediate periphery so that the repair is not inadvertently disrupted. While endoscopy and debridement is a standard procedure in adult postoperative care, this is often not tolerated in pediatric patients, especially in patients younger than 10 to 12 years.[6] For this reason, a low threshold is maintained for re-evaluation under general anesthesia between 5 and 7 days to remove packing, debride crusting, and remove any residual packing or hemostatic material that does not directly overlie the graft or flap (▶ Fig. 34.4).

34.3 Infection Prophylaxis

Prevention of surgical site infection is of paramount importance due to intraoperative communication of the sinonasal cavity and intracranial space. There is no meaningful precedent in the literature to guide use, as evidenced by a recent report stating that no meta-analysis could be performed on the existing literature, as it consisted of only observational studies.[7] As such, expert opinion and goals of prophylaxis are considered in selection of antibiotics in the perioperative period. Typically, antibiotics are administered intraoperatively and continued in the postoperative period for the duration of packing placement to

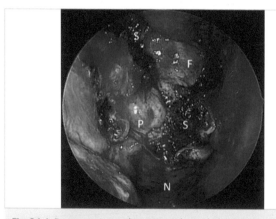

Fig. 34.4 Postoperative endoscopic endonasal photograph at debridement after endonasal resection of a large sellar craniopharyngioma. The nasoseptal flap pedicle (P) is seen on the right of the operative defect and extending superiorly to the flap (f). Absorbable packing material on the periphery of the flap (S) is left in place. The nasopharynx (N) is seen at the inferior aspect of the image.

decrease risk of toxic shock syndrome.[6] It has been standard practice at the authors' institutions to utilize a fourth-generation cephalosporin for *Pseudomonas* coverage and central nervous system penetration and adding vancomycin if preoperative screening or clinical concern for methicillin-resistant *Staphylococcus aureus* (MRSA) is present. Mupirocin ointment can be applied to the nares to further minimize toxic shock syndrome risk and improve MRSA coverage. Avoidance of neomycin-containing ointments is recommended, as a substantial minority of the population is sensitive to this medication.

34.4 Imaging

Imaging in the acute period was reviewed earlier in this chapter. Following the acute period, MRI is typically performed at 6- to 12-month intervals following tumor resection, with the duration of surveillance imaging dependent on pathology (▶ Fig. 34.5). If individual patient or tumor factors such as an aggressive tumor or subtotal resection are noted, the interval may be decreased to 3 months. A CT scan is not routinely obtained after the acute postoperative period unless an additional surgical intervention is planned.

34.5 Cerebrospinal Fluid Leak Prevention and Management

As mentioned previously, a tiered approach to activity is utilized after ESBS to minimize the risk of postoperative CSF leak and maximize skull base repair healing potential. In addition to the measures already discussed, lumbar drain is more frequently used in the pediatric population. Recent reports have cited no difference in outcome with or without lumbar drain placement.[8,9] These reports reviewed the existing literature, which is limited, and focused on adult patients. Despite this, Tien and colleagues do support implementation of CSF diversion in select cases.[9] However, in a series of strictly pediatric ESBS patients, lumbar drain utilization was reported in 19 to 45% of patients.[10,11] In the pediatric population, response to noxious stimuli, avoidance of Valsalva, and adherence to nasal precautions are variable, all potentially challenging the integrity of the repair. For this reason, lumbar drain is frequently utilized for CSF diversion in pediatric patients requiring repair of CSF leak to help mitigate these confounding variables and

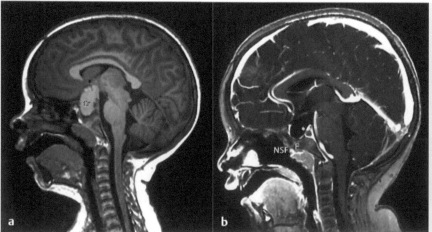

Fig. 34.5 Surveillance imaging following tumor resection. **(a)** Preoperative sagittal T1-weighted MRI revealing sellar craniopharyngioma (Cr) extending into the suprasellar space (*) in a 4-year-old adolescent boy. **(b)** A 6-month postoperative sagittal BRAVO T1-weighted, noncontrasted MRI demonstrating no evidence of disease in the sella (*) and intact nasoseptal flap (NSF). This patient developed postoperative CSF rhinorrhea and his repair was revised and supplemented with an abdominal fat graft (F).

minimize pressure on the skull base repair. In teenage patients or select children who demonstrate the maturity to comply with sinus precautions, lumbar drain should be avoided. If employed, lumbar drainage is typically continued until the time of packing removal, clamping the drain 24 hours before packing removal to allow for evaluation of the integrity of the repair.

If a patient presents with clear fluid drainage despite the aforementioned steps, physical examination with challenge of the reconstruction (tilt test with or without Valsalva) and a noncontrasted CT to evaluate for increased pneumocephalus are required, as described earlier. If obvious, continuous clear fluid is observed, a CSF leak is presumptively diagnosed, and reoperation is indicated. If the amount of fluid is discrete or if no fluid is observed despite previous reports (with or without witnesses), then additional investigation is necessary.[2] This can be achieved by repeating a noncontrast head CT (new or increased pneumocephalus will confirm the leak), testing the nasal discharge for beta-2 transferrin, or even direct bedside nasal endoscopic assessment in older patients as tolerated.

Once confirmed, a CSF leak is managed surgically with immediate reoperation. In the vast majority of cases, the multilayered repair (nasoseptal flap and grafts) is found to be displaced due to improper placement, brain herniation, or Valsalva maneuvering.[2] Simple repositioning of the flap and packing will usually suffice, but occasionally, the reconstruction is reinforced with abdominal fat. This is decided on a case-to-case basis, taking into account factors such as difficulty to perform the reconstruction and defect size.

Table 34.1 Postoperative complications following endonasal skull base surgery (ESBS) with prevention and management strategies

ESBS complications				
Time frame	**Complication**	**Prevalence**	**Prevention**	**Management**
Immediate	Crusting	+++++	• Nasal saline irrigation • Coverage of exposed bone and cartilage with mucosa when available	• Nasal saline irrigation • Endoscopy with debridement
	Epistaxis	+++	• Cautery of base of turbinate after resection • Maintain mucosalization of anterior septum	• Oxymetazoline • Topical hemostatic agents • Endoscopy with cautery
	Anosmia	+	• Ensure patent pathway to cribriform • Preserve 1-cm superior septal mucosa when able	• N/a if from nerve injury • Removal of obstruction if obstructive source
	Cranial nerve injury	+	• Careful dissection in known location of cranial nerves	N/a
	Cerebrovascular accident	Rare	N/a	• Address source of bleeding if hemorrhagic • Restore perfusion and avoid hypotension if ischemic
Anytime	Infection	+	• Prophylactic antibiotics • Copious irrigation during surgery	• Culture-directed antibiotics • Ensure separation of intracranial and sinonasal cavities • Drainage of abscess if present
	Endocrine dysfunction	+	• Careful dissection around sella and suprasellar space	• Identification and hormone replacement
	CSF leak	+	• Robust, vascularized repair • Ensure that flap overlays the demucosalized bone circumferentially	• Rapid identification of presence of leak and site of leak • Surgical repair with flap ± abdominal fat graft
Delayed	Nasal obstruction	+	• Preserve anterior one-third of septum • Avoid inferior turbinate resection	• Assess for septal deflection, empty nose syndrome, or crusting and address as appropriate
	Chronic sinusitis	+	• Ensure unobstructed sinus outflow tracts • Nasal saline irrigations to aid in mucosal clearance	• Treatment of exacerbations • Revision of sinus surgery to allow for adequate mucociliary clearance
	Craniofacial growth restriction	Rare	• Avoid unnecessary septal resection	N/a

Abbreviations: CSF, cerebrospinal fluid; N/a, not available.
Note: Relative prevalence of each complication is also noted, based on previous reports.[10,11]

34.6 Endocrine Management

Endocrine abnormalities are not infrequently encountered following ESBS due to manipulation of the pituitary, instrumentation adjacent to the hypothalamus, or the stress induced by surgical intervention. Certain pathologies, most notably craniopharyngiomas, are highly associated with endocrinopathy following ESBS given their intimate relationship with the hypothalamus and pituitary stalk/gland. There is a high potential for temporary or permanent injury to the surrounding secretory tissues with resultant dysfunction.[10,12] The most frequent endocrinopathy noted following ESBS is DI, characterized by production of copious dilute urine and seen in 15% of pediatric ESBS patients in one series.[10] Focal anterior pituitary dysfunction follows DI in prevalence, affecting 10.5% and characterized as dysfunction of select adenohypophyseal hormones without panhypopituitarism. SIADH is the third most prevalent endocrinopathy, affecting 2.3% in a sample of 133 pediatric skull base surgery patients.[10] In any case involving manipulation of the sella, early endocrinology consultation is appropriate to proactively assess endocrine function and replace or treat as indicated.

34.7 Complications and Morbidity

Appropriate and accurate execution of the surgical effort is only a portion of the care necessary to minimize complications and morbidity in the care of ESBS patients. Potential complications and morbidity, their temporal association with presentation, and measures to prevent and manage the complications are presented in ▶ Table 34.1.

34.8 Adjuvant Therapy

In cases of surgery for neoplasm, postoperative radiation or chemotherapy may be required based on tumor characteristics and completeness of resection. Ensuring that the patient's repair is intact and well healed prior to initiation of therapy decreases the incidence of operative site morbidity. To that end, careful evaluation at the time of debridement is necessary. Following radiation-based adjuvant therapies, crusting may increase, and additional debridement may be indicated. Any endoscopic efforts that are not able to be completed in the office should be coordinated with sedated imaging studies to minimize anesthetic exposure.

34.9 Conclusion

The postoperative care of the pediatric ESBS patients borrows heavily from experiences with adult skull base patients, with several notable variations primarily related to the pediatric patient's potential limited ability to understand and/or comply with the typical restrictions required following ESBS. A thoughtful, patient-centered approach to postoperative care for each patient focused on the patient's insight into what will be expected after surgery allows for appropriate provision of care and best outcomes.

References

[1] Stapleton AL, Tyler-Kabara EC, Gardner PA, Snyderman CH. Endoscopic endonasal surgery for benign fibro-osseous lesions of the pediatric skull base. Laryngoscope. 2015; 125(9):2199–2203

[2] Ditzel Filho LF, Prevedello DM, Kerr EE, Jamshidi AO, Otto BO, Carrau RL. Endonasal resection of craniopharyngiomas: post-operative management. In: Evans JJ, Kenning TJ, eds. Craniopharyngiomas: Comprehensive Diagnosis, Treatments, and Outcomes. Oxford: Elsevier; 2014:271–279

[3] Oliveira NC, Santos JL, Linhares MB. Audiovisual distraction for pain relief in paediatric inpatients: A crossover study. Eur J Pain. 2016

[4] Nadimi S, Caballero N, Carpenter P, Sowa L, Cunningham R, Welch KC. Immediate postoperative imaging after uncomplicated endoscopic approach to the anterior skull base: is it necessary? Int Forum Allergy Rhinol. 2014; 4(12): 1024–1029

[5] Paul M, Dueck M, Kampe S, Petzke F, Ladra A. Intracranial placement of a nasotracheal tube after transnasal trans-sphenoidal surgery. Br J Anaesth. 2003; 91(4):601–604

[6] Tien DA, Stokken JK, Recinos PF, Woodard TD, Sindwani R. Comprehensive postoperative management after endoscopic skull base surgery. Otolaryngol Clin North Am. 2016; 49(1):253–263

[7] Rosen SA, Getz AE, Kingdom T, Youssef AS, Ramakrishnan VR. Systematic review of the effectiveness of perioperative prophylactic antibiotics for skull base surgeries. Am J Rhinol Allergy. 2016; 30(2):e10–e16

[8] Ahmed OH, Marcus S, Tauber JR, Wang B, Fang Y, Lebowitz RA. Efficacy of perioperative lumbar drainage following endonasal endoscopic cerebrospinal fluid leak repair: a meta-analysis. Otolaryngol Head Neck Surg. 2017; 156(1): 52–60

[9] Tien DA, Stokken JK, Recinos PF, Woodard TD, Sindwani R. Cerebrospinal fluid diversion in endoscopic skull base reconstruction: an evidence-based approach to the use of lumbar drains. Otolaryngol Clin North Am. 2016; 49 (1):119–129

[10] Chivukula S, Koutourousiou M, Snyderman CH, Fernandez-Miranda JC, Gardner PA, Tyler-Kabara EC. Endoscopic endonasal skull base surgery in the pediatric population. J Neurosurg Pediatr. 2013; 11(3):227–241

[11] Quon JL, Hwang PH, Edwards MS. Transnasal endoscopic approach for pediatric skull base tumors: a case series. Neurosurgery. 2016; 63 Suppl 1:179

[12] Duff J, Meyer FB, Ilstrup DM, Laws ER, Jr, Schleck CD, Scheithauer BW. Long-term outcomes for surgically resected craniopharyngiomas. Neurosurgery. 2000; 46(2):291–302, discussion 302–305

Index

Note: Page numbers set **bold** or *italic* indicate headings or figures, respectively.